FREE RADICALS AND DISEASES

Edited by **Rizwan Ahmad**

Free Radicals and Diseases
http://dx.doi.org/10.5772/61358
Edited by Rizwan Ahmad

Contributors

Sumitra Miriyala, Mini Chandra, Manikandan Panchatcharam, Daniel R Gonzalez, Ulises Novoa, Adriana Treuer, Adem Kara, Emin Sengul, Semin Gedikli, Volkan Gelen, Seckin Ozkanlar, Martha Cecilia Rosales Hernández, Maricarmen Hernández-Rodriguez, Jessica Elena Mendieta-Wejebe, Jose Correa Basurto, Marc Diederich, Aloran Mazumder, Alejandra Guillermina Miranda-Diaz, Luis Miguel Roman-Pintos, Geannyne Villegas-Rivera, Adolfo Daniel Rodriguez-Carrizalez, Ernesto German Cardona-Muñoz, Fermín Pacheco-Moisés, José Pedraza-Chaverri, Dianelena Eugenio-Pérez, Liliana Yazmín Medina-Fernández, Jennyfer Andrea Saldivar-Anaya, Eduardo Molina-Jijón, Rk Chaitanya, Genaro Gabriel Ortiz, Mario Mireles-Ramírez, J Luis Flores-Alvarado, Héctor González-Usigli, Erica Daniela González-Renovato, Angelica Sánchez-López, Lorenzo Sánchez-Romero, Irma E Velázquez-Brizuela, Bruna Pereira, Carolina Baraldi A. Restini, Tufik Geleilete, Frank Sellke, M. Ruhul Abid, Jalal Pourahmad, Shuichi Ueda, Ayuka Ehara, Cleva Villanueva, Robert Kross, Luis Perez-Astudillo, Ramón Rodrigo, Francesca Ciani, Eugenio Luigi Iorio, Simona Tafuri, Natascia Cocchia, Francesco Landolfi, Salvador Uribe-Carvajal, Monica Rosas Lemus, Cristina Uribe-Alvarez, Martha Contreras-Zentella, Luis A. Luévano Martinez, Natalia Chiquete-Félix, Adriana Muhlia-Almazan, Edgardo Escamilla, Selva Rivas-Arancibia, Erika Rodriguez-Martinez

Published by InTech

Janeza Trdine 9, 51000 Rijeka, Croatia

Publishing Process Manager Iva Lipovic

Technical Editor SPi Global

Cover InTech Design team

First published November, 2016

Printed in Croatia

Additional hard copies can be obtained from orders@intechopen.com

Free Radicals and Diseases, Edited by Rizwan Ahmad

p. cm.

Print ISBN 978-953-51-2746-8
Online ISBN 978-953-51-2747-5

For EU product safety concerns:
IN TECH d.o.o., Prolaz Marije Krucifikse Kozulić 3, 51000 Rijeka, Croatia,
info@intechopen.com or visit our website at intechopen.com.

Meet the editor

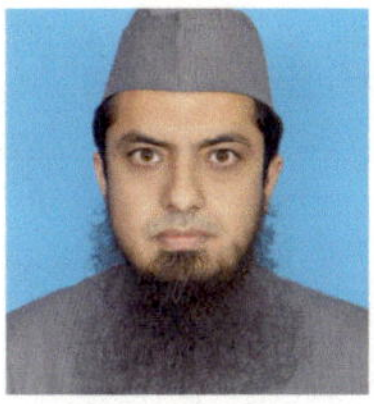

Dr. Rizwan Ahmad is the founding head of the School of Life and Allied Health Sciences at Glocal University, India. He received his MPhil and PhD in Biochemistry from the Faculty of Medicine, Aligarh Muslim University, Aligarh, India. He worked as an associate professor in the Human Function Group at Oman Medical College in partnership with WVU, USA, from 2010 to 2013. He worked as an assistant professor in the Department of Biochemistry, SBS Post Graduate Institute, Dehradun, India, from 2004 to 2010; during this period, more than 30 students completed their postgraduate dissertation under his supervision. He has published several research papers in reputed international journals. His research interest has been on free radicals and their role in autoimmune disorders.

Contents

Preface

Free radicals are natural by-products of ongoing biochemical reactions in the body, including ordinary metabolic processes and immune system responses. Free radical–generating substances can be found in the food we eat, the drugs and medicines we take, the air we breathe, and the water we drink. Bruce Ames, a well-known scientist in the field of free radicals, estimates that just one cell in the human body is hit about 10,000 times a day by a free radical; when multiplied by the trillions of cells in the body, the damage potential is huge.

The past two to three decades have witnessed the remarkable advances in our knowledge about the implication of free radicals in various diseases.

Oxidation is the damage caused by free radicals in the body. Rampaging free radicals react with compounds in the body and oxidize them. The amount of oxidation in the body is the measure of oxidative stress (OS). OS is believed to be the cause of diseases and disorders. This book is a consolidated effort of authors working in the field of oxidative stress to provide comprehensive and up-to-date information on it.

The current opinions on the role of free radical reactions in diabetic cardiomyopathy, polyneuropathy, and neurodegenerative disorders are reported here. Redoxomics and oxidative stress review the "electrophilic stress" as an emerging health risk factor for early aging and many infectious diseases.

This book integrates knowledge in free radical–associated diseases from the basic to the advanced level, and from the bench side to bed side.

The search for effective, nontoxic natural compounds with antioxidative activity has been intensified in recent years. This volume aims to introduce antioxidant activity of herbs. The role of antioxidants in chronic kidney disease is also envisaged. The chapter on novel antioxidant therapy against myocardial ischemia during coronary angioplasty enlightens the knowledge of cardiac interventions.

I would herewith like to thank the publishing team and all the authors for their contribution. I am also indebted to Prof. Sadath Ali for his comments during editorial assignment.

I am sure that the chapters of this book will be of interest to many biomedical researchers and clinicians in the field.

Since the topic of free radicals and diseases needs extensive research, I also hope that this book will draw the attention of many scientists interested in the field of free radicals.

Rizwan Ahmad, MPhil, PhD
Head, School of Life and Allied Health Sciences
Glocal University, India

Chapter 1

Oxygen: From Toxic Waste to Optimal (Toxic) Fuel of Life

Mónica Rosas-Lemus, Cristina Uribe-Alvarez, Martha Contreras-Zentella, Luis Alberto Luévano-Martínez, Natalia Chiquete-Félix, Norma Lilia Morales-García, Emilio Espinosa Simón, Adriana Muhlia-Almazán, Edgardo Escamilla-Marván and Salvador Uribe-Carvajal

Additional information is available at the end of the chapter

http://dx.doi.org/10.5772/63667

Abstract

Some 2.5 billion years ago, the great oxygenation event (GOE) led to a 10^5-fold rise in atmospheric oxygen [O_2], killing most species on Earth. In spite of the tendency to produce toxic reactive oxygen species (ROS), the highly exergonic reduction of O_2 made it the ideal biological electron acceptor. During aerobic metabolism, O_2 is reduced to water liberating energy, which is coupled to adenosine triphosphate (ATP) synthesis. Today, all organisms either aerobic or not need to deal with O_2 toxicity. O_2-permeant organisms need to seek adequate [O_2], for example, aquatic crustaceans bury themselves in the sea bottom where O_2 is scarce. Also, the intestinal lumen and cytoplasm of eukaryotes is a microaerobic environment where many facultative bacteria or intracellular symbionts hide from oxygen. Organisms such as plants, fish, reptiles and mammals developed O_2-impermeable epithelia, plus specialized external respiratory systems in combination with O_2-binding proteins such as hemoglobin or leg-hemoglobin control [O_2] in tissues. Inside the cell, ROS production is prevented by rapid O_2 consumption during the oxidative phosphorylation (OxPhos) of ATP. When ATP is in excess, OxPhos becomes uncoupled in an effort to continue eliminating O_2. Branched respiratory chains, unspecific pores and uncoupling proteins (UCPs) uncouple OxPhos. One last line of resistance against ROS is deactivation by enzymes such as super oxide dismutase and catalase. Aerobic organisms profit from the high energy released by the reduction of O_2, while at the same time they need to avoid the toxicity of ROS.

Keywords: oxygen, ROS, oxidative stress, oxyconformers, oxyregulators, adaptative metabolism

1. At the beginning, all life was anaerobic

The early Earth atmosphere contained high [H_2], [NH_3] and [CH_4], while [O_2] was less than 10^{-5} the present atmospheric level (PAL) [1, 2]. All life forms were anaerobic [3, 4]. Early redox reactions involved electron donors such as H_2, CO_2 or HS [5, 6], while electron acceptors were sulfur and NO_3 [7]. Eukaryotes were present before O_2 rose [8, 9] and contained anaerobic mitochondrion-like organelles [10, 11].

2. The massive increase in [O_2] and the need to counteract its toxicity

Approximately 2.5 billion years ago, the great oxygenation event (GOE) was precipitated by both geological processes [12] and by the photosynthetic activity of cyanobacteria [13, 14]. Today, O_2 is the preferred electron acceptor used by facultative microorganisms and the only one used by aerobes. The highly exergonic reduction of O_2 provided the energy needed for the development of multicellular organisms. In addition, the high energy of activation required for O_2 reduction ensures that this reaction occurs mostly through catalyzed reactions. For instance, oxidases bind their substrate tightly, preventing the liberation of reactive oxygen species (ROS) [15]. At low concentrations, ROS are useful as signaling molecules, while at higher concentrations ROS damage and kill cells. Cells need much less [O_2] than what is found in the atmosphere and thus, to prevent ROS production internal O_2 is kept at a low level [16]. Cells have developed two mechanisms to deal with surplus O_2: (1) avoiding it and (2) rapidly reducing it. Furthermore, cellular O_2 is found mostly bound to proteins such as hemoglobin, leg-hemoglobin and myoglobin. Early oxy-conformer organisms are permanent to O_2, and thus, at different stages in their life cycle, they have to migrate to microaerobic or anaerobic spaces (**Table 1**) to cope with variations in O_2. More evolved oxyregulator organisms from fish to mammals enveloped themselves in an O_2-impermeable epithelium, while at the same time developing highly specialized systems that control tissue [O_2] (**Figure 1**). Oxyconformers and oxyregulators display different strategies to manage O_2-by-product toxicity (**Figure 1**).

In oxyconformers, all cells are exposed to environmental [O_2]. O_2-permeable organisms do have O_2 transport proteins and intracellular O_2-binding proteins, but in addition, they need to implement diverse strategies to deal with changing O_2. These include searching for microaerophilic or anaerobic environments. Arthropoda, the most abundant and widely distributed phylum on Earth, are oxyconformers [17]; it comprises subphyla Chelicerata (spiders), Myriapoda (centi- and millipedes), Hexapoda (Insects) and Crustacea, all of them protected by an exoskeleton. Nonaquatic insects possess a hard waterproof cuticle and branched invaginated tubules forming a specialized respiratory structure that works well at constant

[O_2]. Aquatic organisms, including most of the crustacea, are exposed to highly variant [O_2], which may be 26 times lower than in the atmosphere [18, 19]. In water, [O_2] varies with temperature, depth, mechanical aeration and tidal movements. Only few invertebrates (Plathelmynthes, Nematoda, Molluska, Anellida and Sypuncula) have been thoroughly studied in regard to their mechanisms to deal with fluctuating [O_2] [20, 21]. Remarkably, very few studies on Crustacea are available.

Environment	O_2 concentration (μM)	References
Atmosphere	1000m ASL 256.0 Sea level 1028.0	[88]
Alveoles	143.0	[89]
Arteries	123.0 *Hb bound 120.5* *Not bound 2.5*	[89] [90]
Capillaries	130.0	[89]
Interstitial fluid	55.0	[89]
Tissue cells	31.0	[89]
Veins	59.0	[89]
Mitochondria	Minimal for coupling 0.1 Minimal reported 20.0	[91]
Distilled water	223.0	[92]
Sea water	Surface 198-397.0 250.0 MOZ < 20.0	[93] [34] [94]
Estuaries	Surface 375.0 Bottom 62.5	[95] [96]

Oxygen concentrations reported were modified from partial pressures to micromolar concentration (μM) using Henry's law at 310.15K ASL (above sea level).

Table 1. Oxygen concentrations in different environments.

In order to control the release of ROS oxyconformers reduce aerobic activity during hypoxia/anoxia cycles, marine crustaceans display different responses to hypoxia/anoxia. To avoid hyperoxygenated or anoxic waters, crustaceans migrate between open sea and coastal lagoons (**Figure 2**), or migrate vertically through the water column to flee the O_2 minimum zone (OMZ) and into [O_2] compatible with their metabolic needs [22, 23]. Some shrimp species, such as the burrowing thalassinids *Upogebia major* and *Callianasa japonica,* which commonly inhabit the extremely hypoxic or even anoxic intertidal flats, can reduce their respiratory rate in dugout burrows, surviving up to 5 h of anoxia for *U. major* and 19 h for *C. japonica* [24]. *Artemia franciscana* is well known for its high tolerance to anoxia; the embryos of this species survive without O_2 for years through the complete depression of their metabolic rates [25, 26]. Metabolic rate depression is also observed in ectotherms, which lower their mitochondrial activity in function of temperature adjusting their O_2 consumption machinery accordingly [27]. However, it is not clear how mitochondria from oxyconformers respond to hypoxia, how respiratory activity adapts to reduced metabolic rates and how the cellular redox balance and energetic homeostasis are preserved [28, 29].

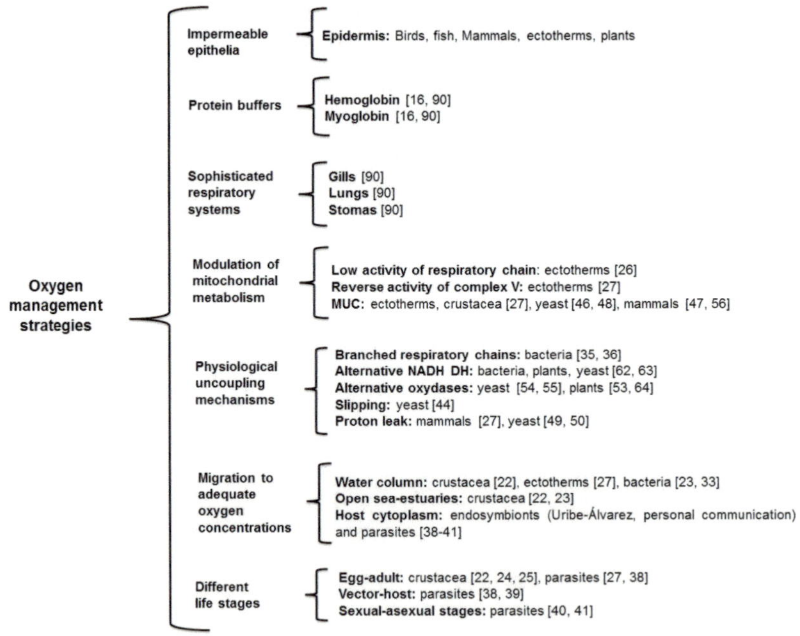

Figure 1. Oxygen management strategies in different organisms. Organisms need to adapt to the O_2 concentration in the environment. Therefore, either they move to environments with adequate O_2 or they engineer different mechanisms to process O_2 at varying rates (electron transport chain (ETC) activity, mitochondrial unspecific channels (MUC), uncoupling proteins (UCPs). Additionally, oxyregulators have developed O_2-excluding mechanisms such as impermeable epithelia, external respiratory systems (lungs, gills, stomas) and O_2-transporting proteins (hemoglobin, myoglobin).

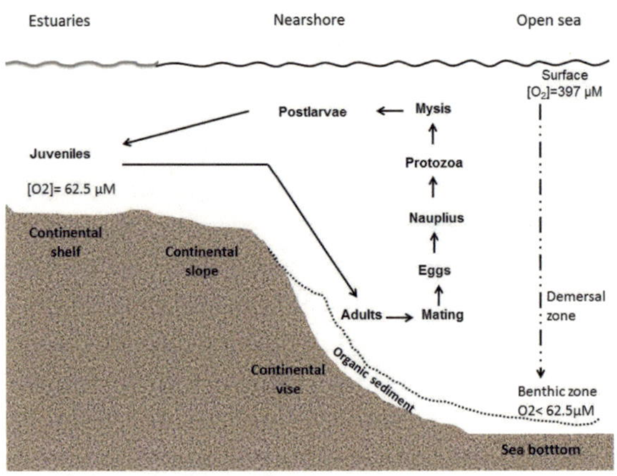

Figure 2. Migration of shrimp during their life cycle. Shrimp spend most of their life in the open sea, where they mate and lay eggs which hatch and undergo different larval stages (Nauplius, Protozoa, Mysis). Once in the postlarval stage, they travel to estuaries where they mature reaching the juvenile stage, and burying themselves in the sand for long periods. Once maturity is reached, they begin the cycle again returning to the open sea. This migration pattern takes shrimp to waters with widely different O_2 concentrations.

Among unicellular organisms, diverse yeast species can survive at almost any $[O_2]$. *Saccharomyces cerevisiae* can thrive at very low $[O_2]$ through fermentation, although it does possess a facultative aerobic metabolism. The anaerobic metabolism of *S. cerevisiae, D. hansenii* and other yeast species is the basis for the fermentation industry of bread, wine and cheese. For example, during wine fermentation, *S. cerevisiae* produces large amounts of ethanol, while *D. hansenii* produces volatile products conferring the characteristic aroma of wine [30]. Also, *S. cerevisiae* participates in cheese fermentation, whereas *D. hansenii* protects against other filamentous fungi during ripening [31, 32]. Yeast and other organisms have developed diverse systems to detoxify oxygen through physiological uncoupling and these are discussed later.

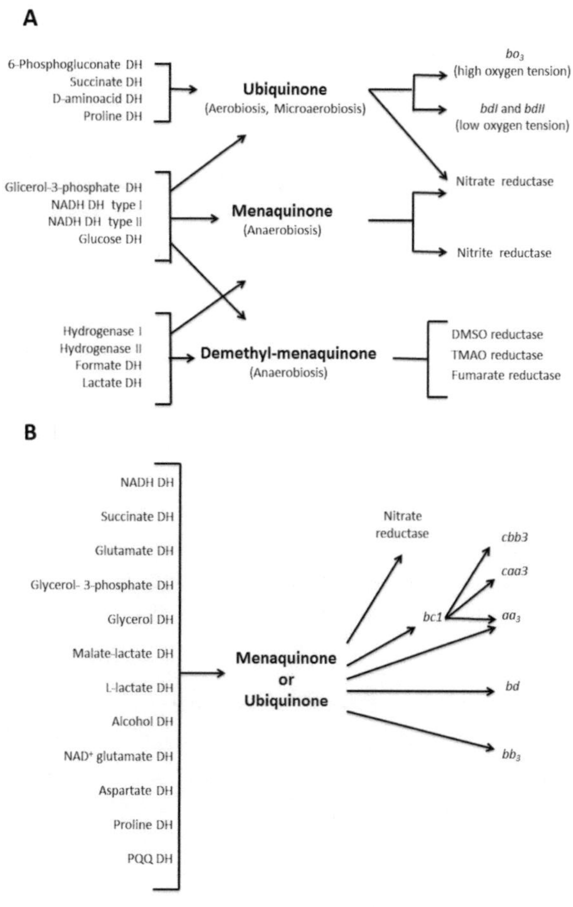

Figure 3. Diversity of bacterial respiratory chains at different $[O_2]$. **A**. The respiratory chain from *Escherichia coli* during aerobiosis, micro-aerobiosis and anaerobiosis. Modified from [35, 36]. Ubiquinone is expressed at high $[O_2]$ and NADH DH type II is overexpressed as compared to the NADH DH type I, which in turn is expressed at low $[O_2]$. The major final oxidase is cytochrome *bo*. During anaerobiosis, the respiratory chain in *Escherichia coli* succinate dehydrogenase is not expressed, whereas fumarate reductase or nitrate reductase may be the final electron acceptors. **B**. Hypothetical respiratory chain of *Wolbachia pipientis* constructed from BLAST and genome sequences reported in [76, 77]. At high $[O_2]$ cytochrome, bc1 and different cytochrome oxidases are expressed. Under microaerobic conditions, cytochrome *bd* is expressed. Then, under anaerobiosis, nitrate reductase is expressed.

Many bacteria are facultative. Among these, *Escherichia coli* is a very illustrative representative that may thrive both in microaerobic environments such as the intestinal lumen and in the external environment in a wide range of [O_2]. Bacteria respond to environmental [O_2] variations or other conditions such as the need to fixate N_2 [33, 34] by varying the composition of their branched respiratory chains (**Figure 3A**), which vectorially transport from 0 to 10 protons, as many as those in orthodox respiratory chains [35, 36]. Still, when motile, bacteria will swim toward environments containing the ideal [O_2].

Obligate endosymbionts, such as *R. prowazekii*, *Wolbachia sp.* or *Sodalis*, live in cytoplasmic vacuoles of multicellular organisms. The cytoplasm is a microaerophilic environment equipped with O_2-consuming organelles and ROS-detoxifying enzymes. Remarkably, most endosymbionts contain a respiratory chain that at least in the case of *Wolbachia* seems to aid host mitochondria to deplete intracellular O_2 (**Figure 3B**).

Many parasites exhibit various life-cycle stages, which have different sensitivities to ROS engineered to endure attacks from macrophages. *Leishmania sp.* undergoes a relatively simple life cycle with two stages: the flagellated mobile promastigote living in the gut of the sand fly vector and the intracellular amastigote within phagolysosomal vesicles of the vertebrate host macrophage [37]. Promastigotes contain respiratory complexes I, II, III and IV, while it is not clear whether amastigotes possess an oxidative phosphorylation (OxPhos) machinery. Strikingly, amastigotes exhibit a succinate-dependent, uncoupler-sensitive transmembrane potential. Differences in sensitivity to oxidants are also observed between them, *in vitro*, promastigotes are more resistant to H_2O_2 than amastigotes [38].

In the bloodstream, *Trypanosoma cruzi* trypomastigotes contain high complex II and III activities. Interestingly, cytochrome *c* oxidase (COX) activity decreases creating an "electron bottleneck" that favors an increase in electron leakage, thus overproducing ROS. The oxidative preconditioning provided by this mechanism confers protection to bloodstream trypomastigotes against ROS liberated by the host immune system. These changes in mitochondrial activity, during the *T. cruzi* life cycle, are probably a key metabolic adaptation for survival in different hosts [39].

Malarial parasites are vulnerable to oxidative stress during their intraerythrocyte life stages. They contain the canonical respiratory chain (complex I, II, III and IV) plus an alternative electron transport pathway. Moreover, malarial mitochondria coordinate the biosynthesis of pyrimidine, heme and coenzyme Q [40]. *Plasmodium falciparum* possesses genes for two different superoxide dismutases (SOD), a cytosolic, Fe^{2+}-dependent, (SOD-1) expressed throughout the intraerythrocytic life of the parasite. The second, SOD-2, is mitochondrial and possesses a reminiscent apicoplast-targeting sequence. The host immune response to malaria involves phagocytosis and the production of nitric oxide and ROS that end up contributing to the pathology of the disease [41].

Regardless the organism studied, cytoplasmic [O_2] can vary widely, so damage control is needed at two levels. Either O_2 is reduced independently of adenosine triphosphate (ATP) production in a process known as physiological uncoupling, or the ROS-handling enzymes are activated. We shall briefly describe only physiological uncoupling as many reviews on

http://dx.doi.org/10.5772/63667

ROS-handling enzymes, such as superoxide dismutase and catalase are found elsewhere [42, 43].

3. Physiological uncoupling as an O_2-depleting mechanism and prevents ROS production

Both in oxyconformers and in oxyregulators, once O_2 enters the cell it has to be reduced at a high rate. When ATP is needed the respiratory chain rapidly catalyzes this reduction. When there is energy surplus, O_2 consumption has to be uncoupled from ATP synthesis with the aim of preventing ROS overproduction [44]. A review on the physiological uncoupling mechanisms observed in mitochondria from different species of yeasts has been published recently [45]. Yeast mitochondrial uncoupling mechanisms may be (a) proton sinks, such as the mitochondrial unspecific channels [46–48] and the uncoupling protein (UCP) [49, 50], or (b) nonpumping redox alternative enzymes found in branched respiratory chains [51–55].

(a). Proton sinks: The opening of the mitochondrial permeability transition pore (MPTP) leads to mitochondrial uncoupling and to the activation of signaling events leading to apoptosis [56], which was first detected in mammalian mitochondria as a response to the disruption of intracellular calcium homeostasis. In crustaceans subjected to hypoxia, mitochondrial functions are downregulated [57, 58, 20] and there is an anoxia-triggered intracellular increase in both calcium and phosphate, while ATP production is inhibited, probably as a result of the opening of a MPTP. In *Artemia franciscana* [26] and in the ghost shrimp *Lepidophthalmus louisianensis* [59], the proteins needed to form the MPTP are present. However, whether these crustaceans possess MPTPs is to be defined. Both in crustacean mitochondria and in other known hypoxia-tolerant invertebrates (mussels, oysters, and cnidarians among others), the role of a putative MPTP is an interesting question.

(b). Branched respiratory chains: Bacteria do not exhibit a permeability transition. This seems to be a mitochondrial trait. Instead, bacteria (and many mitochondria) exhibit branched respiratory chains. Indeed, different species of mitochondria may exhibit from none to three alternative enzymes. In contrast, bacteria may contain as much as twenty electron entry ports and as many exits. Thus, in most prokaryotes, branched respiratory chains seem to be the mechanism of choice to maintain a high rate of O_2 consumption, while adjusting ATP production to the energy requirements of the cell. In this regard, the bioenergetic efficiency for each entry point is defined as the stoichiometry of H^+ pumped per e^- traveling through the respiratory chain [60]. In addition, terminal oxidases are remarkably varied and their active site orientation, to the cytoplasm or to the periplasm determines their pumping efficiency [36].

Alternative oxidoreductases is the term designating all components of the respiratory chain different to the usual complexes I through IV. Most alternative oxidoreductases lack proton-pumping activity and may coexist with, or substitute for the respiratory proton-pumping complexes. Alternative enzymes catalyze the rapid, uncoupled flow of electrons towards O_2. Alternative NADH dehydrogenases may either substitute for (*S. cerevisiae*) or coexist with (bacteria, plants and diverse fungi) complex I [61, 62].

Alternative oxidases (AOXs) catalyze the oxidation of ubiquinol to quinone and the reduction of O_2 to H_2O in the absence of proton translocation [53]. Although highly represented among plants, fungi and protist species, animal AOXs have been predicted to exist only in Molluska, Nematoda and Chordata [63]. Recently, the number of phyla that probably possess AOX has increased including Placozoa, Porifera, Cnidaria, Annelida, Echinodermata, Hemichordata and Chordata. In some marine vertebrates, such as sipunculids, annelids (*Nereis pelagica,* and *Arenicola marina)* and in bivalves (*Arctica islandica),* AOX has been detected [64–66]. However, there are no confirmed reports for AOX in mitochondria from crustaceans [51]. In different plant and animal species, cells lacking AOX show an increased susceptibility to death due to H_2O_2, hypoxia and pathogens [67]. The ultimate decoupling of electron flow occurs when NADH dehydrogenases act in concert with alternative oxidases. The yeast *Yarrowia lipolytica* is a strict aerobic organism for which several biotechnological applications have been developed, such as in the cheese fermentation, obtention of extracellular enzymes [68], production of organic acids [69] and interconversion of fatty acids and alkenes [70]. In *Y. lipolytica,* metabolism occurs in a complex network between compartments, such as peroxisomes, endoplasmic reticulum, lipid bodies and mitochondria [69]. Mitochondria play an important role in ATP production, as well as in the maintenance of the $NADH/NAD^+$ redox ratio [71]. The respiratory chain is composed of the classic complexes: I, II, III and IV, one alternative NADH dehydrogenase external (NADH2) [72] and two isoforms of AOX [73]. During the logarithmic growth phase, NADH2 interacts with supercomplexes III–IV channeling the electrons to oxygen, while pumping protons at both complex III and IV [74]. In contrast, during the stationary growth phase, electrons are directly transferred from alternative NDH2 to AOX, thus uncoupling oxidative phosphorylation and decreasing the production of ROS [54, 55]. This is a very illustrative example, which suggests that physiological uncoupling systems are present in all living organisms. Furthermore, in *Y. lipolytica,* both proton sinks and branched chains are observed [50, 54].

Bacterial cytochrome-containing oxidases are many. These enzymes are differentially expressed in response to different oxygen concentrations and on whether an organism is an obligate aerobic or a facultative species. In addition, oxidases may coexist depending on the species under study and they may play different roles in the cell [75]. In *E. coli,* different oxidases are expressed depending on $[O_2]$. At high O_2, bo3 is expressed, while at low O_2, bd cytochromes are observed. Furthermore, *E. coli* is capable of growth under anaerobiosis, using respiratory chains reminiscent of the early Earth that use ubiquinone, menaquinone or demethylmenaquinone to donate electrons to enzymes that use terminal acceptors different to O_2 (**Figure 3A**) [35, 36]. Branched respiratory chains provide the possibility of consuming O_2 without producing ATP. In the yeast *Y. lipolytica,* in the bacterium *E. coli* and probably in the Rickettsial *Wolbachia sp.,* the arrangement of the respiratory chain varies such that when $[O_2]$ is high, or ATP is needed, high proton pumping efficiency is observed. In contrast, factors such as arrival to the stationary phase or microaerophilic conditions probably trigger overexpression of the alternative NADH dehydrogenase and/or the AOX leading to the futile reduction of O_2 [61]. A possible arrangement of the respiratory chain of *Wolbachia* sp is illustrated (**Figure 3B**) where a large number of possible electron-donating enzymes reduce

http://dx.doi.org/10.5772/63667

menaquinone or ubiquinone that in turn reduce final electron-accepting enzymes that are expressed according to the presence of O_2 in the cytoplasm of the host [76, 77].

4. N-fixating bacteria are a special case

Nitrogen-fixating bacteria may be facultative as *Klebsiella pneumonia* or strict aerobics as *Azotobacter vinelandii* or *Gluconobacter diazotrophicus*. As they contain fragile, oxygen-sensitive nitrogen-fixating enzymes that need to be protected, these bacteria have developed many strategies to detoxify [O_2]. Thus, in N-fixating bacteria, both N-reductases and different oxidases are expressed: *A. vinelandii* contains a highly active respiratory chain and is able to adjust the expression of its three oxidases to a wide range of [O_2]. Among these, cytochrome *bd* has high O_2 affinity (KmO_2= 5 μM) and becomes active during N fixation [15, 78–80]. Indeed, during N fixation the H^+/O index is low, at 1 [81]. In *Ga. diazotrophicus* different periplasmic membrane enzymes such as glucose-, acetaldehyde- or ethanol-dehydrogenase reduce a quinone, which in turn donates its electrons to two different oxidases, *ba* which is coupled to ATP synthesis and bb_3 which is not coupled, but its role is to deplete O_2 in the vicinity of nitrogen reductases [82].

5. ROS detoxification

In spite of the production-prevention mechanisms outlined earlier, ROS may reach high concentrations, for example, during ischemia-reperfusion. The last line of defense is detoxification. Enzymes such as superoxide dismutases (SODs) and catalases deactivate ROS. SODs have been grouped on the basis of the metal cofactor, which can be Fe, Mn, Ni or Cu/Zn [83]. The Fe-SODs are mostly found in microaerophiles and anaerobes. Microorganisms in aerobic environments prefer Mn-SOD [84]. Catalase dismutates hydrogen peroxide to water plus O_2 [85]. Several genes capable of H_2O_2 dismutation evolved from ancestral genomes. The most abundant was heme-containing enzymes spread among bacteria, Archaea and Eukarya [86].

In *Clostridium acetobutylicum*, a strict anaerobic that survives little time when exposed to O_2, no catalases are found [87], and a function has yet to be found for the annotated SODs.

6. Conclusion

During the early paleoproterozoic period, a massive death toll resulted from a 10^5 times rise in atmospheric O_2. In order to survive, organisms had to learn to cope with O_2 toxicity while profiting from the large energy release coupled to its reduction. Several O_2-management strategies are revised here. Among these is hiding away from O_2, moving to adequate O_2

concentrations or excluding O_2 with impermeable epithelia. Once O_2 enters the cell, other mechanisms are designed to handle it. Its reactivity is controlled by O_2-quenching proteins or by rapidly reducing it with specific oxidases. In order to avoid side reactions, the rate of reduction had to be kept at optimal pace, independently of ATP production and thus several mechanisms of physiological uncoupling of oxidative phosphorylation evolved. Physiological uncoupling was achieved either by opening proton sinks or by using O_2 independently of the proton gradient. Today, these mechanisms are expressed in many cells. Proton sinks include unspecific channels and uncoupling proteins, while proton gradient-independent consumption of O_2 involved alternative oxido-reductases found in the branched respiratory chains of fungi, plants and arthropods. In spite of the function of all these O_2-management machines, O_2 can still react unspecifically to form ROS, which destroy the cell through processes such as aging, apoptosis or necrosis. Once formed, ROS may still be eliminated by enzymes such as SOD and catalase, which are reviewed elsewhere [43] O_2 is a great source of energy for the cell, but its high toxicity has to be dealt with, through mechanisms that we are only beginning to understand.

Acknowledgements

Authors thank Ramón Méndez-Franco for technical assistance. Partially funded by the PAPIIT program and DGAPA/UNAM (grant IN202612). MRL, NLMG and CUA are CONACYT fellows enrolled in the Biochemistry Graduate Program at UNAM.

Declaration of Interest. The authors do not have any interests to disclose.

Author details

Mónica Rosas-Lemus[1], Cristina Uribe-Alvarez[1], Martha Contreras-Zentella[2], Luis Alberto Luévano-Martínez[3], Natalia Chiquete-Félix[1], Norma Lilia Morales-García[1], Emilio Espinosa Simón[1], Adriana Muhlia-Almazán[4], Edgardo Escamilla-Marván[5] and Salvador Uribe-Carvajal[1*]

1 Department of Molecular Genetics, Institute of Cellular Physiology, UNAM, CDMX, México

2 Department of Cellular Biology and Development, Institute of Cellular Physiology, UNAM, CDMX, México

3 Department of Biochemistry, Institute of Chemistry, U de Sao Paulo, Sao Paulo, SP, Brazil

4 Laboratory of Bioenergetics and Molecular Genetics CIAD, Hermosillo, Sonora, México

5 Posthumous paper

http://dx.doi.org/10.5772/63667

References

[1] Lane N. Oxygen the molecule that made the world. Oxford: Oxford University Press; 2002. p. 384.

[2] Sessions AL, Doughty DM, Welander PV, Summons RE, Newman DK. The continuing puzzle of the great oxidation event. Current Biology. 2009;19(14):R567–74.

[3] Pavlov AA, Kasting JF. Mass-independent fractionation of sulfur isotopes in Archean sediments: strong evidence for an anoxic Archean atmosphere. Astrobiology. 2002;2(1): 27–41.

[4] Martin W, Rotte C, Hoffmeister M, Theissen U, Gelius-Dietrich G, Ahr S, et al. Early cell evolution, eukaryotes, anoxia, sulfide, oxygen, fungi first (?), and a tree of genomes revisited. IUBMB Life. 2003;55(4–5):193–204.

[5] Nisbet EG, Sleep NH. The habitat and nature of early life. Nature. 2001;409(6823):1083–91.

[6] Martin W, Muller M. The hydrogen hypothesis for the first eukaryote. Nature. 1998;392(6671):37–41.

[7] Castresana J, Saraste M. Evolution of energetic metabolism: the respiration-early hypothesis. Trends in Biochemical Sciences. 1995;20(11):443–8.

[8] Gray MW. Evolution of organellar genomes. Current Opinion in Genetics & Development. 1999;9(6):678–87.

[9] Kurland CG, Andersson SG. Origin and evolution of the mitochondrial proteome. Microbiology and Molecular Biology Reviews. 2000;64(4):786–820.

[10] Hellemond JJv, Klei Avd, Weelden SHv, Tielens AGM. Biochemical and evolutionary aspects of anaerobically functioning mitochondria. Philosophical Transactions of the Royal Society of London Series B: Biological Sciences. 2003;358(1429):205–15.

[11] Mentel M, Martin W. Energy metabolism among eukaryotic anaerobes in light of Proterozoic ocean chemistry. Philosophical Transactions of the Royal Society of London Series B, Biological Sciences. 2008;363(1504):2717–29.

[12] Hayes JM, Waldbauer JR. The carbon cycle and associated redox processes through time. Philosophical Transactions of the Royal Society B: Biological Sciences. 2006;361(1470):931–50.

[13] Holland HD. The oxygenation of the atmosphere and oceans. Philosophical Transactions of the Royal Society of London Series B, Biological Sciences. 2006;361(1470):903–15.

[14] Golblatt C, Lenton TM, Watson AJ. Bistability of atmospheric oxygen and the Great Oxidation. Nature. 2006;443(7112):683–6.

[15] Poole RK, D'Mello R, Hill S, Ioannidis N, Leung D, Wu G. The oxygen reactivity of bacterial respiratory haemoproteins: oxidases and globins. Biochimica et Biophysica Acta. 1994;1187(2):226–31.

[16] Hinton HE. Respiratory systems of insect egg shells. Annual review of entomology. 1969;14:343–68.

[17] Hochachka PW, Somero GN. Biochemical adaptation: mechanism and process in physiological evolution. United States Of America: Oxford University Press; 2002. 467 p.

[18] Hill RW, Wyse GA, Anderson M. Animal physiology. MA, USA: Sinauer Associates Inc. Publishers; 3rd Ed., 2012, P.799.

[19] Abele D. Toxic oxygen: the radical life-giver. Nature. 2002;420(6911):27.

[20] Martinez-Cruz O, Calderon de la Barca AM, Uribe-Carvajal S, Muhlia-Almazan A. The function of mitochondrial F(O)F(1) ATP-synthase from the whiteleg shrimp Litopenaeus vannamei muscle during hypoxia. Comparative Biochemistry and Physiology Part B, Biochemistry & Molecular Biology. 162(4):107–12.

[21] Müller M, Mentel M, van Hellemond JJ, Henze K, Woehle C, Gould SB, et al. Biochemistry and evolution of anaerobic energy metabolism in eukaryotes. Microbiology and Molecular Biology Reviews. 2012;76(2):444–95.

[22] Dall W, Hill BJ, Rothlisberg PC, Sharples DJ. The biology of the Penaeidae. Advances in Marine Biology; 1990. pp 489, 27. CSIRO Marine Laboratories, P.O. Box 120, Cleveland, Qld. 4163, Australia 1990.

[23] Ekau W, Auel H, Pörtner HO, Gilbert D. Impacts of hypoxia on the structure and processes in pelagic communities (zooplankton, macro-invertebrates and fish). Biogeosciences. 2010;7(5):1669–99.

[24] Mukai H, Koike I. Behavior and respiration of the Burrowing Shrimps Upogebia major (de Haan) and Callianassa japonica (de Haan). Journal of Crustacean Biology. 1984;4(2):191–200.

[25] Clegg J. Embryos of Artemia franciscana survive four years of continuous anoxia: the case for complete metabolic rate depression. Journal of Experimental Biology. 1997;200(3):467–75.

[26] Menze MA, Hutchinson K, Laborde SM, Hand SC. Mitochondrial permeability transition in the crustacean Artemia franciscana: absence of a calcium-regulated pore in the face of profound calcium storage. American Journal of Physiology – Regulatory, Integrative and Comparative Physiology. 2005;289(1):R68–76.

[27] Galli GJ, Richards J. Mitochondria from anoxia-tolerant animals reveal common strategies to survive without oxygen. Journal of Comparative Physiology B. 2014;184(3):285–302.

[28] Strahl J, Dringen R, Schmidt MM, Hardenberg S, Abele D. Metabolic and physiological responses in tissues of the long-lived bivalve Arctica islandica to oxygen deficiency. Comparative Biochemistry and Physiology Part A, Molecular & Integrative Physiology. 2011;158(4):513–9.

[29] Buttemer WA, Abele D, Costantini D. From bivalves to birds: oxidative stress and longevity. Functional Ecology. 2010;24(5):971–83.

[30] Rosi I, Vinella M, Domizio P. Characterization of beta-glucosidase activity in yeasts of oenological origin. The Journal of Applied Bacteriology. 1994;77(5):519–27.

[31] Roostita R, Fleet GH. Growth of yeasts in milk and associated changes to milk composition. International Journal of Food Microbiology. 1996;31(1–3):205–19.

[32] Eliskases-Lechner F, Ginzinger W, Rohm H, Tschager E. Raw milk flora affects composition and quality of Bergkäse. 1. Microbiology and fermentation compounds. Lait. 1999;79(4):385–96.

[33] Baracchini O, Sherris JC. The chemotactic effect of oxygen on bacteria. The Journal of Pathology and Bacteriology. 1959;77(2):565–74.

[34] Ulloa O, Canfield DE, DeLong EF, Letelier RM, Stewart FJ. Microbial oceanography of anoxic oxygen minimum zones. Proceedings of the National Academy of Sciences of the United States of America. 2012;109(40):15996–6003.

[35] Ingledew WJ, Poole RK. The respiratory chains of Escherichia coli. Microbiological Reviews. 1984;48(3):222–71.

[36] Unden G, Bongaerts J. Alternative respiratory pathways of Escherichia coli: energetics and transcriptional regulation in response to electron acceptors. Biochimica et Biophysica Acta. 1997;1320(3):217–34.

[37] Chakraborty B, Biswas S, Mondal S, Bera T. Stage specific developmental changes in the mitochondrial and surface membrane associated redox systems of Leishmania donovani promastigote and amastigote. Biochemistry Biokhimiia. 2010;75(4):494–518.

[38] Van Assche T, Deschacht M, da Luz RA, Maes L, Cos P. Leishmania-macrophage interactions: insights into the redox biology. Free Radical Biology & Medicine. 2011;51(2):337–51.

[39] Gonçalves RL, Barreto RF, Polycarpo CR, Gadelha FR, Castro SL, Oliveira MF. A comparative assessment of mitochondrial function in epimastigotes and bloodstream trypomastigotes of Trypanosoma cruzi. Journal of Bioenergetics and Biomembranes. 2011;43(6):651–61.

[40] Krungkrai J. The multiple roles of the mitochondrion of the malarial parasite. Parasitology. 2004;129(Pt 5):511–24.

[41] Muller S. Redox and antioxidant systems of the malaria parasite Plasmodium falciparum. Molecular Microbiology. 2004;53(5):1291–305.

[42] McCord JM, Keele BB, Jr., Fridovich I. An enzyme-based theory of obligate anaerobiosis: the physiological function of superoxide dismutase. Proceedings of the National Academy of Sciences of the United States of America. 1971;68(5):1024–7.

[43] D'Autreaux B, Toledano MB. ROS as signalling molecules: mechanisms that generate specificity in ROS homeostasis. Nature Reviews Molecular Cell Biology. 2007;8(10):813–24.

[44] Kadenbach B. Intrinsic and extrinsic uncoupling of oxidative phosphorylation. Biochimica et Biophysica Acta. 2003;1604(2):77–94.

[45] Guerrero-Castillo S, Araiza-Olivera D, Cabrera-Orefice A, Espinasa-Jaramillo J, Gutierrez-Aguilar M, Luevano-Martinez LA, et al. Physiological uncoupling of mitochondrial oxidative phosphorylation. Studies in different yeast species. Journal of Bioenergetics and Biomembranes. 2011;43(3):323–31.

[46] Manon S, Roucou X, Guerin M, Rigoulet M, Guerin B. Characterization of the yeast mitochondria unselective channel: a counterpart to the mammalian permeability transition pore? Journal of Bioenergetics Biomembranes. 1998;30(5):419–29.

[47] Bernardi P. The mitochondrial permeability transition pore: a mystery solved? Frontiers in Physiology. 2013;4:95.

[48] Uribe-Carvajal S, Luevano-Martinez LA, Guerrero-Castillo S, Cabrera-Orefice A, Corona-de-la-Pena NA, Gutierrez-Aguilar M. Mitochondrial unselective channels throughout the eukaryotic domain. Mitochondrion. 2011;11(3):382–90.

[49] Nicholls DG, Rial E. A history of the first uncoupling protein, UCP1. Journal of Bioenergetics and Biomembranes. 1999;31(5):399–406.

[50] Luevano-Martinez LA, Moyano E, de Lacoba MG, Rial E, Uribe-Carvajal S. Identification of the mitochondrial carrier that provides Yarrowia lipolytica with a fatty acid-induced and nucleotide-sensitive uncoupling protein-like activity. Biochimica et Biophysica Acta. 2010;1797(1):81–8.

[51] McDonald AE, Vanlerberghe GC, Staples JF. Alternative oxidase in animals: unique characteristics and taxonomic distribution. Journal of Experimental Biology. 2009;212(Pt 16):2627–34.

[52] McDonald AE, Vanlerberghe GC. Alternative oxidase and plastoquinol terminal oxidase in marine prokaryotes of the Sargasso Sea. Gene. 2005;349:15–24.

[53] Vanlerberghe GC, McIntosh L. Alternative oxydase: from gene to function. Annual Review of Plant Physiology and Plant Molecular Biology. 1997;48:703–34.

[54] Guerrero-Castillo S, Cabrera-Orefice A, Vazquez-Acevedo M, Gonzalez-Halphen D, Uribe-Carvajal S. During the stationary growth phase, Yarrowia lipolytica prevents the overproduction of reactive oxygen species by activating an uncoupled mitochondrial respiratory pathway. Biochimica et Biophysica Acta. 2012;1817(2):353–62.

[55] Cabrera-Orefice A, Chiquete-Felix N, Espinasa-Jaramillo J, Rosas-Lemus M, Guerrero-Castillo S, Pena A, et al. The branched mitochondrial respiratory chain from Debaryomyces hansenii: components and supramolecular organization. Biochimica et Biophysica Acta. 2013;1837(1):73–84.

[56] Bernardi P. Mitochondrial transport of cations: channels, exchangers, and permeability transition. Physiological Reviews. 1999;79(4):1127–55.

[57] Kwast KE, Hand SC. Acute depression of mitochondrial protein synthesis during anoxia: contributions of oxygen sensing, matrix acidification, and redox state. The Journal of Biological Chemistry. 1996;271(13):7313–9.

[58] Eads BD, Hand SC. Mitochondrial mRNA stability and polyadenylation during anoxia-induced quiescence in the brine shrimp Artemia franciscana. The Journal of Experimental Biology. 2003;206(Pt 20):3681–92.

[59] Holman JD, Hand SC. Metabolic depression is delayed and mitochondrial impairment averted during prolonged anoxia in the ghost shrimp, Lepidophthalmus louisianensis (Schmitt, 1935). Journal of Experimental Marine Biology and Ecology. 2009;376(2):85–93.

[60] Borisov VB, Murali R, Verkhovskaya ML, Bloch DA, Han H, Gennis RB, et al. Aerobic respiratory chain of Escherichia coli is not allowed to work in fully uncoupled mode. Proceedings of the National Academy of Sciences. 2011;108(42): 17320–4.

[61] Kerscher SJ. Diversity and origin of alternative NADH:ubiquinone oxidoreductases. Biochimica et Biophysica Acta (BBA) - Bioenergetics. 2000;1459(2â€"3):274–83.

[62] Büschges R, Bahrenberg G, Zimmermann M, Wolf K. Nadh: Ubiquinone oxidoreductase in obligate aerobic yeasts. Yeast. 1994;10(4):475–9.

[63] McDonald A, Vanlerberghe G. Branched mitochondrial electron transport in the Animalia: presence of alternative oxidase in several animal phyla. IUBMB Life. 2004;56(6):333–41.

[64] Tschischka K, Abele D, Portner HO. Mitochondrial oxyconformity and cold adaptation in the polychaete Nereis pelagica and the bivalve Arctica islandica from the Baltic and White Seas. The Journal of Experimental Biology. 2000;203(Pt 21):3355–68.

[65] Buchner T, Abele D, Portner HO. Oxyconformity in the intertidal worm Sipunculus nudus: the mitochondrial background and energetic consequences. Comparative Biochemistry and Physiology Part B, Biochemistry & Molecular Biology. 2001;129(1): 109–20.

[66] Hildebrandt TM, Grieshaber MK. Three enzymatic activities catalyze the oxidation of sulfide to thiosulfate in mammalian and invertebrate mitochondria. FEBS Journal. 2008;275(13):3352–61.

[67] Vanlerberghe GC, Robson CA, Yip JY. Induction of mitochondrial alternative oxidase in response to a cell signal pathway down-regulating the cytochrome pathway prevents programmed cell death. Plant Physiology. 2002;129(4): 1829–42.

[68] Beckerich JM, Boisrame-Baudevin A, Gaillardin C. Yarrowia lipolytica: a model organism for protein secretion studies. International Microbiology: The Official Journal of the Spanish Society for Microbiology. 1998;1(2):123–30.

[69] Otto C, Holz M, Barth G. Production of Organic Acids by Yarrowia lipolytica. In: Barth G, editor. Yarrowia lipolytica: Biotechnological Applications. Berlin, Heidelberg: Springer Berlin Heidelberg; 2013. p. 137–49.

[70] Darvishi Harzevili F. Yarrowia lipolytica: An Overview. Chapter 1, Biotechnological Applications of the Yeast Yarrowia lipolytica. SpringerBriefs in Microbiology, Springer International Publishing; 2014. p. 1–16.

[71] Kerscher S, Dröse S, Zwicker K, Zickermann V, Brandt U. Yarrowia lipolytica, a yeast genetic system to study mitochondrial complex I. Biochimica et Biophysica Acta (BBA) – Bioenergetics. 2002;1555(1–3):83–91.

[72] Kerscher SJ, Okun JG, Brandt U. A single external enzyme confers alternative NADH:ubiquinone oxidoreductase activity in Yarrowia lipolytica. Journal of Cell Science. 1999;112(Pt 14):2347–54.

[73] Medentsev AG, Arinbasarova AY, Golovchenko NP, Akimenko VK. Involvement of the alternative oxidase in respiration of Yarrowia lipolytica mitochondria is controlled by the activity of the cytochrome pathway. FEMS Yeast Research. 2002;2(4):519–24.

[74] Guerrero-Castillo S, Vazquez-Acevedo M, Gonzalez-Halphen D, Uribe-Carvajal S. In Yarrowia lipolytica mitochondria, the alternative NADH dehydrogenase interacts specifically with the cytochrome complexes of the classic respiratory pathway. Biochimica et Biophysica Acta. 2009;1787(2):75–85.

[75] Cook GM, Poole RK. Oxidase and periplasmic cytochrome assembly in Escherichia coli K-12: CydDC and CcmAB are not required for haem-membrane association. Microbiology. 2000;146(Pt 2):527–36.

[76] Wu M, Sun LV, Vamathevan J, Riegler M, Deboy R, Brownlie JC, et al. Phylogenomics of the reproductive parasite Wolbachia pipientis wMel: a streamlined genome overrun by mobile genetic elements. PLoS Biology. 2004;2(3):E69.

[77] Klasson L, Walker T, Sebaihia M, Sanders MJ, Quail MA, Lord A, et al. Genome evolution of Wolbachia strain wPip from the Culex pipiens group. Molecular Biology and Evolution. 2008;25(9):1877–87.

[78] Haddock BA, Jones CW. Bacterial respiration. Bacteriological Reviews. 1977;41(1):47–99.

[79] Jones K. Acetilene reduction by mats of blue-green algae in sub-tropical grassland: possible contribution by other micro-organisms. New Phytologist. 1977;78(2):437–40.

[80] Ng TCN, Laheri AN, Maier RJ. Cloning, sequencing, and mutagenesis of the cytochrome c4 gene from Azotobacter vinelandii: characterization of the mutant strain and a proposed new branch in the respiratory chain. Biochimica et Biophysica Acta (BBA) – Bioenergetics. 1995;1230(3):119–29.

[81] Bertsova YV, Bogachev AV, Skulachev VP. Two NADH:ubiquinone oxidoreductases of Azotobacter vinelandii and their role in the respiratory protection. Biochimica et Biophysica Acta. 1998;1363(2):125–33.

[82] González PJ, Correia C, Moura I, Brondino CD, Moura JJG. Bacterial nitrate reductases: molecular and biological aspects of nitrate reduction. Journal of Inorganic Biochemistry. 2006;100(5â€"6):1015–23.

[83] Whittaker MM, Whittaker JW. A glutamate bridge is essential for dimer stability and metal selectivity in manganese superoxide dismutase. The Journal of Biological Chemistry. 1998;273(35):22188–93.

[84] Cannio R, Fiorentino G, Morana A, Rossi M, Bartolucci S. Oxygen: friend or foe? Archaeal superoxide dismutases in the protection of intra- and extracellular oxidative stress. Frontiers in Bioscience: A Journal and Virtual Library. 2000;5:D768–79.

[85] Klotz MG, Loewen PC. The molecular evolution of catalatic hydroperoxidases: evidence for multiple lateral transfer of genes between prokaryota and from bacteria into eukaryota. Molecular Biology and Evolution. 2003;20(7):1098–112.

[86] Zamocky M, Furtmuller PG, Obinger C. Evolution of catalases from bacteria to humans. Antioxidants & Redox Signaling. 2008;10(9):1527–48.

[87] Nölling J, Breton G, Omelchenko MV, Makarova KS, Zeng Q, Gibson R, et al. Genome sequence and comparative analysis of the solvent-producing bacterium Clostridium acetobutylicum. Journal of Bacteriology. 2001;183(16):4823–38.

[88] Peacock AJ. ABC of oxygen: oxygen at high altitude. British Medical Journal. 1998;317(7165):1063–6.

[89] Hall JE, Guyton AC. Unit VII Respiration. In: Hall J, editor. Textbook of Medical Physiology. 12. Philadelphia, PA, USA: Elsevier; 2012.

[90] Popel AS. Theory of oxygen transport to tissue. Critical Reviews in Biomedical Engineering. 1989;17(3):257–321.

[91] Wilson DF, Rumsey WL, Green TJ, Vanderkooi JM. The oxygen dependence of mitochondrial oxidative phosphorylation measured by a new optical method for measuring oxygen concentration. The Journal of Biological Chemistry. 1988;263(6):2712–8.

[92] Geng M, Duan Z. Prediction of oxygen solubility in pure water and brines up to high temperatures and pressures. Geochimica et Cosmochimica Acta. 2010;74(19):5631–40.

[93] Chapelle G, Peck LS. Amphipod crustacean size spectra: new insights in the relationship between size and oxygen. Oikos. 2004;106(1):167–75.

[94] Beman JM, Carolan MT. Deoxygenation alters bacterial diversity and community composition in the ocean's largest oxygen minimum zone. Nature Communications. 2013;4:2705.

[95] Borsuk ME, Stow CA, Luettich Jr RA, Paerl HW, Pinckney JL. Modelling oxygen dynamics in an intermittently stratified estuary: estimation of process rates using field data. Estuarine, Coastal and Shelf Science. 2001;52(1):33–49.

[96] Engle V, Summers JK. Refinement, validation, and application of a benthic condition index for Northern Gulf of Mexico estuaries. Estuaries. 1999;22(3):624–35.

Chapter 2

Oxidative Stress in Invertebrate Systems

R.K. Chaitanya, K. Shashank and P. Sridevi

Additional information is available at the end of the chapter

http://dx.doi.org/10.5772/64573

Abstract

Invertebrates have been valuable research models in the discovery of many scientific principles owing to the numerous advantages they provide. Throughout the life cycle, many of them thrive in pathogen-rich environments, manage harsh weathers, exposed to a number of allochemicals, and adapt well to both terrestrial and marine ecosystems. Their remarkable ability to cope up with the enormous oxidative stress generated in all these circumstances, make them attractive models in this field of research. Endocrine control of oxidative stress in insects is recently emerging. Adipokinetic hormone, glucagon, ecdysteroids and juvenile hormone have been implicated in antioxidative protective role in insects. *Drosophila* and *Caenorhabditis elegans* have provided the largest body of evidence addressing the free radical theory of ageing. Oxidative stress is also induced by pesticides/insecticides. In mollusks, pesticides exert their biological effects via generation of ROS. Oxidative stress has been shown to be associated with exposure to several organophosphorous compounds and different classes of pyrethroids. Malathion is a potential hazard to the environment. Adverse effects induced by malathion in earthworms and insects have been reported. Information is now available in great detail on the role of ROS in modulating insect immunity during parasite invasion and bacterial infection. In *Drosophila melanogaster* ROS are actively produced in the midgut at a basal level in the presence of commensal microbiota and highly generated upon bacterial challenge. The involvement of reactive oxygen species (ROS) in mosquito immunity against bacteria and *Plasmodium* was investigated in the malaria vector *Anopheles gambiae*. The concentration of ROS increased in sand fly midguts after they fed on the insect pathogen *Serratia marcescens*. Elevated oxidative stress was previously reported for a mosquito line experimentally infected with *Wolbachia,* indicating that oxidative stress may be important for *Wolbachia*-mediated antiviral protection. In a nutshell, this chapter highlights the current advances of oxidative stress in invertebrate model systems and its implications.

Keywords: oxidative stress, invertebrates, reactive oxygen species, antioxidative system

1. Oxidative stress: an introduction

Oxidative stress can be defined as a disturbance in the balance between the production of reactive oxygen species and antioxidant defenses [1]. Reactive oxygen species (ROS) are free radicals, which are important for the cellular functions generated in different biological processes. A free radical is unstable and highly reactive and contains one or more unpaired electrons. These free radicals are involved in the regulation of various mechanisms and intercellular signaling and act as bactericidal agents [2]. ROS can also induce cellular senescence, apoptosis, and cell growth regulatory pathways [3]. ROS are generated as a by-product of the aerobic respiration where the superoxide anion (O_2^-) and H_2O_2 are formed when molecular oxygen chemically oxidizes electron carriers. Cellular sources of ROS are produced by the action of different oxidative enzymes, which include plasma membrane nicotinamide adenine dinucleotide phosphate (NADPH) oxidase, intracellular cytosolic xanthine oxidase, peroxisomal oxidases, endoplasmic reticular oxidases, and mitochondrial electron transport components [4]. Apart from this, auto-oxidation of catecholamines, ubihydroquinone, hemoproteins, and flavin enzymes also produces ROS [5]. In response to nutrient stress, cells enter autophagy that can lead to adaptation or death. Starvation-induced autophagy results in reactive oxygen species (ROS) production, DNA damage, and PARP-1 activation, leading to the inhibition of mTOR.

In all these cases, the generation of free radicals is implied.

2. Biological factors of oxidative stress in invertebrates

Reactive oxygen species are naturally produced in all cells and organisms. Modifications of normal conditions alter reactive species generation and may result in oxidative stress. In this chapter, we have discussed the role of the most important causes of the ROS generation in the invertebrate systems.

2.1. Blood feeding

Insects like mosquitoes which feed on human blood face severe oxidative stress due to the release of iron from hemoglobin which in turn can potentially induce oxidative damage and eventually death [6]. To face such odd situation, blood-feeding insects evolved with strong defense mechanisms against the stress. Mosquitoes protect themselves by secretion of the peritrophic matrix (PM) [7] in the midgut which is made up of chitin and a protein-containing layer. It also has a role in protecting the insect from invasive pathogens [8]. The direct contact of the gut epithelium with intermediates of hemoglobin digestion induces oxidative stress in sand fly and *Aedes aegypti* [9].

2.2. Xenobiotic degradation

A source of ROS in the honeybee is the microsomal oxidation of xenobiotics. Microsomes contain enzymes of cytochrome P450 (CYP) system, which catalyzes polyvalent oxidation of xenobiotics with simultaneous generation of O_2^- and other ROS. The CYP hydroxylase system includes flavoproteins and a family of hemoproteins which are localized on the membranes of the endoplasmic reticulum. Different isoforms of CYP are involved in metabolism of various xenobiotics [10, 11]. CYP groups are distinguished based on the metabolism of endogenous and exogenous substances. Microsomal glutathione S-transferase (GST) is closely linked with the CYP system, which contributes to rapid inactivation of active metabolites produced during the metabolism of xenobiotics.

2.3. Dopamine synthesis

In the insect nervous system, ROS-mediated decline of neuron survival can be observed. The dopamine-producing neurons show the highest sensitivity to oxidative stress as the dopamine production machinery is linked to an endogenous production of high amounts of ROS, thus making these cells prone to damages caused by ROS. These high levels of ROS lead to the development of Parkinson's disease-like phenotypes [12]. It is a suitable mechanism to induce neurodegenerative processes using ROS as typically seen in Parkinson's disease. One of the most reproducible ways to do this is through hyperoxia, which consequently is able to induce these phenotypes enabled *Drosophila* as a model for Parkinson's disease [13]. In an Alzheimer's disease model, based on tau activation in the nervous system, ROS has been shown to modulate the sensitivity, thus demonstrating that oxidative stress plays a major role in the development of Alzheimer's disease.

2.4. Microbiome

The intestinal microbiome is one of the densest populations on earth. Thus, attaining a homeostatic balance between fight against potential pathogens and maintenance of the microbial community within the intestinal tract is a major challenge for the gut immune system [14]. Fighting pathogens is achieved via enzymes producing ROS. Dual oxidase (DUOX) is a member of nicotinamide adenine dinucleotide phosphate oxidase (NADPH oxidase) family and the most important enzyme secreted from enterocytes in response to pathogen contact [11, 15]. It is independent of classical immune response pathways such as the Toll [16] or the IMD pathway [17]. The killing mechanism of DUOX comprises the production of H_2O_2, which is a typical feature of DUOX enzymes in general [18]. The fly phenol oxidases (POs) are another enzyme set that produces a melanin coat surrounding invaders of different nature. These enzymes are able to produce a locally high concentration of ROS, which may be one of the major effectors of the prophenoloxidase (PPO) system. This melatonin production is triggered by the recognition of bacterial patterns including peptidoglycans [19].

Airway infection is one of the well-studied areas in fruit fly [20]. In addition to classical aspects of an antibacterial response including antimicrobial peptide genes, some of these enzymatic antioxidants are strongly upregulated. The antioxidant system of the airway epithelium contains both producers of ROS and protectors against them.

2.5. Oxidative burst in macrophages

Motile cells of the innate immune system use production of highly effective ROS which is a versatile method to fight pathogens. The oxidative burst produced by macrophages is the most impressive example highlighting this strategy. Reactive oxygen species (ROS) is generated by many phagocytic cells in response to membrane perturbations such as receptor-ligand interactions and phagocytosis [16, 21], which defend these cells against infectious diseases by virtue of their antimicrobial properties. Initially, superoxide anion (O_2^-) is produced which is spontaneously or enzymatically converted to hydrogen peroxide (H_2O_2), subsequently giving rise to even more toxic products, such as hydroxyl radical ($^{\bullet}OH$), hypochlorous acid (HOCl), and singlet oxygen (IO_2). ROS are either directly toxic or exert increased antimicrobial activity in synergism with lysosomal hydrolases and/or reactive nitrogen species (RNS), plasma membrane-bound enzyme complexes, and the NADPH oxidase (NOX) system [22].

Leishmania parasite manages both to survive and proliferate within the mature phagolysosomal compartment of the macrophages [21]. Trypanosomatids do not express essential antioxidant enzymes like catalase and selenium-containing glutathione (GSH) peroxidases [23]. Defense system of the *Leishmania* parasite contains several mechanisms, which include trypanothione (N1, N8-bis(glutathionyl)spermidine adduct) [24, 25]. It is the primary thiol in these parasites and adopts the metabolic role of glutathione. Along with this, ovothiol A acts as a nonenzymatic scavenger of H_2O_2 though it is much less efficient than trypanothione [26]. Trypanothione reductase (TR) is a member of the disulfide reductase family, which is the enzyme responsible for maintaining trypanothione in its reduced form [27]. Tryparedoxin peroxidases or peroxiredoxins are a family of peroxidases that reduce H_2O_2 and alkyl hydroperoxides to water and alcohol, respectively, with the use of reducing equivalents provided by thiol-containing proteins [28]. The enzyme arginase is a part of the host as well as parasite defense. Phagocytosis of promastigotes leads toward the two opposing forms of classical and alternative activation of host macrophages which results in differential L-arginine metabolism [29, 30]. Being effective in modulating macrophage signaling and antimicrobial function, *Leishmania* parasites possess surface protein kinases which phosphorylate members of complement system, thus inactivating cellular cascades. This helps the parasite to evade the innate immune responses and ensure a safe environment for its proliferation [31].

Parasites can inhibit the activation of several inflammatory cytokines like interleukin-12 (involved in T-cell activation), interferon gamma, interleukin-1, and tumor necrosis factor-alpha that strengthens parasite survival. Few species induce heterologous population of host inflammatory cells, such as neutrophils and monocytes/macrophages, which are effective in controlling/clearing infections. The T helper cell type 1 (Th1) response as a result decreased expression of induced nitric oxide synthase and reduced activity of NK cells [32].

Selenocysteine is analogous to a cysteine residue but has sulfur substituted by selenium. Selenoprotein families, some with antioxidant properties, such as glutathione peroxidase

(GPx) and thioredoxin glutathione reductase (TGR) appear to be essential in flatworms and in *Plasmodium falciparum* and other *Plasmodium* species [33, 34].

Ascorbate peroxidase is another antioxidant, which is a heme peroxidase identified in the inner mitochondrial membrane of the *Leishmania* parasite. Overexpression of this enzyme confers tolerance to oxidative stress-mediated cardiolipin oxidation and thus protects the parasites from extensive protein damage. *Leishmania* promastigotes inhibit phagolysosome biogenesis via lipophosphoglycan (LPG), which causes periphagosomal accumulation of F-actin and impaired assembly of nicotinamide adenine dinucleotide phosphate (NADPH) oxidase complex and exclusion of vesicular proton ATPase from phagosomes [35].

2.6. Respiration

The major task of airway epithelial cells is enabling an effective oxygen transport and exchange. These cells react to different stimuli with appropriate responses including massive responses if pathogens are experienced. In principal, all oxygen transport systems are prone to damage caused by high oxidative stress because these cells have direct contact with the air and large volumes of air pass over their surface during the process of gas exchange.

3. Nonbiological factors of oxidative stress in invertebrates

3.1. Effect of pollutants

Environment has a major role in the production of stress because of different pollutants like air, soil, and water. The compounds used in industry and agriculture include metals, metalloids, and numerous other organic compounds. Majority of these compounds have been shown to induce oxidative stress by generating ROS in nontarget species including invertebrates [36].

3.2. Effect of phytochemicals, herbicides, and insecticides

Plant phenolic compounds, such as flavonoids and tannins, which are involved in plant defense mechanism, can produce free radical in herbivorous insects [37]. The midgut of insect is a highly oxidizing environment. Hence in lepidopteran larvae, *Helicoverpa zea* and *Spodoptera littoralis* with phenolic acids were found to increase various indicators of oxidative stress in gut tissues [38, 39]. Additionally, furanocoumarins in some plants and herbicides like paraquat are well known to generate oxidative stress in insect species [36]. Insect growth regulator (IGR) is a substance (chemical) that inhibits the life cycle of an insect and has been used to control the insect pests. Hormonal IGRs typically work by mimicking or inhibiting the juvenile hormone (JH) or ecdysone. Studies on the IGRs like Applaud (buprofezin) as a chitin synthesis inhibitor and Admiral (pyriproxyfen) as juvenile hormone analog (JHA) in the larval body of the cotton leaf worm, *S. littoralis,* resulted in the occurrence of lipid peroxidation in the larval tissues which enhanced different antioxidant defensive systems to overcome its effect like malondialdehyde (MDA) and glutathione reduction [40].

3.3. Effect of metal ions

Disruption of metal ion homeostasis may lead to oxidative stress, a state where increased formation of reactive oxygen species (ROS) overwhelms body antioxidant protection and subsequently induces symptoms for numerous diseases, involving cancer, cardiovascular disease, diabetes, atherosclerosis, neurological disorders (Alzheimer's disease, Parkinson's disease), chronic inflammation, and others [41].

Metals, such as iron (Fe), copper (Cu), chromium (Cr), and cobalt (Co), induce the formation of the superoxide and hydroxyl radicals (mainly through Fenton reaction) and other ROS, which ultimately leads to the production of malondialdehyde (MDA), 4-hydroxynonenal (HNE), and other exocyclic DNA adducts that are carcinogenic and mutagenic. On the other hand, the redox-inactive metals, such as cadmium (Cd), arsenic (As), and lead (Pb), induce toxicity through bonding to sulphydryl groups of proteins and depletion of glutathione. Zinc (Zn) is a redox-inert metal, which is an essential component of numerous proteins involved in the defense against oxidative stress. In addition, Zn possesses neuroprotective properties. Depletion of Zn may enhance DNA damage through impairments of DNA repair mechanisms. Cellular antioxidants (ascorbic acid (vitamin C), alpha-tocopherol (vitamin E), glutathione (GSH), carotenoids, flavonoids, and other antioxidants) and chelate metal ions reduce their catalytic activity to form ROS. A novel therapeutic approach to suppress oxidative stress is based on the development of dual function antioxidants which comprise of chelating and scavenging agents [39, 40].

4. ROS production in marine invertebrates

Oxidative stress is highly prevalent in marine invertebrates, particularly bivalve mollusks, due to the degradation of marine ecosystems, massive aquaculture productions, climate change, and pathogenic infections. Mollusk hemocytes produce ROS and RNS as part of their basal metabolism as well as in response to both endogenous and exogenous stimuli. However, sources, pathways, and mechanistic aspects of these reactive species production are currently poorly deciphered. Unique pathways seem to exist in marine bivalves [42].

High oxygen solubility in cold water is responsible for an elevated level of antioxidant protection in marine ectotherms from polar environments. However, tissue oxidative stress is a function of elevated or variable pO_2, rather than of an elevated tissue oxygen level [43].

To counteract or to regulate the free radical production, several antioxidant mechanisms were evolved (**Figure 1**) [44].

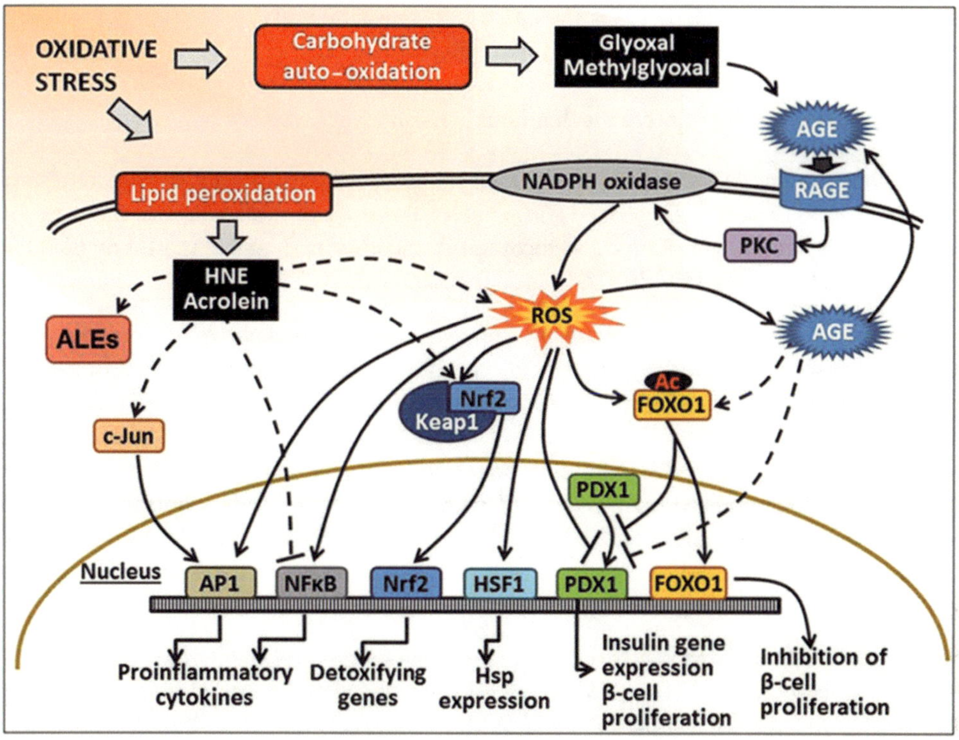

Figure 1. Schematic representation of the pathways activated by the oxidative stress on macromolecules like lipids and carbohydrates leads to the signal transduction through ROS-dependent and ROS-independent mechanisms. Glyoxal and methylglyoxal formed by the oxidation of the carbohydrates were detected by the AGE and activate cell surface molecule RAGE. It passes signal to NADPH oxidase through PKC, which activates the ROS. ROS activates several transcription factors such as AP-1; NF-kB: pro-inflammatory cytokines; Nrf2: detoxifying genes; HSF1: Hsp expression; and FOXO1: inhibition of B-cell proliferation. It also inhibits the PDX1 transcription factor which activates insulin gene expression and B-cell proliferation. In ROS-independent pathway, AGE can directly activate FOXO1 and inhibits PDX1. In lipid peroxidation, 4-hydroxynonenal (HNE) and acrolein-mediated signaling activate AP-1 through c-Jun and Nrf2. It blocks NF-kB–mediated transcription activation apart from the ROS-activated signaling.

5. Antioxidants

Oxidative stress arises when there is a marked imbalance between the production and removal of reactive oxygen and nitrogen species. Free radical production is normally controlled by the antioxidant defense mechanisms [2]. Antioxidative defenses could essentially be divided broadly into two main mechanisms: one is enzymatic and the other is nonenzymatic.

5.1. Enzymatic antioxidative mechanisms

Insects, like other animals, possess a suite of enzymes that are directed toward the removal of various radicals [45–48]. These include superoxide dismutase present in cytosol and mitochondria, catalase present in peroxisomes, ascorbate peroxidase [49], glutathione S-transferase peroxidase, thioredoxin/thioreductase system [50], and so on.

5.2. Nonenzymatic antioxidative mechanisms

In addition to the classical antioxidant enzyme systems, a number of small molecules also play a significant role in scavenging ROS, and some of these small molecules are plant derived, whereas others such as carotenoids, α-tocopherol, ascorbic acid, and glutathione (GSH) can be synthesized by insects [45, 50–52].

In addition to the antioxidant mechanisms and systems described above, insects also possess several water-soluble molecules (uric acid, carbohydrates, and polyols) and iron-binding proteins (ferritin and transferrin) that serve crucial antioxidant functions [45]. Antioxidant properties of vitellogenin are specified by its Zn-binding capacity [53] and preferential oxidative carboxylation under oxidative stress in honeybees [54]. With respect to these properties, vitellogenin is compared to Cu/ZnSOD, a key metal-binding antioxidant enzyme that undergoes preferential carbonylation [55], and serum albumin, a metal-binding protein, that can function as free radical acceptors and reduce oxidative marker levels such as protein carbonylation [56].

Responses to oxidative stress induced by a blood meal were investigated in *A. aegypti* [7]. In female mosquitoes, higher levels of ferritin were observed after repeated blood meals. Ferritin is a sensitive defense mechanism against oxidative stress induced by blood meal [57]. An increase of secreted ferritin due to the induced synthesis of ferritin heavy chain homologue (HCH) was observed [58].

6. Regulation of defenses against oxidative stress

Oxidative stress triggers a range of responses in insect cells which could be physiological, pathological, and adaptive. A large number of signaling pathways are involved in response to oxidative stress. *Drosophila melanogaster* is a well-studied organism in the field of oxidative stress. Among these signaling pathways, in fruit fly, PI3-kinase pathway is one of the important responses to oxidative stress by activating the transcription factor FOXO [13], and an alternative signaling is represented by the Nrf2/Keap1 pathway which is required for a proper and efficient expression of genes associated with an increase in oxidative stress resistance [41]. Other signaling systems include activator protein-1 (AP-1), nuclear factor-kB (NF-kB), protein kinase C (PKC), protein 53 (p53), and redox regulation by redox factor-1 and the nuclear factor erythroid 2–related factor 2 (Nrf2)-mediated antioxidant response. Nrf2 belongs to a group of specialized transcription factors termed xenobiotic-activated receptors (XARs). These recognize specific xenobiotics and coordinate the transcription of batteries of genes.

Honeybees possess only about half the genes of GST, CYP, and carboxyl/cholinesterases as in other insects [17–19]. This deficit can contribute to insufficient resistance to oxidative stress caused by incomplete microsomal oxidation of xenobiotics [59]. These insects have more genes of class sigma GST [60], which has a high affinity to the products of lipid peroxidation localized in the thorax muscle of flies to protect these tissues against oxidative stress by-products [61].

The idea behind one of the first theories of aging was oxidative stress-induced damage [42]. Enzymes which regulate the oxidative stress are responsible for the longevity that was supported by shortened life span in flies lacking a functional thioredoxin-2 [60]. Peroxiredoxin of type 2, named Jafrac1 [61], and other peroxiredoxins, especially those present in mitochondria, are also relevant for life span, as their downregulation has a significant impact on this aspect of life [62] along with other enzymes like glutathione reductase [63], SODs, and catalase [64–66].

Intriguingly, genes belonging to the family of antimicrobial peptide genes are obviously relevant for this adaptation to extreme oxygen concentrations and therewith to higher levels of oxidative stress [67, 68]. In insects, compared to vertebrates, genes encoding glutathione reductase (GR) and glutathione peroxidase (GPX) are absent. Their functions are performed by homologous genes that encode thioredoxin reductase (TrxR) [52] and thioredoxin peroxidase (TPx) [67]. In addition, insects' genes encode enzymes of antioxidant defense that act as peroxidases: phospholipid-hydroperoxide GPx homologues with TPx activity (GTPx) [69] and GST [70, 71]. Thus, the secondary antioxidant enzymes in insects that act on ROS indirectly include TrxR, which converts both Trx and GSH, and methionine sulfoxide reductases (MsrA and MsrB), which are involved in protein repair by catalyzing the Trx-dependent conversion of methionine sulfoxide to methionine [72, 73].

In the nervous system, the dopamine metabolism produces high ROS concentration leading to the SOD overexpression. Increase in the glutathione S-transferase activity in the nervous system protects these dopaminergic neurons [74]. However, this ROS-based mechanism of neurodegenerative diseases is not applicable for Huntington's disease. Neither overexpression of enzymatic antioxidants nor supplementation with nonenzymatic antioxidants decreased the lethality in this model [61].

The intestinal microbiome regulation DUOX plays a crucial role with killing mechanism by production of H_2O_2 [31]. To protect the gut tissue from the action of ROS, an enzymatic antioxidant, immune-regulated catalase (IRC), is produced [29].

Previous microarray studies in *Drosophila* suggested that IRC is the only catalase to be induced upon infection and may be regulated by the Toll pathway. The IMD pathway could be another candidate for regulation of antioxidants including IRC, since it is induced systemically by Gram-negative bacteria and in turn activates the JNK pathway.

Malpighian tubules also perform crucial roles in stress sensing and response [75]. At molecular level, multiple cell-specific signaling pathways including cAMP, cGMP, and calcium modulate the tissue and, hence, organism responds to various stress, such as detoxification and xenobiotic handling, and stress sensing of oxidative, osmotic (ionic/salt) and immune challenges [76–78].

7. ROS-dependent biological processes in insects

7.1. Autophagy

In the regulation of intestinal microbiome, apart from the ROS-induced OS regulation of pathogens, ROS production induces a JNK-triggered autophagy in the enterocytes in *D. melanogaster* [59].

7.2. Differentiation of hemocytes

Motile cells of the innate immune system use oxidative burst to control invading pathogens. Apart from that, ROS play an important role in the differentiation of hemocytes. In *Drosophila,* multipotent hematopoietic progenitors react to different ROS levels with a speeding up or arresting of their differentiation [79]. Both the JNK and the FOXO pathways are involved in the transduction of ROS levels into developmental signals [80].

8. Hormonal regulation of oxidative stress

8.1. Adipokinetic hormones (AKHs): stress hormones of insects

The insect endocrine system produces three main groups of hormones [81] including (a) ecdysteroids, (b) juvenile hormones (JHs), and (c) neurohormones. Out of these, a group of neurohormones belonging to the AKH/RPCH family (adipokinetic hormone/red pigment-concentrating hormone family) is associated with stress responses [82, 83]. Recently, it has been found that AKHs are also involved in the control of oxidative stress (OS) in insects [79]. The balance between the OS and its control by AKHs was attained by feedback regulation between an oxidative stressor and AKH actions. The effect is reported for paraquat [84, 85], *Galanthus nivalis* agglutinin and *Bacillus thuringiensis* toxin [84] and also for endosulfan and malathion [86] insecticides with an OS effect. Reports are available for the elevation of AKH in stress other than OS [53–56]. It was suggested that the activation of protective anti-oxidative mechanisms is derived from the effect of oxidative stressors on AKH level in the insect body.

Not only have AKHs been implicated to be involved in hormonal control of antioxidative protective reactions in insects, but other hormones such as glucagon, ecdysteroids, and JHs have also been suggested to be involved in antioxidative protective mechanisms. Analogous to vertebrates [87–89], it was suggested for insects that glucagon could play a role in defense against OS. Ecdysteroids were shown to be involved in the control of OS by inhibiting the oxidation of cholesterol and the peroxidation of polyunsaturated fatty acids in the lipoproteins, microsomes, and other components of biological systems [90].

8.2. 20-Hydroxyecdysone (20E)

In *D. melanogaster*, ecdysone-induced methionine sulfoxide reductase A enhances resistance to hydrogen peroxide [91]. It also regulates the methionine sulfoxide reductase [92, 93] enzyme

http://dx.doi.org/10.5772/64573

expression via the ecdysone receptor (EcR-UPS) complex [54]. Treatment with insect 20E protected mammals against cerebral ischemia injury by inhibiting production of ROS/RNS and modulating OS-induced signal transduction pathways. Treatment of B35 rat neuroblastoma cells with hydrogen peroxide led to OS-induced apoptosis, mitochondrial membrane potential dissipation, neuronal injury, generation of intracellular ROS/RNS, decrease of cellular antioxidant potential, and increase of lipid peroxidation, all of which were significantly eliminated by 20E [54, 94–97].

8.3. Juvenile hormone

JHs are synthesized and secreted in/from the corpora allata in the insect brain. Recent studies have implicated that lack of JH may confer resistance to OS. The elimination of JH synthesis extended the survival of flies exposed to hydrogen peroxide. The survival times returned to those in control when the knockout flies were treated with JH analog methoprene. Moreover, another JH analog, pyriproxyfen, induced OS in the wax moth *Galleria mellonella,* as the antioxidative enzyme activities, CAT and SOD, increased after the pyriproxyfen application. Similarly, pyriproxyfen increased the activity of enzymes CAT and GST, as well as the accumulation of MDA and GSH, in larvae of *S. littoralis*. JHs are also involved in the control of antioxidative reactions albeit indirectly via the regulation of vitellogenin and transferrin synthesis [54, 94–97].

9. Summary

This chapter summarizes current knowledge on pro- and antioxidant processes in invertebrates particularly insects. Reactive oxygen species (ROS) formation and their adaptations in different organisms were discussed in the context of the usage of invertebrates as a model organism in the field of OS to study the OS-mediated diseases in humans.

Author details

R.K. Chaitanya[1*], K. Shashank[1] and P. Sridevi[2]

*Address all correspondence to: chaitanyark@gmail.com

1 School of Basic & Applied Sciences, Central University of Punjab, Bhatinda, India

2 Department of Biotechnology, Indira Gandhi National Tribal University, Amarkantak, India

References

[1] Betteridge, D.J., What is oxidative stress? Metabolism, 2000. 49(2 Suppl 1): p. 3–8.

[2] Evans, P. and B. Halliwell, Free radicals and hearing. Cause, consequence, and criteria. Ann N Y Acad Sci, 1999. 884: p. 19–40.

[3] Valko, M., et al., Free radicals, metals and antioxidants in oxidative stress-induced cancer. Chem Biol Interact, 2006. 160(1): p. 1–40.

[4] Uday B. et al., Reactive oxygen species: oxidative damage and pathogenesis. Curr Sci, 1999. 77(5–10).

[5] Ahmad, S. and R.S. Pardini, Mechanisms for regulating oxygen toxicity in phytophagous insects. Free Radic Biol Med, 1990. 8(4): p. 401–13.

[6] Kirkinezos, I.G. and C.T. Moraes, Reactive oxygen species and mitochondrial diseases. Semin Cell Dev Biol, 2001. 12(6): p. 449–57.

[7] Saeaue, L., et al., Antioxidative systems defense against oxidative stress induced by blood meal in *Aedes aegypti*. Southeast Asian J Trop Med Public Health, 2011. 42(3): p. 542–9.

[8] Bhatnagar, R.K., et al., Synthetic propeptide inhibits mosquito midgut chitinase and blocks sporogonic development of malaria parasite. Biochem Biophys Res Commun, 2003. 304(4): p. 783–7.

[9] Araújo A.P., et al., Disruption of the peritrophic matrix by exogenous chitinase feeding reduces fecundity in *Lutzomyia longipalpis* females. Mem Inst Oswaldo Cruz 2012 107(4): 543–45.

[10] Tellam, R.L., G. Wijffels, and P. Willadsen, Peritrophic matrix proteins. Insect Biochem Mol Biol, 1999. 29(2): p. 87–101.

[11] Zhao, H.W., et al., Experimental selection for Drosophila survival in extremely high O_2 environments. PLoS One, 2010. 5(7): p. e11701.

[12] Ha, E.M., et al., A direct role for dual oxidase in Drosophila gut immunity. Science, 2005. 310(5749): p. 847–50.

[13] Chaudhuri, A., et al., Interaction of genetic and environmental factors in a Drosophila parkinsonism model. J Neurosci, 2007. 27(10): p. 2457–67.

[14] Gruenewald, C., et al., Hyperoxia-induced neurodegeneration as a tool to identify neuroprotective genes in *Drosophila melanogaster*. Free Radic Biol Med, 2009. 46(12): p. 1668–76.

[15] Kounatidis, I. and P. Ligoxygakis, Drosophila as a model system to unravel the layers of innate immunity to infection. Open Biol, 2012. 2(5): p. 120075.

[16] Wagner, C., et al., Molecular architecture of the fruit fly's airway epithelial immune system. BMC Genomics, 2008. 9: p. 446.

[17] Ha, E.M., et al., An antioxidant system required for host protection against gut infection in Drosophila. Dev Cell, 2005. 8(1): p. 125–32.

[18] Ha, E.M., et al., Regulation of DUOX by the Galphaq-phospholipase Cbeta-Ca^{2+} pathway in Drosophila gut immunity. Dev Cell, 2009. 16(3): p. 386–97.

[19] Ryu, J.H., E.M. Ha, and W.J. Lee, Innate immunity and gut-microbe mutualism in Drosophila. Dev Comp Immunol, 2010. 34(4): p. 369–76.

[20] Bidla, G., M.S. Dushay, and U. Theopold, Crystal cell rupture after injury in Drosophila requires the JNK pathway, small GTPases and the TNF homolog Eiger. J Cell Sci, 2007. 120(Pt 7): p. 1209–15.

[21] McConville, M.J., et al., Living in a phagolysosome; metabolism of Leishmania amastigotes. Trends Parasitol, 2007. 23(8): p. 368–75.

[22] Koppenol, W.H., et al., Peroxynitrite, a cloaked oxidant formed by nitric oxide and superoxide. Chem Res Toxicol, 1992. 5(6): p. 834–42.

[23] Castro, H., et al., Complementary antioxidant defense by cytoplasmic and mitochondrial peroxiredoxins in *Leishmania infantum*. Free Radic Biol Med, 2002. 33(11): p. 1552–62.

[24] Henderson, G.B., et al., Biosynthesis of the trypanosomatid metabolite trypanothione: purification and characterization of trypanothione synthetase from *Crithidia fasciculata*. Biochemistry, 1990. 29(16): p. 3924–9.

[25] Krauth-Siegel, R.L. and M.A. Comini, Redox control in trypanosomatids, parasitic protozoa with trypanothione-based thiol metabolism. Biochim Biophys Acta, 2008. 1780(11): p. 1236–48.

[26] Ariyanayagam, M.R. and A.H. Fairlamb, Ovothiol and trypanothione as antioxidants in trypanosomatids. Mol Biochem Parasitol, 2001. 115(2): p. 189–98.

[27] Dumas, C., et al., Disruption of the trypanothione reductase gene of Leishmania decreases its ability to survive oxidative stress in macrophages. EMBO J, 1997. 16(10): p. 2590–8.

[28] Rhee, S.G., et al., Peroxiredoxin, a novel family of peroxidases. IUBMB Life, 2001. 52(1–2): p. 35–41.

[29] Kropf, P., et al., Signaling through the T1/ST2 molecule is not necessary for Th2 differentiation but is important for the regulation of type 1 responses in nonhealing Leishmania major infection. Infect Immun, 2003. 71(4): p. 1961–71.

[30] Iniesta, V., L.C. Gomez-Nieto, and I. Corraliza, The inhibition of arginase by N(omega)-hydroxy-l-arginine controls the growth of Leishmania inside macrophages. J Exp Med, 2001. 193(6): p. 777–84.

[31] Forget, G., et al., Role of host phosphotyrosine phosphatase SHP-1 in the development of murine leishmaniasis. Eur J Immunol, 2001. 31(11): p. 3185–96.

[32] Campos-Neto, A., What about Th1/Th2 in cutaneous leishmaniasis vaccine discovery? Braz J Med Biol Res, 2005. 38(7): p. 979–84.

[33] Maiorino, M., et al., A selenium-containing phospholipid-hydroperoxide glutathione peroxidase in *Schistosoma mansoni*. Eur J Biochem, 1996. 238(3): p. 838–44.

[34] Williams, D.L., et al., Molecular cloning and sequencing of glutathione peroxidase from *Schistosoma mansoni*. Mol Biochem Parasitol, 1992. 52(1): p. 127–30.

[35] Das, S., et al., The complex world of cellular defense in the Leishmania parasite. Proc Ind Natl Sci Acad, 2015. 81(3): p. 629–41.

[36] Ahmad, S., Oxidative stress from environmental pollutants. Arch Insect Biochem Physiol, 1995. 29(2): p. 135–57.

[37] Sakihama, Y., et al., Plant phenolic antioxidant and prooxidant activities: phenolics-induced oxidative damage mediated by metals in plants. Toxicology, 2002. 177(1): p. 67–80.

[38] Krishnan, N. and F. Sehnal, Compartmentalization of oxidative stress and antioxidant defense in the larval gut of *Spodoptera littoralis*. Arch Insect Biochem Physiol, 2006. 63(1): p. 1–10.

[39] Jomova, K. and M. Valko, Advances in metal-induced oxidative stress and human disease. Toxicology, 2011. 283(2–3): p. 65–87.

[40] Nedal M.F., Impact of two insect growth regulators on the enhancement of oxidative stress and antioxidant efficiency of the cotton leaf worm, *Spodoptera littoralis* (Biosd.). Egypt Acad J Biolog Sci, 2012. 5(1): p. 137–49.

[41] Hybertson, B.M., et al., Oxidative stress in health and disease: the therapeutic potential of Nrf2 activation. Mol Aspects Med, 2011. 32(4–6): p. 234–46.

[42] Donaghy, L., et al., The known and unknown sources of reactive oxygen and nitrogen species in haemocytes of marine bivalve molluscs. Fish Shellfish Immunol, 2015. 42(1): p. 91–7.

[43] Abele, D. and S. Puntarulo, Formation of reactive species and induction of antioxidant defence systems in polar and temperate marine invertebrates and fish. Comp Biochem Physiol A Mol Integr Physiol, 2004. 138(4): p. 405–15.

[44] Jaganjac, M., et al., Reactive aldehydes—second messengers of free radicals in diabetes mellitus. Free Radic Res, 2013. 47 Suppl 1: p. 39–48.

[45] Felton, G.W. and C.B. Summers, Antioxidant systems in insects. Arch Insect Biochem Physiol, 1995. 29(2): p. 187–97.

[46] Krishnan, N. and D. Kodrik, Antioxidant enzymes in *Spodoptera littoralis* (Boisduval): are they enhanced to protect gut tissues during oxidative stress? J Insect Physiol, 2006. 52(1): p. 11–20.

[47] Krishnan, N., et al., Stage-specific distribution of oxidative radicals and antioxidant enzymes in the midgut of *Leptinotarsa decemlineata*. J Insect Physiol, 2007. 53(1): p. 67–74.

[48] Krishnan, N., et al., 20-Hydroxyecdysone prevents oxidative stress damage in adult *Pyrrhocoris apterus*. Arch Insect Biochem Physiol, 2007. 65(3): p. 114–24.

[49] Mathews, M.C., C.B. Summers, and G.W. Felton, Ascorbate peroxidase: a novel antioxidant enzyme in insects. Arch Insect Biochem Physiol, 1997. 34(1): p. 57–68.

[50] Krishnan, N., et al., Glutathione-ascorbic acid redox cycle and thioredoxin reductase activity in the digestive tract of *Leptinotarsa decemlineata* (Say). Insect Biochem Mol Biol, 2009. 39(3): p. 180–8.

[51] Yu, B.P., Cellular defenses against damage from reactive oxygen species. Physiol Rev, 1994. 74(1): p. 139–62.

[52] Kanzok, S.M., et al., Substitution of the thioredoxin system for glutathione reductase in *Drosophila melanogaster*. Science, 2001. 291(5504): p. 643–6.

[53] Amdam, G.V., et al., Hormonal control of the yolk precursor vitellogenin regulates immune function and longevity in honeybees. Exp Gerontol, 2004. 39(5): p. 767–73.

[54] Seehuus, S.C., et al., Reproductive protein protects functionally sterile honey bee workers from oxidative stress. Proc Natl Acad Sci U S A, 2006. 103(4): p. 962–967.

[55] Choi, J., et al., Oxidative modifications and aggregation of Cu,Zn-superoxide dismutase associated with Alzheimer and Parkinson diseases. J Biol Chem, 2005. 280(12): p. 11648–55.

[56] Quinlan, G.J., G.S. Martin, and T.W. Evans, Albumin: biochemical properties and therapeutic potential. Hepatology, 2005. 41(6): p. 1211–9.

[57] Sanders, H.R., et al., Blood meal induces global changes in midgut gene expression in the disease vector, *Aedes aegypti*. Insect Biochem Mol Biol, 2003. 33(11): p. 1105–22

[58] Geiser, D.L., D. Zhang, and J.J. Winzerling, Secreted ferritin: mosquito defense against iron overload? Insect Biochem Mol Biol, 2006. 36(3): p. 177–87

[59] Wu, H., M.C. Wang, and D. Bohmann, JNK protects *Drosophila* from oxidative stress by trancriptionally activating autophagy. Mech Dev, 2009. 126(8–9): p. 624–37.

[60] Dias-Santagata, D., et al., Oxidative stress mediates tau-induced neurodegeneration in *Drosophila*. J Clin Invest, 2007. 117(1): p. 236–45.

[61] Bahadorani, S. and A.J. Hilliker, Antioxidants cannot suppress the lethal phenotype of a *Drosophila melanogaster* model of Huntington's disease. Genome, 2008. 51(5): p. 392–5.

[62] Tettweiler, G., et al., Starvation and oxidative stress resistance in *Drosophila* are mediated through the eIF4E-binding protein, d4E-BP. Genes Dev, 2005. 19(16): p. 1840–3.

[63] Zhang, D.D., Mechanistic studies of the Nrf2-Keap1 signaling pathway. Drug Metab Rev, 2006. 38(4): p. 769–89.

[64] Harman, D., Aging: a theory based on free radical and radiation chemistry. J Gerontol, 1956. 11(3): p. 298–300.

[65] Svensson, M.J. and J. Larsson, Thioredoxin-2 affects lifespan and oxidative stress in *Drosophila*. Hereditas, 2007. 144(1): p. 25–32.

[66] Lee, F.K., et al., The role of ubiquitin linkages on alpha-synuclein induced-toxicity in a *Drosophila* model of Parkinson's disease. J Neurochem, 2009. 110(1): p. 208–19.

[67] Radyuk, S.N., et al., Mitochondrial peroxiredoxins are critical for the maintenance of redox state and the survival of adult *Drosophila*. Free Radic Biol Med, 2010. 49(12): p. 1892–902.

[68] Mockett, R.J., R.S. Sohal, and W.C. Orr, Overexpression of glutathione reductase extends survival in transgenic *Drosophila melanogaster* under hyperoxia but not normoxia. FASEB J, 1999. 13(13): p. 1733–42.

[69] Missirlis, F., et al., A putative glutathione peroxidase of Drosophila encodes a thioredoxin peroxidase that provides resistance against oxidative stress but fails to complement a lack of catalase activity. Biol Chem, 2003. 384(3): p. 463–72.

[70] Tang, A.H. and C.P.D. Tu, Biochemical-characterization of *Drosophila* glutathione S-transferases D1 and D21. J Biol Chem, 1994. 269(45): p. 27876–84.

[71] Toba, G. and T. Aigaki, Disruption of the microsomal glutathione S-transferase-like gene reduces life span of *Drosophila melanogaster*. Gene, 2000. 253(2): p. 179–87.

[72] Moskovitz, J., H. Weissbach, and N. Brot, Cloning and expression of a mammalian gene involved in the reduction of methionine sulfoxide residues in proteins. Proc Natl Acad Sci U S A, 1996. 93(5): p. 2095–9.

[73] Kumar, R.A., et al., Reaction mechanism, evolutionary analysis, and role of zinc in Drosophila Methionine-R-sulfoxide reductase. J Biol Chem, 2002. 277(40): p. 37527–35.

[74] Whitworth, A.J., et al., Increased glutathione S-transferase activity rescues dopaminergic neuron loss in a *Drosophila* model of Parkinson's disease. Proc Natl Acad Sci U S A, 2005. 102(22): p. 8024–9.

[75] Davies, S.A., et al., Cell signalling mechanisms for insect stress tolerance. J Exp Biol, 2014. 217(Pt 1): p. 119–28.

[76] Chintapalli, V.R., J. Wang, and J.A. Dow, Using FlyAtlas to identify better *Drosophila melanogaster* models of human disease. Nat Genet, 2007. 39(6): p. 715–20.

[77] Dow, J.A., Insights into the Malpighian tubule from functional genomics. J Exp Biol, 2009. 212(Pt 3): p. 435–45.

[78] Wang, J., et al., Function-informed transcriptome analysis of *Drosophila* renal tubule. Genome Biol, 2004. 5(9): p. R69.

[79] Owusu-Ansah, E. and U. Banerjee, Reactive oxygen species prime *Drosophila* haematopoietic progenitors for differentiation. Nature, 2009. 461(7263): p. 537–41.

[80] Radyuk, S.N., et al., Peroxiredoxin 5 modulates immune response in Drosophila. Biochim Biophys Acta, 2010. 1800(11): p. 1153–63.

[81] Orr, W.C. and R.S. Sohal, Extension of life-span by overexpression of superoxide dismutase and catalase in *Drosophila melanogaster*. Science, 1994. 263(5150): p. 1128–30.

[82] Scarborough, R.M., et al., Isolation and primary structure of two peptides with cardioacceleratory and hyperglycemic activity from the corpora cardiaca of *Periplaneta americana*. Proc Natl Acad Sci U S A, 1984. 81(17): p. 5575–9.

[83] Goldsworthy, G., K. Opoku-Ware, and L. Mullen, Adipokinetic hormone enhances laminarin and bacterial lipopolysaccharide-induced activation of the prophenoloxidase cascade in the African migratory locust, *Locusta migratoria*. J Insect Physiol, 2002. 48(6): p. 601–8.

[84] Kodrik, D., N. Krishnan, and O. Habustova, Is the titer of adipokinetic peptides in *Leptinotarsa decemlineata* fed on genetically modified potatoes increased by oxidative stress? Peptides, 2007. 28(5): p. 974–80.

[85] Vecera, J., et al., Adipokinetic hormone-induced enhancement of antioxidant capacity of *Pyrrhocoris apterus* hemolymph in response to oxidative stress. Comp Biochem Physiol C Toxicol Pharmacol, 2007. 146(3): p. 336–42.

[86] Velki, M., et al., Oxidative stress elicited by insecticides: a role for the adipokinetic hormone. Gen Comp Endocrinol, 2011. 172(1): p. 77–84.

[87] Lu, S.C., et al., Hormonal regulation of glutathione efflux. J Biol Chem, 1990. 265(27): p. 16088–95.

[88] Lu, S.C., et al., Hormone-mediated down-regulation of hepatic glutathione synthesis in the rat. J Clin Invest, 1991. 88(1): p. 260–9.

[89] Alquicer, G., et al., Activation of insect anti-oxidative mechanisms by mammalian glucagon. Comp Biochem Physiol B Biochem Mol Biol, 2009. 152(3): p. 226–33.

[90] Lacort, M., et al., Protective effect of estrogens and catecholestrogens against peroxidative membrane damage in vitro. Lipids, 1995. 30(2): p. 141–6.

[91] Roesijadi, G., et al., Ecdysone induction of MsrA protects against oxidative stress in Drosophila. Biochem Biophys Res Commun, 2007. 354(2): p. 511–6.

[92] Weissbach, H., L. Resnick, and N. Brot, Methionine sulfoxide reductases: history and cellular role in protecting against oxidative damage. Biochim Biophys Acta, 2005. 1703(2): p. 203–12.

[93] Hu, X., L. Cherbas, and P. Cherbas, Transcription activation by the ecdysone receptor (EcR/USP): identification of activation functions. Mol Endocrinol, 2003. 17(4): p. 716–31.

[94] Jamroz, R.C., et al., Transferrin in a cockroach: molecular cloning, characterization, and suppression by juvenile hormone. Proc Natl Acad Sci U S A, 1993. 90(4): p. 1320–4.

[95] Harizanova, N., et al., *Aedes aegypti* transferrin. Gene structure, expression pattern, and regulation. Insect Mol Biol, 2005. 14(1): p. 79–88.

[96] Andrus, P.K., et al., Protein oxidative damage in a transgenic mouse model of familial amyotrophic lateral sclerosis. J Neurochem, 1998. 71(5): p. 2041–8.

[97] Kodrik, D., et al., Hormonal regulation of response to oxidative stress in insects—an update. Int J Mol Sci 2015, 16, 25788–816.

Chapter 3

Oxidative Stress and Autophagy

Adem Kara, Semin Gedikli, Emin Sengul,
Volkan Gelen and Seckin Ozkanlar

Additional information is available at the end of the chapter

http://dx.doi.org/10.5772/64569

Abstract

Free radical production related with many stress factors including radiation, drugs, ageing and trauma plays a key role in cell death. Notwithstanding, free radicals can cause pathology in a variety of diseases through oxidative stress: Under oxidative stress, excessive production of free radicals can trigger cell death by primarily DNA and all cellular macromolecule damages. Also, excessive free radicals have a role in early inducers of autophagy cell death upon nutrient deprivation. Autophagy is physiologic process of eukaryotic systems, which have significant role in adaptation to oxidative stress by degradation of metalloproteins and oxidatively damaged macromolecules. By oxidizing, membrane injuries allow the leakage of enzymes and contribute to cell damage. However, recent publications demonstrate the protecting role of lysosome system during excessive reactive oxygen species (ROS) production by the elimination of damaged proteins or organelles. Activation of autophagic or lysosomal system can eliminate the oxidizing components of cell in oxidative stress response. This chapter aims to provide the novel insight data for oxidative damage-mediated autophagy as well as their metabolic networks.

Keywords: oxidative stress, free radicals, autophagy, cell death

1. Introduction

The number of studies on oxidative stress has been increasing for the last 30 years and its effects on many illnesses' pathogenesis have been investigated. In this chapter, we focused the cellular injuries that are caused by the oxidant agents in the cell and potential relationships between oxidative stress and autophagy, that is, both cells' method of saving itself from death and its death mechanism at the same. We also aimed to enable the new therapeutic intervention to break oxidative stress-mediated cell injuries and promote cell surviving.

Free radicals are a molecule or atom species and they have free electron charges [1]. These free electrons show a high reactivity towards unstable agents. Free radicals are produced both in physiological conditions and in pathological conditions. Overproduced free radicals can cause injuries by reacting to the organelles such as cell membrane and DNA which are the components of cells [1, 2]. The production of the oxidant agents, which are produced in the cell and which carry free electron pairs that are able to damage cell, is balanced by the antioxidant system [2, 3]. The imbalance between antioxidant and oxidant system is called 'oxidative stress' [1].

The reactive oxygen species (ROS) in biological systems including superoxide anion ($^2O_2$), hydroxyl radical (HO), nitric oxide (NO), peroxyl radical (ROO) and non-radical hydrogen peroxide (H_2O_2) compose the most important components of oxidative stress [4]. The primary source of ROS is the mitochondrial-carrying system in the cell [5]. Electrons, which weaken in the mitochondrion, turn into oxygen (O^{-2}) atoms and then turn into H_2O_2 by spontaneous or superoxide dismutase (SOD) catalysis. In this stage, the mitochondrial ROS amount is at the rate of 1–2% of the total oxygen consumption. Although this amount seems to be low, it is equal to one billion molecules when the intracellular ROS amount that every single cell of the body produces is calculated [6]. When it is thought that there are about 100 trillion cells in the human body, the physiological ROS amount being produced increases more. In some cases, with the effect of factors such as exceeding of energy need, decreasing of mitochondrial activity (ageing), exogenous (UV, radiation) and endogenous (oxidase and oxygenase), ROS is produced in the body in an excess quantity [7]. In addition to mitochondria, sarcolemma, sarcoplasmic reticulum and transverse tubules are of the strongest sources of ROS due to the existence of NADH/NADPH oxidase (Nox) [8]. Moreover, endoplasmic reticulum (ER), peroxisomes, plasma membrane, polymorph nuclear cells and macrophages are known as the places in which ROS is produced [9]. In the cell, the ROS produced must be kept in balance with the antioxidant system [10].

2. Oxidative stress

Oxidative stress plays an important role in the pathophysiology of many diseases. For this reason, the medical importance of the oxidative stress is being understood even better day by day. Especially, along with the inseparable process between oxidative stress and inflammation with molecular interactions makes this subject be more and more attractive researched area [10, 11]. Today, for the development of new treatment options, antioxidant treatment strategies are being increasingly researched. The aim of this review is to enlighten the relation between oxidative stress and inflammation, which has a role in the physiopathogenesis of many diseases.

The production of ROS may increase in the beginning phase of the defence response of the cells during inflammation [12]. The Nox system, which settled in the plasma membranes of cells, contributes to ROS production by being activated during phagocytosis. Moreover, it is stated that the Nox is the primary factor contributing to the oxidative stress in the mitochondrial redox system [13, 14]. In addition to Nox, arachidoriic acid (AA) mechanism, nitric oxide and xanthine oxidase (XO) cause ROS production, as well [15]. AA is produced by the activation of phospholipase A2 and this may cause increase in ROS production [16]. At the same time, AA cyclooxygenase increases ROS production by activating various enzymes such as cytochrome P-450-dependent monooxygenase XO [17]. Xanthine oxidase is an ROS indicator, which causes more oxygen to be free as a result of hypoxanthine's degradation [18].

3. Redox biology

Eukaryotic cells make gene expression through multiple metabolic pathways with environmental stimulations. In the cell, ROS-sensitive transcription factors and oxidative response give the cellular warning according to the redox condition [19]. These signal proteins are two signal pathways belonging to two different families. The first of these pathways is mitogen-activated protein (MAP) kinase family and in this pathway phosphorescence occurs starting from cytoplasm and continuing to nucleus by the activities of extracellular signal regulator kinases, which are c-jun N terminal kinase and p38 MAP kinase. The second family is redox-sensitive signal pathway and cytoplasmic signal factor includes thioredoxin reductase, thioredoxin, nuclear factor Ref-1 and a few transcription factors (AP-1, nuclear factor kappa B (NF-kB), Nfr-1 and Egr-1). When these redox-sensitive 'sulphydryl switches' are stimulated, by passing from cytoplasm to nucleus, they trigger the transcription factors and enable the expression of specific genes [20, 21].

Oxidative stress has a role in many illnesses' pathogenesis such as ischaemia/reperfusion injury, Alzheimer, Parkinson and diabetes mellitus [22]. For example, the ROS amounts effecting to the cell in cancer may result in the expression of some genes via the redox-sensitive signal pathway by causing DNA damage. These redox-sensitive signal factors play roles in many processes such as cell division, cell cycle and the survival of the cell. On the other side, it is the potential molecular target of anticancer agents. This redox-sensitive sulphydryl switches signal pathways have important characteristics for potential cancer treatment. Their characteristics are firstly being overexpressed in tumours, secondly the depression of prosurvival signal pathways when they are inhibited, thirdly the entrance of cell cycle to the arrest when this signal pathway is depressed and lastly the increase of anticancer agents' activities parallel to their inhibition [21].

4. The importance of oxidative stress in cell biology

It is known that ROS have both beneficial and harmful effects on the cell. Its very low concentrations can perform as the second runner in some signal transmission ways [23]. However, they can cause many oxidative injuries in many vital structures when they are extremely produced. In the cell, there is a dynamic relation between ROS production and antioxidant capacity. Some oxidation processes such as cysteine oxidation play roles in the dynamic regulator system inside the cell [24]. It is shown that transcriptional factors such as NF-kB, p53 and AP-1 are regulated by oxygen types [25]. For this reason, sublethal ROS production can be blocked by signal transmission ways. Especially H_2O_2 is actually the second runner for various physiological stimulations such as angiotensin inflammatory cytokines and growth factors or transforming factors [26]. There is a contradiction between the reactive oxygen types such as superoxide radicals and their physiological/pathophysiological roles. It is considered that the production of superoxide radicals can be activated by neutrophils and other phagocytes [27]. When the redox homeostasis changes, the cell is exposed to oxidative stress. As a result of the mitochondrial function disorder in case of oxidative stress, a significant decrease in the cellular energy occurs, and due to this decrease apoptosis is activated. The damages in cells occur only when ROS overcomes the biochemical defence system of the cell. ROS, especially hydroxyl radicals, can react with all biological macromolecules such as lipids, proteins, nucleic acids and carbohydrates [28]. Multiple unsaturated fatty acids continuously threaten the cellular integrity and functions for oxidative injury [28, 29]. It is known that iron, which is a transition metal, has a vital role in the beginning of new lipid radical chain reactions [30]. Lipid peroxidation is a significant biological result of ageing and oxidative damages [29]. Chemotherapy agents, radiation and numerous neurodegenerative illnesses are some sources of ROS [31]. In brief, whereas oxidative stress is a positive status in processes such as cellular proliferation and activation, it is a negative status in terms of lipid peroxidation, DNA injury and the inhibition of cell growth or in terms of its causing cell deaths.

5. Antioxidant system

The antioxidant enzyme system in the cell is responsible for the scavengers of ROS (O_2^-, H_2O^2 and peroxides), which consists of superoxide dismutase, catalase (CAT) and glutathione (GSH-Px or GPx) enzymes [10, 32]. Also, antioxidant defence system is responsible for the scavengers of reactive nitrogen species (RNS). Peroxynitrite ($ONOO^-$) is a really dangerous molecule [33] and nitrite oxide is a high reactive gas radical and it is water soluble and it can pass the cell membrane by diffusion [33, 34]. As in ROS, excessive production of oxidant types originating from NO in the cell leads to imbalance between oxidants and antioxidants, which causes irreversible damage in the cells' biomolecules and causes cell death [10].

When thioredoxin, which is an intracellular enzyme, is overexpressed, it blocks oxidative stress in the cell. It is stated that there is a dynamic relation between thioredoxin enzyme and antioxidant components, and various oxygen types [35]. It has been determined in different studies that the difference in cysteine modification can affect thioredoxin function [36].

6. Oxidative stress and DNA damage

Lipids in DNA, which is a stable molecule, can have oxidative injuries just like carbohydrates and proteins [37, 38]. All changes in the structural integrity of genetic material occurring as a result of the endogenous or exogenous factors are described as DNA damage. The integrity of the genomic DNA is constantly under threat with the effect of environmental factors. Changes in the structure of DNA may occur endogenously during cellular events such as DNA replication and DNA recombination [39, 40].

It is believed that the DNA damages can be caused by oxidative stress result in mutation in the cell DNA and that it is a major reason for cancer [41, 42]. As a result of oxidative DNA damage, a decrease in the cascade signal occurs, which is effective in cancer development, and gene expression, a discontinuation in transcription, genomic instability and replication failure. Oxidative DNA damage plays important roles in the development of tumourigenesis, which is related to inflammation as well as increasing the risk of cancer development [43]. Moreover, it has been reported as a result of various studies conducted that the genomic damage has important roles in cases such as chronic illnesses, cardiovascular illnesses, neurodegenerative illnesses, inflammation/infection and ageing [44]. Oxidative DNA damage is rather dangerous for cell in terms of its causing mutation in cell, affecting the cell cycle and causing cancer [45].

It is stated that oxidative damage occurs in mitochondrial DNA (mtDNA) along with the nucleus DNA. It has been determined that the oxidative damage is greater in mitochondrial DNA compared to the nucleus DNA. Among the reasons for this situation, we can count that the mitochondrial DNA is quite close to the areas that produce free radicals in mitochondria and that it is not protected by histones. What is more, factors such as that the DNA damage repair system is insufficient compared to nucleus DNA and that there is an increase in mutations according to the age cause mitochondrial DNA to get more damage [46]. The damage occurred in the DNA is seen in low levels thanks to the DNA's ability to be repaired. There is an increase in oxidative DNA damage as a result of the increase in the reactive oxygen types, decrease in the antioxidant enzyme levels and the insufficiency of DNA repair mechanisms. Depending upon the oxidative damage, single- and double-chain fractures, abasic areas and base modifications can originate or cross-linking between the DNA molecule and proteins can occur [47].

Oxide DNA base damages are generally removed in two ways. These are base excision repair and damaged oligonucleotide excision repair [48]. Nearly more than 20 major damage products, which originate as a result of oxidative DNA damage, have been determined [49]. DNA product radicals give more reaction via different mechanisms to form the last product. The type of the originating DNA modification product depends on reaction conditions such as the redox potential of the substance to react, the radical production system and the existence of oxygen. Radicals can be oxidation and reduction depending on their redox potentials and the reacting substances. Although 8-hydroxypurines and formapyrimidines can originate in both presence and absence of oxygen, they better prefer to originate in an environment with oxygen. These compounds are hemiorthoamids and they can turn into each other easily [50].

The most commonly used for the last products of ROS-mediated DNA damage biomarker is 8-hydroxy-2′-deoxyguanosine (8-OHdG) [51]. 8-OHdG is a mutagen that reacts with DNA during the excessive ROS production. As Cu^{+2} ions are found in a high level in areas rich for guanine-cytosine, the base which is most exposed to the oxidative damage is guanine. OH radical composes DNA product radicals as a result of the reaction with the atoms of guanine in positions numbered 4, 5 and 8. OH product radicals of the fourth and fifth carbon atoms are dehydrated and the imidazole ring of the eighth carbon OH product radicals is exposed to the opening. Other DNA base damage products have less mutagenic effects. For this reason, the most commonly measured 8-OHdG base damage product is a parameter that is widely used to determine the DNA damage [52, 53].

For the first time, it was determined that 8-OHdG is an indicator of the DNA damage in 1984 by Kasai and Nishimura. Analysis of 8-OHdG, which is the major oxidation product of DNA, was reported in 1989 for the first time. There are two approaches for the analysis method of 8-OHdG. The first of these, direct approach, is isolation of the DNA lesion by using physical and chemical methods and making DNA extraction and hydrolysation. The second method, indirect approach, includes the saving of DNA structure and seeing the formation of lesion in site. In this approach, measurement is made by using antibodies that have low specific features or via the activity of specific DNA repair enzymes [54, 55].

7. Autophagy: apoptosis interaction

In addition to the studies of Swhweichel and Merker, who researched cell death mechanism morphologically for the first time, Clarke mentioned three basic cell morphology in cell death and described apoptosis as type I, autophagy as type II and cell death, which is not lysosomal, as type III programmed cell death [56, 57]. Apoptosis is an event characterized by cell shrinkage and chromatin condensation and cell divides into pieces called 'apoptotic bodies' in the end of the process. It has been determined that, in this type of cell death, the morphological changes occurring in the cell take place as a result of cutting DNA and proteins by proteases called caspase. The apoptotic bodies arising as a result of these fractures are resolved by lysosomes [57].

In autophagy, which is a mechanism in which intracellular macromolecules and organelles are directed to lysosomes in sachets and broken up in this mechanism, the short-lived proteins are broken up inside ubiquitin-proteasome system, intracellular organelles and long-lived proteins are benefited from as they are destroyed in autophagy system and decomposed into the building stones similar to amino acids to be used again inside the cell [58, 59]. In the autophagic cell death, there are organelles such as cytoplasm parts, which are inside two or more layered (lipid bilayer) membrane-covered sachets, and/or mitochondria, endoplasmic reticulum. In the end, autophagy sachets form a compound with lysosome and make it possible for the material inside them to be broken up by the lysosomal enzymes [60].

Either apoptosis or autophagy, no matter what the death type is, it is known that these processes are regulated by molecular mechanisms. In the same cell, as different death cell mechanisms can take action even simultaneously, these mechanisms can involve each other and they cannot be distinguished easily all the time. It is difficult to describe whether the morphological changes, which come into light with the cell death mechanisms, are due to apoptosis or autophagy [61]. The reason for this can be that different cell death mechanisms have different main goals. The main goal of autophagic cell death is mainly cytoplasm, while the main goal of apoptosis is cell nucleus. Apoptosis can be sufficient for the disposal of cells with small cytoplasm. However, in cells with large cytoplasm, more than one mechanism may have to take action together. In other words, while mechanisms dispose the nucleus, cytoplasm and organelles are cleaned by the autophagy event and the cell death can be accelerated. In literature, there are studies supporting this view [62, 63].

7.1. Apoptotic signals

Caspases playing a role in apoptosis are classified in two ways:

1. Caspases starting the apoptotic signals (caspases 2, 8, 9, 10).

2. Lethal caspases that have a role in the breaking up of g-proteins (caspases 3, 6 and 7).

Along with the caspase-dependent mechanisms that control the cell death, some cell deaths are reported to be caspase-free [64]. Caspase-dependent pathway triggers cell death by activating in two ways: extrinsic and intrinsic factors. In the extrinsic pathway, tumour necrosis factor- α (TNF-α), which is on the surface of cell membrane, connects to TNF-like ligands such as FasL or TRAIL, and causes procaspase-8 or procaspase-10 to be triggered and finally the apoptotic process starts [65].

In the intrinsic pathway, the failure of mitochondria results in cytochrome-C expression and then begins activations of caspases 9, 7 and 3. Another protein family having a role in the mitochondrial pathway is Bcl-2 family. It is decided whether the cell will enter apoptotic phase as a result of the interaction between Bcl-2 family members and pro-apoptotic signal molecules. The members of the Bcl-2 family are divided into three groups:

1. Anti-apoptotic group including Bcl-2, Bcl-xL and Mcl-1.

2. Group triggering apoptosis that includes Bax and Bak.

3. Group that has pro-apoptotic activity including Bad, Bik, Bid, Bim, NOXA and Puma ç.

The extrinsic pathway, also called death receptor, is a mechanism which contains cell surface receptors that generate the start of apoptosis and the formation of the death-inducing signalling complex (DISC) that is a multi-protein complex [66]. With the connection of ligand, an adaptor protein called FADD, which brings caspase 8 to DISC, becomes a part of the activity [67–69]. In the activated caspase 8, either effector caspases such as caspase 3, directly activate the apoptosis pathway or intrinsic apoptosis pathway [70]. An apoptosis pathway can be activated when the endoplasmic reticulum is under stress [71].

7.2. The molecular connections between apoptosis and autophagy

As autophagy can block apoptosis and cell death occurs as a result of both of these events, it is believed that the regulation of these mechanisms is made in coordination. Previously, it was considered that the same proteins control both of these processes. However, the latest data show that it is not true. p53 is a strong apoptosis inductive and it can also induce autophagy by increasing the expression of DRAM that is the direct p53 target gene [72]. Similarly, the activation of a well-known apoptosis inhibitor, PI3 kinase/Akt pathway, inhibits autophagy at the same time [73]. In this way, it was understood that important signal pathways could increase or decrease both apoptosis and autophagy, simultaneously. In brief, central components proteins directly regulated both apoptosis and autophagy mechanisms [74].

Beclin-1/Atg-6 is a part of the type III PI3 kinase complex, which is necessary for the formation of autophagic vesicles and the interaction with Beclin-1 can block the induction of autophagy. Beclin-1 is described as a protein that can interact with Bcl-2, as well [74]. This case shows that an apoptosis regulator physically interacts with an autophagy regulator. Beclin-1 interacts with other major anti-apoptotic Bcl-2 family (Bcl-xL) proteins, either [75]. In the regulation of these mechanisms, depending on the presence of Bcl-2 in mitochondria and endoplasmic reticulum, in other words depending on its condition in the subcellular localization, there may be differences. The inhibition of the autophagy with Bcl-2 function takes place only in the endoplasmic reticulum, and mitochondrial-directed Bcl-2, which is a strong inhibitor of many apoptotic stimuli, cannot inhibit autophagy [75, 76]. Another mechanism that is able to control the autophagy via Bcl-2 was located in endoplasmic reticulum [77]. In this method, Bcl-2 blocks calcium passage in endoplasmic reticulum instead of interacting with Beclin-1. Calcium activates Ca^{2+}/calmoduline-dependent kinase, kinase-β and adenosine monophosphate (AMP)-activator protein kinase. This case causes mTOR inhibition to activate autophagy. By this way, permission was given to Bcl-2 for autophagy inhibition instead of apoptosis inhibition in two completely different mechanisms [78].

Extrinsic death pathway, which is one of the best-described key components of apoptosis process, can control autophagy, as well. The connection of FADD adaptor protein to the ligand-dependent death receptor is a necessary step for the formation of DISC. DISC accompanies death receptor signals with FADD, which acts as a platform in which caspase 8 dimerization and activation take place. FADD includes two protein areas, one death area and one death effector area, which interact with each other. The death area of the FADD can, unexpectedly, induce a new cell death mechanism, which includes really high levels of autophagy in normal epithelium cells. Actually, as FADD death area does not have catalytic activity, it is possible that it induces autophagy by interacting with other proteins. The interesting point is that autophagy response can be observed more easily when apoptosis stops and this case supports that the apoptosis and autophagy in normal epithelium cells are simultaneously induced by FADD death area [79].

These cases, mentioned above, show that the components of the apoptosis mechanism, which are regulated by intrinsic and extrinsic pathways, could control autophagy, as well. Contrary to this case, there are studies expressing that autophagy regulators control apoptosis. These experiments, which analyse autophagic cell death originating from interferon and Atg-5, show that FADD can interact with Atg-5 [80]. The conducted study showed that this interaction ends with cell death only in a way that requires FADD and caspases, without the formation of autophagic vesicles. From this study, the conclusion that Atg-5 can regulate extrinsic apoptosis pathway components is drawn. Another mechanism, which is about the ability of Atg-5 for regulating apoptosis, was described. The key step in this mechanism is to provide the activation of intrinsic apoptosis pathway that can be blocked by Bcl-2 and to compose a protein form, which is translocated to mitochondria in order to start the cytochrome-C oscillation. To be able to realize this, Atg-5 must be cut by calpain. The general importance of this mechanism is supported by the information that Atg-5 knock-down protects tumour cells against a kind of apoptosis stimulation. This case can still be complex and as the cutting of Atg-5 by calpain can cause a formation of protein, which is not able to activate autophagy, it is possible for calpain activity to increase or decrease autophagy [81]. There are some studies showing that calpain activity is necessary for autophagy, which is induced by the lack of rapamycin and amino acid [79].

7.3. Autophagy: type II cell death

Autophagy is a death mechanism characterized by the degradation of cellular components, and plays roles in the pathophysiology of many diseases' [82, 83]. The damaged cellular components and contents are removed by lysosomal autophagy. In case of increasing the autophagic effect with oxidative stress or physiological stimulations, protein synthesis and

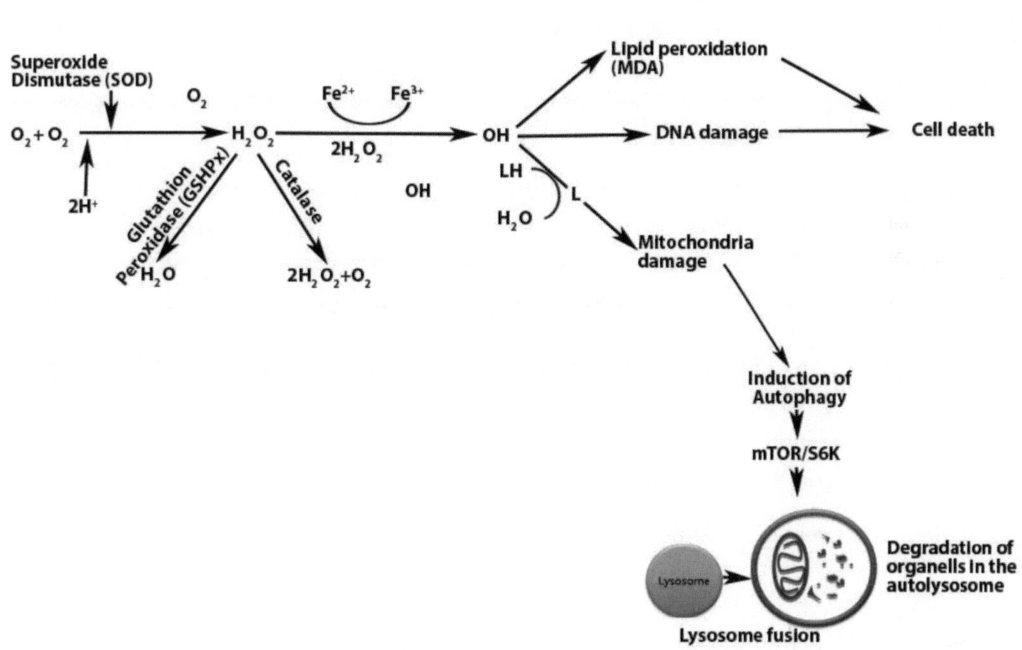

Figure 1. Oxidative stress-mediated cell damages in the cell: Excessive ROS production can lead to damages in mitochondria, which can cause cell death or oxidative-damaged cell components are degraded by autophagy and promote cell survival.

energy output pathways, cell organelles and proteins are disrupted in the cells. Also, under limited food intake, autophagy provides internal energy sources [82, 83]. With this effect of lysosomal autophagy, cell can survive in case of oxidative stress. This survival system occurring in the cell is stimulated by stress factors such as hunger, hyperthermia and hypoxia [84]. mTOR (mammalian target of rapamycin), which is a factor playing important role in autophagic activation, is a kinase signal pathway. This signal pathway is classically activated in case of hunger, hypoxia or stress condition [83].

In eukaryotic cells, the first step of the oxidative damage is antioxidant defence system and the second step is lysosomal autophagy [85]. In the second step, damaged cell components such as proteins, organelles or DNA are removed with lysosomal autophagy [82]. This defence system provides degradation of these components and cell surviving. In the third defence step, there is type II cell death (autophagy). Severe damaged and not repaired cells are removed by autophagy and the organ's integrity is ensured [86] (**Figure 1**).

Autophagy is also activated in many cases of metabolic and therapeutic stress such as the lack of growth factor in the cell, signal inhibition of receptor tyrosine kinase/Akt/mTOR metabolic pathway, ischaemia/reperfusion, intracellular calcium accumulation and endoplasmic reticulum stress [87, 88]. Increased production of ROS stimulates the initiation of autophagy in association with stress signal pathways. For this, cysteine protease Atg-4 inactivation is made with ROS accumulation in the cell. This inactivation results in Atg-4 phosphoethanolamine precursor accumulation, which is also necessary for the beginning of autophagosome [89]. In this way, under stress condition, oxidative damaged cell components are degraded by autophagy and continue its life by this way. There is a complex relation between cell death and stress adaptation [90]. The molecular relationship between cell death and autophagy has not been completely understood nowadays.

While autophagic cell death is the main cell death seen during the development, it has been reported in recent studies that apoptosis-induced cell death can be connected or related to autophagy [78, 91]. The signal cross-talk between apoptosis and autophagy can be related to Bcl-2 gene family. Moreover, it has been shown that Bcl-2 family proteins inhibit the apoptosis and autophagy [75, 92]. The association between the anti-apoptotic Bcl-2 protein and the autophagic Beclin-1 protein has an important role in the point of convergence of the apoptotic and autophagic cell death. In the autophagic process, Bcl-2 protein has an important role in autophagosome formation via Beclin-1 network [75]. Also, anti-apoptotic Bcl-2 proteins inhibit the Beclin-1-dependent autophagic cell death [93].

The antioxidant effect of anti-apoptotic Bcl-2 proteins has been reported. This anti-apoptotic protein decreases the production of reactive oxidants and inhibits the apoptotic cell death [94]. By this way, the overexpressed Bcl-2 and decreasing ROS level probably cause the repression of cytochrome-C from mitochondrion and the prevention of death cell [95]. As mentioned above, ROS creates a connection between cellular stress and the starting of autophagy, and autophagosome formation is started by stimulating Atg-8-phosphoethanolamine precursor accumulation [89].

http://dx.doi.org/10.5772/64569

8. Summary and future perspective

Endogenous and exogenous stress factors that cells are exposed to trigger the ROS production in the cell, which causes damages in cellular organelles. Oxidative response is a part of normal cellular physiology and halts the organelles' damages in the cells and promotes cell surviving. While autophagy is a type II cell death, it is also an alternative defence system that cell chooses to be able to survive in cells which are exposed to oxidative damage. Autophagy can provide the removal of damaged organelles with lysosomal autophagy and ensures cell to survive. Autophagy plays an important role in both detecting oxidative stress and removing oxidatively damaged proteins and organelles, as well as the cellular machineries responsible for excessive ROS/RNS production. Investigations into the specific molecular targets of ROS in the autophagy pathway and the specific signalling mechanisms will be important for our understanding of biology and diseases.

Author details

Adem Kara[1*], Semin Gedikli[1], Emin Sengul[2], Volkan Gelen[3] and Seckin Ozkanlar[4]

*Address all correspondence to: ademkara36@gmail.com

1 Faculty of Veterinary, Department of Histology and Embryology, Ataturk University, Erzurum, Turkey

2 Faculty of Veterinary, Department of Physiology, Ataturk University, Erzurum, Turkey

3 Faculty of Veterinary, Department of Physiology, Kafkas University, Kars, Turkey

4 Faculty of Veterinary, Department of Biochemistry, Ataturk University, Erzurum, Turkey

References

[1] Halliwell B. Free radicals and other reactive species in disease. New York, John Wiley & Sons, Ltd, eLS. 2005.

[2] Kara A, Akman S, Ozkanlar S, et al. Immune modulatory and antioxidant effects of melatonin in experimental periodontitis in rats. Free Radical Biology and Medicine. 2013;55:21–6.

[3] Kara A, Yücel A, Yücel N, Özcan H, Selli J and Ünal D. Evaluation of the combined treatment with cisplatin and melatonin on neuroblastoma cell viability and antioxidant capacity. Journal of Experimental and Clinical Medicine. 2014;31.

[4] Babior BM. Phagocytes and oxidative stress. The American Journal of Medicine. 2000;109:33–44.

[5] Chance B, Sies H and Boveris A. Hydroperoxide metabolism in mammalian organs. Physiological Reviews. 1979;59:527–605.

[6] Wagner BA, Venkataraman S and Buettner GR. The rate of oxygen utilization by cells. Free Radical Biology and Medicine. 2011;51:700–12.

[7] Filomeni G, Rotilio G and Ciriolo M. Disulfide relays and phosphorylative cascades: partners in redox-mediated signaling pathways. Cell Death and Differentiation. 2005;12:1555–63.

[8] Powers SK and Jackson MJ. Exercise-induced oxidative stress: cellular mechanisms and impact on muscle force production. Physiological Reviews. 2008;88:1243–76.

[9] Samoylenko A, Hossain JA, Mennerich D, Kellokumpu S, Hiltunen JK and Kietzmann T. Nutritional countermeasures targeting reactive oxygen species in cancer: From mechanisms to biomarkers and clinical evidence. Antioxidants and Redox Signaling. 2013;19:2157–96.

[10] Filomeni G, De Zio D and Cecconi F. Oxidative stress and autophagy: the clash between damage and metabolic needs. Cell Death and Differentiation. 2015;22:377–88.

[11] Hensley K, Robinson KA, Gabbita SP, Salsman S and Floyd RA. Reactive oxygen species, cell signaling, and cell injury. Free Radical Biology and Medicine. 2000;28:1456–62.

[12] Taverne YJ, Bogers AJ, Duncker DJ and Merkus D. Reactive oxygen species and the cardiovascular system. Oxidative Medicine and Cellular Longevity. 2013;2013.

[13] Kuroda J, Ago T, Matsushima S, Zhai P, Schneider MD and Sadoshima J. NADPH oxidase 4 (Nox4) is a major source of oxidative stress in the failing heart. Proceedings of the National Academy of Sciences. 2010;107:15565–70.

[14] Dale DC, Boxer L and Liles WC. The phagocytes: neutrophils and monocytes. Blood. 2008;112:935–45.

[15] Pou S, Keaton L, Surichamorn W and Rosen GM. Mechanism of superoxide generation by neuronal nitric-oxide synthase. The Journal of Biological Chemistry. 1999;274:9573–80.

[16] Davis LM, Rho JM and Sullivan PG. UCP-mediated free fatty acid uncoupling of isolated cortical mitochondria from fasted animals: correlations to dietary modulations. Epilepsia. 2008;49:117–9.

[17] Zuo L, Christofi FL, Wright VP, Bao S and Clanton TL. Lipoxygenase-dependent superoxide release in skeletal muscle. Journal of Applied Physiology. 2004;97:661–8.

[18] Nanduri J, Vaddi DR, Khan SA, Wang N, Makerenko V and Prabhakar NR. Xanthine oxidase mediates hypoxia-inducible factor-2alpha degradation by intermittent hypoxia. PLoS One. 2013;8:e75838.

[19] Chuang Y-YE, Chen Y, Chandramouli V, et al. Gene expression after treatment with hydrogen peroxide, menadione, or t-butyl hydroperoxide in breast cancer cells. Cancer Research. 2002;62:6246–54.

[20] Hirota K, Matsui M, Murata M, et al. Nucleoredoxin, glutaredoxin, and thioredoxin differentially regulate NF-kB, AP-1, and CREB activation in HEK293 cells. Biochemical and Biophysical Research Communications. 2000;274:177–82.

[21] Cook JA, Gius D, Wink DA, Krishna MC, Russo A, Mitchell JB. Oxidative stress, redox, and the tumor microenvironment. Semin Radiat Oncol. 2004;14(3):259–66. Review.

[22] Kannan K and Jain SK. Oxidative stress and apoptosis. Pathophysiology. 2000;7:153–63.

[23] Suzuki YJ, Forman HJ and Sevanian A. Oxidants as stimulators of signal transduction. Free Radical Biology and Medicine. 1997;22:269–85.

[24] Pennisi E. Superoxides relay Ras protein's oncogenic message. Science. 1997;275:1567–8.

[25] Morel Y and Barouki R. Repression of gene expression by oxidative stress. Biochemical Journal. 1999;342:481–96.

[26] Ushio-Fukai M, Alexander RW, Akers M and Griendling KK. p38 mitogen-activated protein kinase is a critical component of the redox-sensitive signaling pathways activated by angiotensin II role in vascular smooth muscle cell hypertrophy. Journal of Biological Chemistry. 1998;273:15022–9.

[27] Babior BM. Oxygen-dependent microbial killing by phagocytes. New England Journal of Medicine. 1978;298:659–68.

[28] Jaeschke H. Mechanisms of oxidant stress-induced acute tissue injury. Experimental Biology and Medicine. 1995;209:104–11.

[29] Reiter RJ, Guerrero JM, Garcia JJ and Acuña-Castroviejo D. Reactive oxygen intermediates, molecular damage, and aging: relation to melatonin. Annals of the New York Academy of Sciences. 1998;854:410–24.

[30] Sies H. Biochemistry of oxidative stress. Angewandte Chemie International Edition in English. 1986;25:1058–71.

[31] Kannan K, Holcombe RF, Jain SK, et al. Evidence for the induction of apoptosis by endosulfan in a human T-cell leukemic line. Molecular and Cellular Biochemistry. 2000;205:53–66.

[32] Flohé L. Changing paradigms in thiology: from antioxidant defense toward redox regulation. Methods in Enzymology. 2010;473:1–39.

[33] Di Giacomo G, Rizza S, Montagna C and Filomeni G. Established principles and emerging concepts on the interplay between mitochondrial physiology and S-(de) nitrosylation: implications in cancer and neurodegeneration. International Journal of Cell Biology. 2012;2012.

[34] Stamler JS, Singel DJ and Loscalzo J. Biochemistry of nitric oxide and its redox-activated forms. Science-New York Then Washington. 1992;258:1898.

[35] Casagrande S, Bonetto V, Fratelli M, et al. Glutathionylation of human thioredoxin: a possible crosstalk between the glutathione and thioredoxin systems. Proceedings of the National Academy of Sciences. 2002;99:9745–9.

[36] Haendeler J, Hoffmann J, Tischler V, Berk BC, Zeiher AM and Dimmeler S. Redox regulatory and anti-apoptotic functions of thioredoxin depend on S-nitrosylation at cysteine 69. Nature Cell Biology. 2002;4:743–9.

[37] Wang C, Li Z, Zhang Q, Zhao M and Liu W. Enantioselective induction of cytotoxicity by o, p′-DDD in PC12 cells: implications of chirality in risk assessment of POPs metabolites. Environmental Science and Technology. 2013;47:3909–17.

[38] Doganlar O and Doganlar ZB. Effects of a mixture of volatile organic compounds on total DNA and gene expression of heat shock proteins in *Drosophila melanogaster*. Archives of Environmental Contamination and Toxicology. 2015;68:395–404.

[39] Kulaksız G and Sancar A. Nükleotid eksizyon onarımı ve kanser (Nucleotide excision repair and cancer). Türk Biyokimya Dergisi (Turkish Journal of Biochemistry). 2007;32:104–11.

[40] Yan S, Sorrell M and Berman Z. Functional interplay between ATM/ATR-mediated DNA damage response and DNA repair pathways in oxidative stress. Cellular and Molecular Life Sciences. 2014;71:3951–67.

[41] Hussain SP, Hofseth LJ and Harris CC. Radical causes of cancer. Nature Reviews Cancer. 2003;3:276–85.

[42] Hosoya N and Miyagawa K. Targeting DNA damage response in cancer therapy. Cancer Science. 2014;105:370–88.

[43] Bartsch H and Nair J. Chronic inflammation and oxidative stress in the genesis and perpetuation of cancer: role of lipid peroxidation, DNA damage, and repair. Langenbeck's Archives of Surgery. 2006;391:499–510.

[44] Kawanishi S and Inoue S. (Damage to DNA by reactive oxygen and nitrogen species). Seikagaku The Journal of Japanese Biochemical Society. 1997;69:1014–7.

[45] Dryden Jr GW, Deaciuc I, Arteel G and McClain CJ. Clinical implications of oxidative stress and antioxidant therapy. Current Gastroenterology Reports. 2005;7:308–16.

[46] Lim KS, Jeyaseelan K, Whiteman M, Jenner A and Halliwell B. Oxidative damage in mitochondrial DNA is not extensive. Annals of the New York Academy of Sciences. 2005;1042:210–20.

[47] Ercan N and Fidanci UR. Oxidative DNA damage products and diseases (Oksidatif DNA Hasar Ürünleri ve Hastalıklar). Dicle Univ Vet Fak Derg. 2012;2:40–57.

[48] Evans MD, Dizdaroglu M and Cooke MS. Oxidative DNA damage and disease: induction, repair and significance. Mutation Research/Reviews in Mutation Research. 2004;567:1–61.

[49] de Souza Machado AA, Hoff MLM, Klein RD, et al. Oxidative stress and DNA damage responses to phenanthrene exposure in the estuarine guppy *Poecilia vivipara*. Marine Environmental Research. 2014;98:96–105.

[50] Dizdaroglu M, Jaruga P and Rodriguez H. Measurement of 8-hydroxy-2′-deoxyguanosine in DNA by high-performance liquid chromatography-mass spectrometry: comparison with measurement by gas chromatography-mass spectrometry. Nucleic Acids Research. 2001;29:e12.

[51] Lu X and Yu C. Enantiomer-specific profenofos-induced cytotoxicity and DNA damage mediated by oxidative stress in rat adrenal pheochromocytoma (PC12) cells. Journal of Applied Toxicology. 2014;34:166–75.

[52] Barroso MF, De-Los-Santos-Alvarez N, Delerue-Matos C and Oliveira MBPP. Towards a reliable technology for antioxidant capacity and oxidative damage evaluation: electrochemical (bio) sensors. Biosensors and Bioelectronics. 2011;30:1–12.

[53] Wang C, Yang J, Lu D, Fan Y, Zhao M and Li Z. Oxidative stress-related DNA damage and homologous recombination repairing induced by N, N-dimethylformamide. Journal of Applied Toxicology. 2015; 936–945.

[54] Valavanidis A, Vlachogianni T and Fiotakis C. 8-hydroxy-2′-deoxyguanosine (8-OHdG): a critical biomarker of oxidative stress and carcinogenesis. Journal of Environmental Science and Health Part C. 2009;27:120–39.

[55] Collins AR, Rašlová K, Somorovská M, et al. DNA damage in diabetes: correlation with a clinical marker. Free Radical Biology and Medicine. 1998;25:373–7.

[56] Schweichel JU and Merker HJ. The morphology of various types of cell death in prenatal tissues. Teratology. 1973;7:253–66.

[57] Clarke PG. Developmental cell death: morphological diversity and multiple mechanisms. Anatomy and Embryology (Berlin). 1990;181:195–213.

[58] Ohsumi Y. Molecular dissection of autophagy: two ubiquitin-like systems. Nature Reviews Molecular Cell Biology. 2001;2:211–6.

[59] Shintani T and Klionsky DJ. Autophagy in health and disease: a double-edged sword. Science. 2004;306:990–5.

[60] Levine B and Yuan J. Autophagy in cell death: an innocent convict? Journal of Clinical Investigation. 2005;115:2679–88.

[61] Betin VM and Lane JD. Caspase cleavage of Atg4D stimulates GABARAP-L1 processing and triggers mitochondrial targeting and apoptosis. Journal of Cell Science. 2009;122:2554–66.

[62] Kroemer G, Marino G and Levine B. Autophagy and the integrated stress response. Molecular Cell. 2010;40:280–93.

[63] Mehrpour M, Esclatine A, Beau I and Codogno P. Overview of macroautophagy regulation in mammalian cells. Cell Research. 2010;20:748–62.

[64] Pradelli LA, Beneteau M and Ricci JE. Mitochondrial control of caspase-dependent and -independent cell death. Cell Molecular Life Science. 2010;67:1589–97.

[65] Schrader K, Huai J, Jockel L, Oberle C and Borner C. Non-caspase proteases: triggers or amplifiers of apoptosis? Cell Molecular Life Science. 2010;67:1607–18.

[66] Thorburn A. Death receptor-induced cell killing. Cellular Signalling. 2004;16:139–44.

[67] Thomas LR, Johnson RL, Reed JC and Thorburn A. The C-terminal tails of tumor necrosis factor-related apoptosis-inducing ligand (TRAIL) and Fas receptors have opposing functions in Fas-associated death domain (FADD) recruitment and can regulate agonist-specific mechanisms of receptor activation. Journal of Biological Chemistry. 2004;279:52479–86.

[68] Chinnaiyan AM, O'Rourke K, Tewari M and Dixit VM. FADD, a novel death domain-containing protein, interacts with the death domain of Fas and initiates apoptosis. Cell. 1995;81:505–12.

[69] Boatright KM, Renatus M, Scott FL, et al. A unified model for apical caspase activation. Molecular Cell. 2003;11:529–41.

[70] Luo X, Budihardjo I, Zou H, Slaughter C and Wang X. Bid, a Bcl2 interacting protein, mediates cytochrome C release from mitochondria in response to activation of cell surface death receptors. Cell. 1998;94:481–90.

[71] Boyce M and Yuan J. Cellular response to endoplasmic reticulum stress: a matter of life or death. Cell Death Differentiation. 2006;13:363–73.

[72] Crighton D, Wilkinson S, O'Prey J, et al. DRAM, a p53-induced modulator of autophagy, is critical for apoptosis. Cell. 2006;126:121–34.

[73] Arico S, Petiot A, Bauvy C, et al. The tumor suppressor PTEN positively regulates macroautophagy by inhibiting the phosphatidylinositol 3-kinase/protein kinase B pathway. The Journal of Biological Chemistry. 2001;276:35243–6.

[74] Liang XH, Jackson S, Seaman M, et al. Induction of autophagy and inhibition of tumorigenesis by Beclin 1. Nature. 1999;402:672–6.

[75] Pattingre S, Tassa A, Qu X, et al. Bcl-2 antiapoptotic proteins inhibit Beclin 1-dependent autophagy. Cell. 2005;122:927–39.

[76] Zhu W, Cowie A, Wasfy GW, Penn LZ, Leber B and Andrews DW. Bcl-2 mutants with restricted subcellular location reveal spatially distinct pathways for apoptosis in different cell types. The EMBO Journal. 1996;15:4130–41.

[77] Høyer-Hansen M, Bastholm L, Szyniarowski P, et al. Control of macroautophagy by calcium, calmodulin-dependent kinase kinase-beta, and Bcl-2. Molecular Cell. 2007;25:193–205.

[78] Shimizu S, Kanaseki T, Mizushima N, et al. Role of Bcl-2 family proteins in a non-apoptotic programmed cell death dependent on autophagy genes. Nature Cell Biology. 2004;6:1221–8.

[79] Thorburn A. Apoptosis and autophagy: regulatory connections between two supposedly different processes. Apoptosis. 2008;13:1–9.

[80] Pyo JO, Jang MH, Kwon YK, et al. Essential roles of Atg5 and FADD in autophagic cell death: dissection of autophagic cell death into vacuole formation and cell death. The Journal of Biological Chemistry. 2005;280:20722–9.

[81] Yousefi S, Perozzo R, Schmid I, et al. Calpain-mediated cleavage of Atg5 switches autophagy to apoptosis. Nature Cell Biology. 2006;8:1124–32.

[82] Cuervo AM. Autophagy: in sickness and in health. Trends in Cell Biology. 2004;14:70–7.

[83] Levine B. Eating oneself and uninvited guests: autophagy-related pathways in cellular defense. Cell. 2005;120:159–62.

[84] Moore MN, Allen JI and McVeigh A. Environmental prognostics: an integrated model supporting lysosomal stress responses as predictive biomarkers of animal health status. Marine Environmental Research. 2006;61:278–304.

[85] Moore MN. Diet restriction induced autophagy: a lysosomal protective system against oxidative-and pollutant-stress and cell injury. Marine Environmental Research. 2004;58:603–7.

[86] Lockshin RA and Zakeri Z. Apoptosis, autophagy, and more. The International Journal of Biochemistry and Cell Biology. 2004;36:2405–19.

[87] Lum JJ, Bauer DE, Kong M, et al. Growth factor regulation of autophagy and cell survival in the absence of apoptosis. Cell. 2005;120:237–48.

[88] Ogata M, Hino S, Saito A, et al. Autophagy is activated for cell survival after endoplasmic reticulum stress. Molecular and Cellular Biology. 2006;26:9220–31.

[89] Scherz-Shouval R, Shvets E, Fass E, Shorer H, Gil L and Elazar Z. Reactive oxygen species are essential for autophagy and specifically regulate the activity of Atg4. The EMBO Journal. 2007;26:1749–60.

[90] Fulda S, Gorman AM, Hori O and Samali A. Cellular stress responses: cell survival and cell death. International Journal of Cell Biology. 2010;2010.

[91] Yu L, Alva A, Su H, et al. Regulation of an ATG7-beclin 1 program of autophagic cell death by caspase-8. Science. 2004;304:1500–2.

[92] Akar U, Chaves-Reyez A, Barria M, et al. Silencing of Bcl-2 expression by small interfering RNA induces autophagic cell death in MCF-7 breast cancer cells. Autophagy. 2008;4:669–79.

[93] Pattingre S and Levine B. Bcl-2 inhibition of autophagy: a new route to cancer? Cancer Research. 2006;66:2885–8.

[94] Chen ZX and Pervaiz S. BCL-2: pro-or anti-oxidant? Front Bioscience (Elite Ed). 2009;1:263–8.

[95] Mirkovic N, Voehringer DW, Story MD, McConkey DJ, McDonnell TJ and Meyn RE. Resistance to radiation-induced apoptosis in Bcl-2-expressing cells is reversed by depleting cellular thiols. Oncogene. 1997;15:1461–70.

Chapter 4

Natural Compound-Generated Oxidative Stress: From Bench to Bedside

Aloran Mazumder and Marc Diederich

Additional information is available at the end of the chapter

http://dx.doi.org/10.5772/64183

Abstract

Oxidants are constantly generated in a biological system as a result of physiological processes. However, an imbalance between oxidants and antioxidants can lead to a pathophysiological condition known as oxidative stress. Natural compounds as inducers of oxidative stress are able to modulate physiological functions of cancer cells leading to cell death or survival. This chapter aims at providing an overview of pro- and antioxidant activities of natural compounds related to cancer and related therapies.

Keywords: natural compounds, cancer, oxidative stress, clinical use

1. Natural compound anticancer agents

In the search of improved cytotoxic agents against cancer, natural compounds possess advantages with regard to availability, low toxicity, and suitability for oral application and metabolite likeliness [1]. Moreover, new technologies of combinatorial chemistry and high-throughput screening are used to design different synthetic drugs with natural compounds that serve as templates for development of novel molecules with enhanced biological properties.

In 1960, the National Cancer Institute (NCI) began a large-scale screening program for anti-tumor agents, and 35,000 plant species samples were tested primarily on mouse leukemia cells [2, 3]. The most promising drug to emerge from this program was paclitaxel, a microtubule disruptive agent obtained from the bark of the Pacific yew *Taxus brevifolia*. This finding served as the springboard for further investigations with natural compounds, and in the late 1960s, vinblastine and vincristine were reported from *Catharanthus roseus*. Both drugs majorly contributed to long-term remission and cures for childhood leukemia, Hodgkin's lymphoma, testicular teratoma, etc. Other anticancer agents to enter clinics, which are derived from natural sources, include etoposide, which has been proven as an effective treatment against testicular teratoma and small cell lung cancer, whereas teniposide was shown to be effective against acute lymphocytic leukemia (ALL) and neuroblastoma in children and non-Hodgkin's lymphoma [1]. A comprehensive study published on new medicines approved by US Food and Drug Administration between 1981 and 2010 revealed that 34% of those medicines based on small molecules were either natural products or a direct derivative which mainly included statins, immunosuppressant, and tubulin-binding anticancer drugs [4, 5].

Natural compound constituents demonstrated anticancer activity according to a combination of epidemiological and experimental studies [6]. Mechanistic insights underlined that the chemotherapeutic potential of these agents may be a combination of antioxidant, anti-inflammatory, immune-promoting, cytostatic, differentiating, and cytotoxic effects. Altogether, natural compounds efficiently prevent initiation, promotion, and progression of cancer development thus interfering with all 10 hallmarks and enabling characteristics of cancer [7–10].

Increasing technological advancements led to the development of better purification techniques with defined molecular assays, which can efficiently exclude "distracting molecules" such as tannins and saponins, thereby increasing the chances of identifying the critical agent with specific anticancer activity. The diverse bioactivity potential of natural compounds can be related to the huge structural diversity existing in nature. This compound repertoire is available for further modifications to improve the therapeutic potential of lead compounds. In addition, combinatorial biosynthesis further modulates the functional groups of lead compounds and can be complemented with high-throughput screening, computational chemistry,

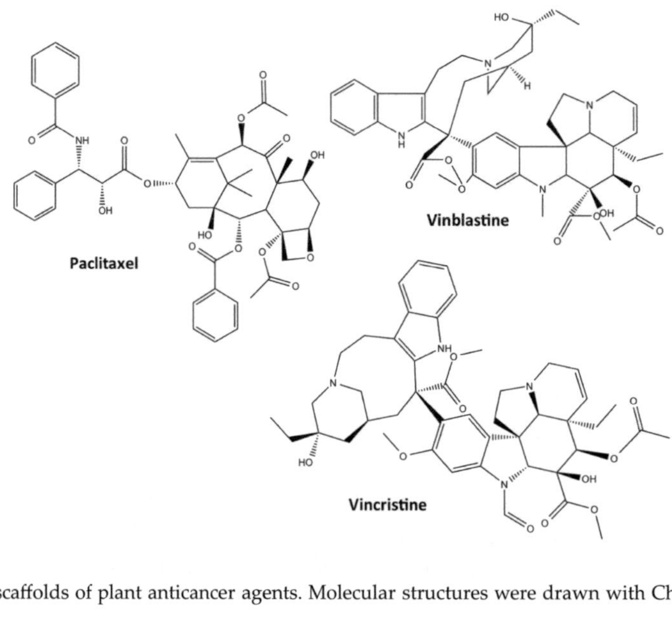

Figure 1. Molecular scaffolds of plant anticancer agents. Molecular structures were drawn with ChemDraw13 (Perkin Elmer).

and bioinformatics to generate structural analogues with improved pharmacological activity and reduced toxicity [1] (**Figure 1**).

2. Natural compounds as scavengers of free radicals

Oxidants are constantly generated in a biological system as a result of physiological processes. However, an imbalance between oxidants and antioxidants can lead to a pathophysiological condition known as oxidative stress [11]. In light of this knowledge, oxidative stress has been defined as perturbations in redox homeostasis. Broadly, the cellular redox level is regulated by three different systems, two of which are dependent on glutathione that includes glutathione (GSH), glutathione reductase (GR), glutathione peroxidases (GPX), and glutathione *S*-transferases (GST) [12–14]. Glutathione undergoes oxidation to form glutathione disulfide (GSSG), thereby reducing the disulfide bonds of cytoplasmic proteins to cysteine and protects the cell against oxidative stress [15]. Under normal conditions, GSH exists in reduced form due to constitutive activity of GR. GSTs act as detoxifying enzymes that conjugate GSH to various electrophilic compounds [16].

Reactive oxygen species (ROSs) have been reported in both solid and hematopoietic cancers where they are associated with tumor development and progression [17, 18]. However, cancer cells also express antioxidant proteins to detoxify ROS, suggesting that the fine-tuning of intracellular ROS signaling is critical for cancer. Therefore, understanding the susceptibility of cancer cells to oxidative signals could open new therapeutic window for rational design of new anticancer agents [19]. In addition to their well-characterized effects on cell division and viability, cytotoxic agents can induce oxidative stress by modulating levels of ROS such as the superoxide anion radical, hydrogen peroxide, and hydroxyl radicals. Eukaryotic cells have highly organized pathways to orchestrate the many extracellular stimuli received and convert them into specific physiological processes. This classical cascade also termed as signal transduction pathways includes a series of events occurring constitutively and initiated by interaction of a ligand with its receptor on the cell membrane. ROS in this cascade have been proposed as second messengers in the activation of signaling events that lead to survival or death [20]. Moreover, redox-sensitive cysteine residues are known to sense and transduce changes in cellular redox status caused by ROS production and the presence of oxidized thiols. Various dietary phytochemicals have been shown to exhibit beneficial effects including the prevention of cancer by modulating the cellular redox status by acting as either an antioxidant or pro-oxidant. They function as detoxifying enzyme inducers, which mainly include phenolic and sulfur-containing compounds. Phenolic compounds are classified as polyphenols or flavonoids, whereas sulfur-containing compounds may be classified into isothiocyanates and organosulfur compounds. Epigallocatechin-3-gallate (EGCG) from green tea, curcumin [21–24] from turmeric, and resveratrol [25, 26] from grapes are the classical examples of polyphenols, whereas flavonoids include quercetin from citrus fruits [26–28] and genistein from soya. Isothiocyanates represent a group of compounds such as sulforaphane from broccoli and phenethyl isothiocyanate from turnips. Organosulfur compounds mainly include diallyltetrasulfide derived from garlic [29–34]. Cells respond to these phytochemicals by a non-classical receptor-sensing mechanism of electrophilic chemical stress characterized as "thiol-modulated cellular signaling" events leading to gene expression commending the pharmacological activity (**Figure 2**).

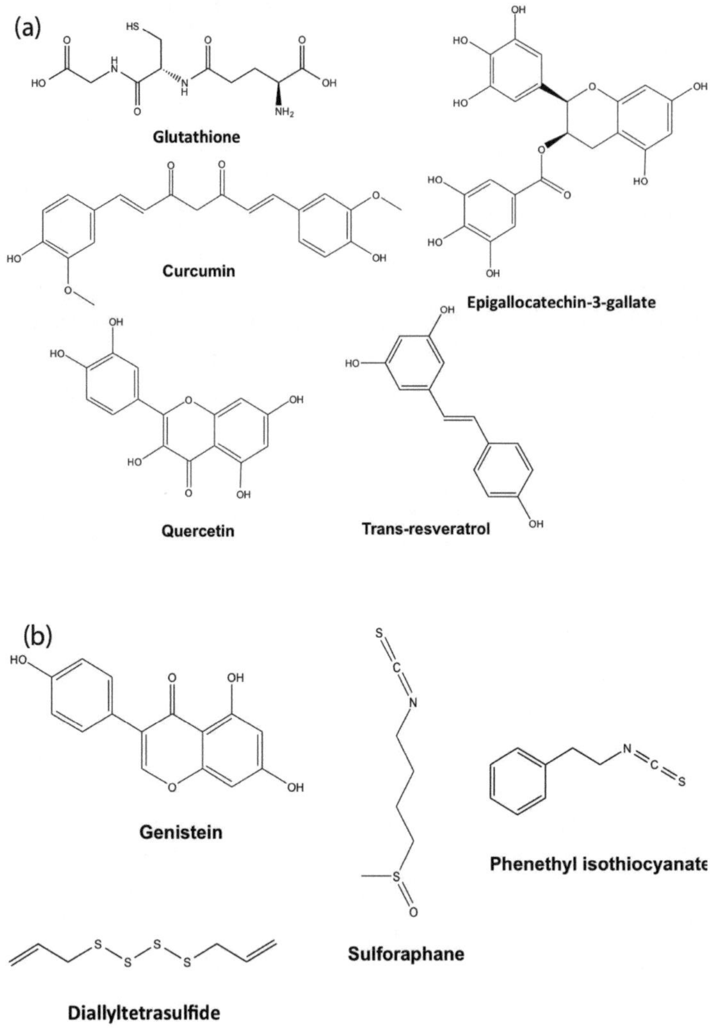

Figure 2. Natural compounds as scavengers of free radicals. Molecular structures were drawn with ChemDraw13 (Perkin Elmer).

3. Survival pathways activated by free radicals

ROSs are tumorigenic as elevated levels of ROS-sensitive signaling pathways have been implicated in various cancers where they are involved in sustenance of cell growth, prolifer-

http://dx.doi.org/10.5772/64183

ation, survival, migration, and by inducing DNA damage leading to formation of genetic lesions initiating tumorigenesis [35, 36]. Low levels of hydrogen peroxide (H_2O_2) stimulation have been shown to propagate cell proliferation in an array of cancer cell types. Role of hormones in endocrine cancers is well documented. In hormone-dependent breast cancer cells, one of the functions of estrogen is to translocate to mitochondria, thereby initiating mitochondrial ROS production that can be impaired by inhibition of mitochondrial uniporter, which prevents estrogen-induced cell proliferation [37, 38]. Sodium arsenic in MCF-7 was shown to mimic the effect of estrogen and potentiated S phase progression and proliferation by inducing ROS production and ROS-related depolarization of the mitochondrial membrane [39]. Moreover, estrogen-induced cell proliferation of MCF-7 was strongly inhibited by antioxidants such as *N*-acetyl-L-cysteine (NAC) or mitochondrial blockers of protein synthesis such as chloramphenicol [40]. ROS generation was shown to augment G1/S transition by increasing the expression levels of cyclins D1, D3, E1, E2, and B2 [41]. In contingent to these finding, cytochrome P450B1-mediated conversion of estrogen to a putative carcinogenic metabolite 4-hydroxyestradiol in human mammary epithelial cells MCF-10 leads to intracellular ROS production and neoplastic transformation. ROS overproduction was shown to activate IκB kinase (IKK) signaling with increased nuclear translocation and NF-κB activity [42].

Since deregulation of NF-κB is related to increased cell survival, proliferation, and development of drug resistance in different cancers, series of work conducted in this direction showed that NF-κB is a redox-regulated sensor for oxidative stress and is activated by low doses of H_2O_2 [43, 44]. In MCF-7 cells, interleukin (IL)-1β stimulation of NF-κB is partially regulated by H_2O_2-mediated activation of NF-κB inducing kinase (NIK)-mediated phosphorylation of IKKα [45]. Moreover, overexpression of manganese superoxide dismutase (MnSOD) in MCF-7 cells completely abolished tumor necrosis factor (TNF) α-mediated NF-κB activation, IκBα degradation, p65 nuclear translocation, and NF-κB-dependent reporter gene expression [40]. In other forms of cancer such as oral squamous carcinoma, a mild difference in endogenous ROS functions as a physiological signaling modulator of the NF-κB signaling cascades through its ability to activate NIK [46]. Besides solid tumors, redox regulation of NF-κB has also been implicated in hematopoietic cancers. Our group for the first time reported that in U937 cells, melatonin a pineal hormone might induce ROS generation, which ultimately is involved in transactivation of NF-κB-promoting survival of these cells [47–50]. Moreover, myeloid leukemia, which often maintains a high intracellular ROS level and uses redox signal for survival, is sensitive to NF-κB inhibition since NF-κB is involved in moderating the ROS level, which prevent activation of c-Jun N-terminal kinase (JNK) and cell death [51–54] (**Figure 3**).

Apart from NF-κB, ROS-mediated regulation of tyrosine phosphatases, protein tyrosine kinases, and receptor tyrosine kinases, which is critical for cell survival and cancer such as mitogen-activated protein (MAP) kinase/extracellular-regulated kinase (Erk) cascade and phosphoinoside-3-kinase (PI3K)/Akt-regulated signaling cascade, is well documented in the literature [55, 56]. Activation of MAPK/Erk1/2, which is mediated through growth factors, and K-ras is functionally linked to increased cell proliferation. Several studies have shown how ROS activate Erk1/2 pathway by modulating and activating its upstream target such as Ras. For instance, oxidative modification at its cysteine 118 residue leads to the inhibition of GDP/

GTP exchange [57]. Moreover, ROS activates p90^{RSK} that acts as an upstream kinase of Erk1/2 [58, 59]. In ovarian cancer, sustained Erk1/2 activity was linked to increased concentration of endogenous ROS resulting from ubiquitination and loss of endogenous mitogen-activated protein kinase phosphatase 3 (MKP3), which negatively regulates Erk1/2 [58, 59].

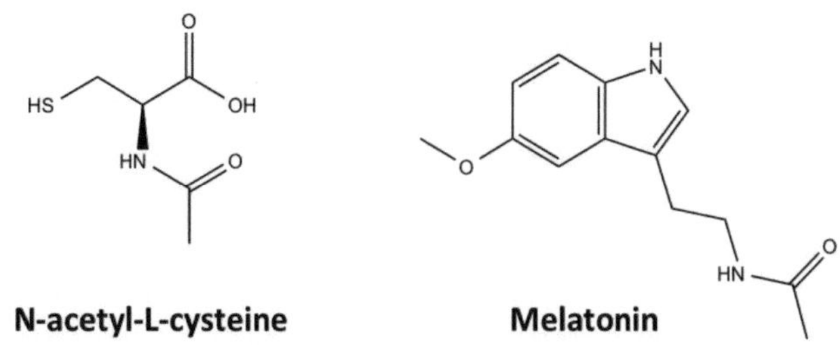

Figure 3. Molecular scaffolds of physiological antioxidants Molecular structures were drawn with ChemDraw13 (Perkin Elmer).

Oxidative stress regulation of PI3K/Akt pathway has been implicated in different cancers. In ovarian cancers, H_2O_2 produced in response to epithelial growth factor signaling (EGF) activates Akt and p70 S6k1, a substrate of Akt involved in regulating protein synthesis [60]. In pancreatic cancer PANC-1 cells, NADPH oxidase (NOX)-4-mediated generation of intracellular ROS was related to survival of these cells, which undergo apoptosis in response to diphenylene iodonium (DPI), an inhibitor of NOX that inhibited superoxide production and impaired levels of phosphorylated Akt [61]. Moreover, benzo(a)pyrene (BaP), a known mammary carcinogen in rodents, increased cell proliferation in human mammary epithelial cells MCF-10A through H_2O_2 generation and activation of epidermal growth factor receptor (EGFR), Akt, and ERK phosphorylation, which was strongly inhibited by NAC treatment [62].

4. Reactive oxygen species contribute in tumor progression

Intracellular redox status aids tumor progression by modulating the processes of metastasis, angiogenesis, survival of cells under hypoxic conditions, and maintenance of cancer stem cell (CSC) subpopulation [63]. Decreased cell adhesion to extracellular matrix, anchorage-independent survival, and invasion of tumor cells are well documented to be influenced by ROS [64]. Perturbation of mitochondrial respiratory chain in breast cancer cells leads to generation of a cellular subpopulation with increased levels of ROS, which are highly metastatic and maintain increased invasive property in vivo [65]. ROS induction was shown to influence overexpression of chemokine CXCL14 through the activator protein (AP)-1-signaling pathway and promote cell motility through elevation of cytosolic Ca^{2+} by binding to the inositol 1,4,5 triphosphate receptor on the endoplasmic reticulum [65]. DNA methylation and histone modification leading to epigenetic silencing of superoxide dismutase (SOD)-2 alter the expression of antioxidant enzyme MnSOD, which promotes invasion of breast cancers [66].

Moreover, a decreased MnSOD level was also associated with increased pancreatic tumor invasion [67]. Degradation of the extracellular matrix (ECM) and activated matrix metalloproteinases (MMPs) are a prerequisite of cancer cell migration and invasion. Binding of several integrins to the ECM results in increased expression of several MMP proteins. Since integrins signal by a vast array of kinases, phosphatases, GTPases, and transcription factors, it is likely that an elevated level of ROS has an effect on integrin-mediated signaling. Several studies reported the inactivation of critical phosphatases such as protein tyrosine phosphatase (PTP)-PEST (PTPN12), SHP-2 (Src homology 2 [SH2] domain-containing non-transmembrane PTP), and low molecular weight protein tyrosine phosphatases (LMW-PTPs) by oxidation [68]. Catalase, a H_2O_2 scavenger, binds SHP-2 and growth factor receptor-bound protein-2 (Grb2) adapter protein upon integrin ligand binding and therefore protects them against H_2O_2-mediated oxidation [69]. In non-transformed intestinal epithelial cells, elevated ROS increased the expression of α2β1-integrin, which subsequently increased the levels of cyclooxygenase-2 (COX-2) and promoted cell migration [64]. These results also suggest a mechanism where ROS-induced modulation of ECM promotes cancer formation in intestinal epithelial cells. ROSs have also been implicated in promoting tumor progression by modulating the processes involved in epithelial mesenchymal transition (EMT). Several transcription factors, which promote metastasis such as AP-1, Ets, Smad, and Snail, are regulated by ROS, inducing an effect on upstream target molecules involved in activation of these transcription factors such as protein kinase (PK) C and PTPs [70].

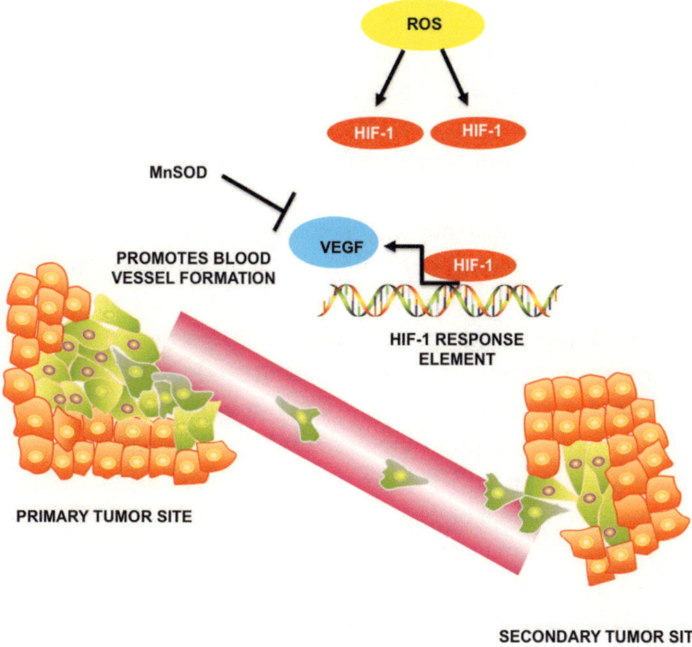

Figure 4. Molecular mechanisms of hypoxia affected by natural compounds. Scheme was drawn with ScienceSlides Suite 2105 (Visiscience).

In a given tumor mass, cancer cells often are exposed to an environment with reduced levels of tissue oxygen, a condition known as hypoxia. Prolonged limitation in oxygen supply can result in cell death. Therefore, cancer cells often undergo genetic and adaptive changes that contribute to a malignant phenotype and adopt characteristics of an aggressive tumor. Cancer cells mimic a phenomenon known as the "Warburg effect" that is to switch to anaerobic glycolysis when adequate oxygen supply is absent [71]. ROSs have been implicated to facilitate the tumor survival under hypoxic conditions by modulating different transcription factors involved. Hypoxia inducible transcription factor (HIF)-1 is most widely studied for its role in tumor promotion under hypoxic conditions. HIF-1 is a heterodimer that consists of hypoxic response factor HIF-1α and constitutively expressed aryl hydrocarbon receptor nuclear translocator (ARNT) also known as HIF-1β [72]. Under reduced oxygen levels, HIF-1 binds to hypoxia response elements, thereby activating hypoxia response genes such as the pro-angiogenic vascular endothelial growth factor (VEGF) [73]. Moreover, HIF-1 has been shown to regulate expression of all enzymes of the glycolysis pathway as well as glucose transporters GLUT1 and GLUT3 [74]. In human breast carcinoma, increased MnSOD activity is reported to inhibit HIF-1α along with suppression VEGF protein that impaired tumor metastasis [75]. Suppression of endogenous ROS by NADPH oxidase inhibitor DPI and mitochondrial electron chain inhibitor rotenone decreased HIF-1 induction and VEGF expression in ovarian and prostate cancer cells [75]. Moreover, growth factor such as epidermal growth factor (EGF)-induced ROS production may lead to activation of AKT/p70S6K1 pathway resulting in increased expression of VEGF stimulating tumor angiogenesis [60] (**Figure 4**).

In any given tumor, subpopulations of cells have the ability to self-renew and drive tumorigenesis. This population of cells is termed as cancer stem cells (CSCs), which are isolated from most cancers such as hematopoietic, breast, lung, colon, etc. CSCs are characterized by the expression of specific stem cell markers and are of clinical relevance as they are highly drug resistant and mostly initiate recurrence after chemo- or radiotherapy [76]. Studies have shown that normal hematopoietic and epithelial stem cells maintained a lower level of ROS than mature progeny to prevent cellular differentiation and maintain long-term cellular self-renewable. Similarly, CSCs unlike cancer cells have reduced level of ROS. Moreover, compared to tumor cell counterparts, CSCs showed increased expression of enzymes, which are associated with ROS scavenging [76]. Particularly, glutathione synthetase that is involved in glutathione synthesis is upregulated along with Forkhead transcription factor (FOXO)-1 to confer resistance to oxidative stress in hematopoietic stem cells [77]. Also, activation of antioxidant response that is frequently reported in CSCs prevents DNA damage in these cells exposed to ionizing radiations, thereby protecting CSCs against irradiation-induced cell death [78]. Based on these findings, it is widely accepted that cancer recurrence in response to withdrawal of conventional therapies is majorly dependent on existence of a resistant CSC subpopulation within the patients. Therefore, further identification of key molecular drivers that regulate the redox balance in CSCs might provide a possibility to eliminate these cells, which may contribute in overcoming the limitations of cancer relapse in future.

5. Cell death pathways activated by reactive oxygen species

As mentioned above, cancer cells in particular generate increased ROS levels; now severe accumulation of cellular ROS in response to chemotherapy may induce cell cycle arrest, senescence, or lethal toxicity inducing apoptosis [79]. Electrons leaking from the respiratory complexes in mitochondria are a major source for ROS production [80]. For instance, As_2O_3 which impair the function of respiratory chain increases the production of superoxide ions [65]. Alternatively, drugs, which act as redox cyclers such as anthracyclines daunorubicin and doxorubicin, react with cytochrome p450 reductase and NAD(P)H dehydrogenase [quinone] 1(NQO1) in the presence of reduced NADPH to generate superoxide in the presence of oxygen [81].

Apoptosis is linked to an increase in mitochondrial oxidative stress that causes a series of hallmark events such as release of cytochrome c followed by caspases activation ultimately leading to cell death. Sodium salicylate and non-steroidal anti-inflammatory drugs were reported to induce apoptosis in cancers such as colon, breast prostate, and leukemia through ROS production and activation of intrinsic cell death pathway measured by cleavage of caspase-9 and caspase-3 [82]. However, apoptosis was subsequently that a Rac1-NADPH oxidase-dependent pathway is activated in response to treatments that produce ROS and triggers apoptosis [82]. Mitochondrial release of H_2O_2 has been associated with activation of different stress kinases such as c-Jun N-terminal kinase (JNK) and p38. In response to ROS production, JNK mediates phosphorylation and downregulation of anti-apoptotic proteins B-cell lymphoma (Bcl)-2 and Bcl-extra large (xL) [79]. Moreover, several studies reported that both Bcl-2 and Bcl-xL antagonize ROS generation and protect cells against apoptosis [44, 83]. p38 MAPKs are also implicated in apoptosis induction in response to increased ROS production [84]. p38 is activated through apoptosis signal regulating kinase (Ask)-1. Activity of Ask-1 is dependent on a redox-regulated protein thioredoxin that in its reduced form binds to and conserves Ask-1 in an inactivated form. Increased ROS production uncouples thioredoxin from Ask-1 leading to its activation and phosphorylation of p38 required for TNFα-mediated apoptosis [84]. Studies conducted on L929 fibrosarcoma cells revealed that mitochondrial ROS play a key role in inducing TNFα cytotoxicity presumably by ROS-mediated caspase activation and cell death [85]. Moreover, TNF receptor associated factor 4 (TNFR4), a component of the TNF signaling chain, binds to NADPH and activates JNK suggesting different mechanisms by which death receptors induce ROS activation in cells [86]. Additionally, different studies have reported the significance of ROS-mediated signaling pathway regulated by protein kinase D1. PDK1 is activated by direct binding to Src and by phosphorylation, which promotes proliferation [35]. Inhibition of this pathway sensitizes cancer cells to ROS. Furthermore, beyond the conventional therapy to induce cytotoxicity to cancer cells and overcome the limitations associated with therapy resistance and risk of developing metastatic phenotype, recent advancement is made to explore the phenomenon of senescence, which inhibits the proliferation of cancer cells and restricts them in a dormant phase [87]. Senescence in cancer cells is mainly characterized by increased activity of β-galactosidase along with modulation of several cell cycle regulators such as cyclin-dependent kinases (CDKs), p16, and p27 [87]. Different polyphenolic compounds extracted from artichokes (*Cynara cardunculus*) or ginseng (*Panax ginseng*) were described to trigger ROS-dependent senescence.

6. Pathological alterations triggered by free radicals

Intracellular ROS generation may lead to damage of cellular macromolecules such as DNA, proteins, and lipid bilayer. Studies have indicated that H_2O_2 is not very reactive towards DNA; however, the damage to DNA is mainly caused by hydroxyl ions that are generated by the Fenton reaction where transition metals such as iron or copper donate or accept free electrons during intracellular reactions [88]. H_2O_2 acts as a catalyst in the reaction in the formation of free radicals. The generated hydroxyl ions are highly diffusible and lead to DNA damage like oxidation, single-, and double-strand breakage. Under normal physiological conditions, such DNA defects are repaired by base excision repair (BER) or nucleotide excision repair (NER). Cells unable to repair the DNA lesions undergo apoptosis to ensure that the mutations are not passed on during cell division. However, failure in either process of DNA repair or apoptosis may harbor the possibility of formation of cancerous growth.

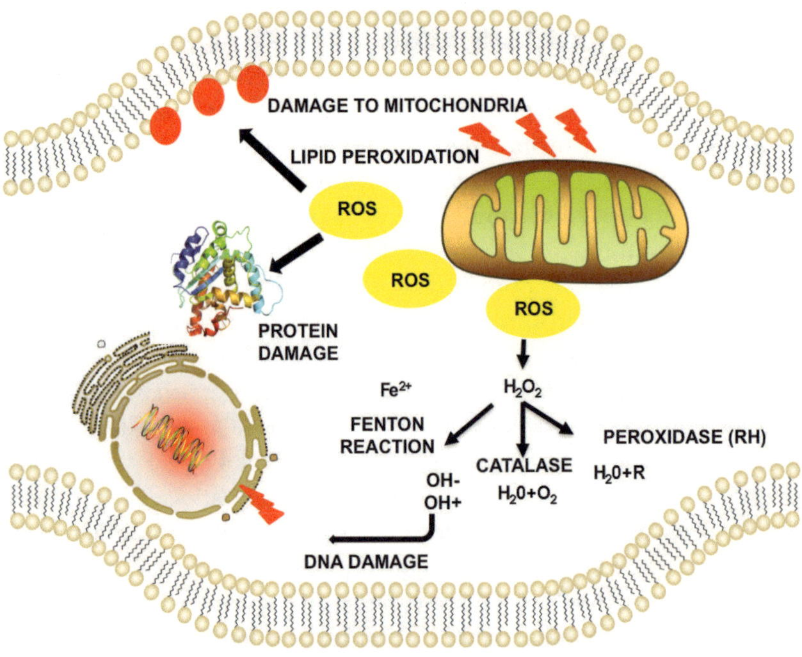

Figure 5. Molecular mechanisms of ROS-induced macromolecule damage. Scheme was drawn with ScienceSlides Suite 2105 (Visiscience).

ROS-mediated damage of proteins is mainly associated with modifications in specific amino acid residues leading to altered function [89]. Beside, some ROS-mediated modifications of protein also includes increased protein carbonylation, nitration of tyrosine and phenylalanine residues or formation of cross-linked and glycated proteins [89]. The oxidized amino acid residues in proteins may influence their activity in a signal transduction pathway. For instance, oxidation of phosphatases within the catalytic sites impairs their enzymatic activity [90].

Moreover, ROSs react with polyunsaturated or polyunsaturated fatty acids to trigger lipid peroxidation that has also been used as a tumor biomarker in clinical studies [91]. For instance, in colorectal cancer patients, the presence of thiobarbituric acid reactivates has been linked to high levels of lipid peroxidation [63] (**Figure 5**).

7. Natural compounds as pharmacological antioxidants

It has been reported in several studies that dietary phytochemicals can interfere with every stage of cancer development. Therefore, antioxidant functions of phytonutrients have been investigated thoroughly for their role in pathophysiology associated with cancer. Dietary antioxidant compounds with significant anticancer activity mainly include anthocyanidins (and their glycosides termed anthocyanins) from berries [92], catechins from green tea, curcumin from turmeric, genistein from soy, resveratrol from grapes and red wine, all-trans lycopene from tomatoes [93], indole-3-carbinol from broccoli, sulforaphane from asparagus, quercetin from red onions and apples. Beside this, carotenoids, flavonoids, and isothiocyanates have also exhibited strong antioxidant properties.

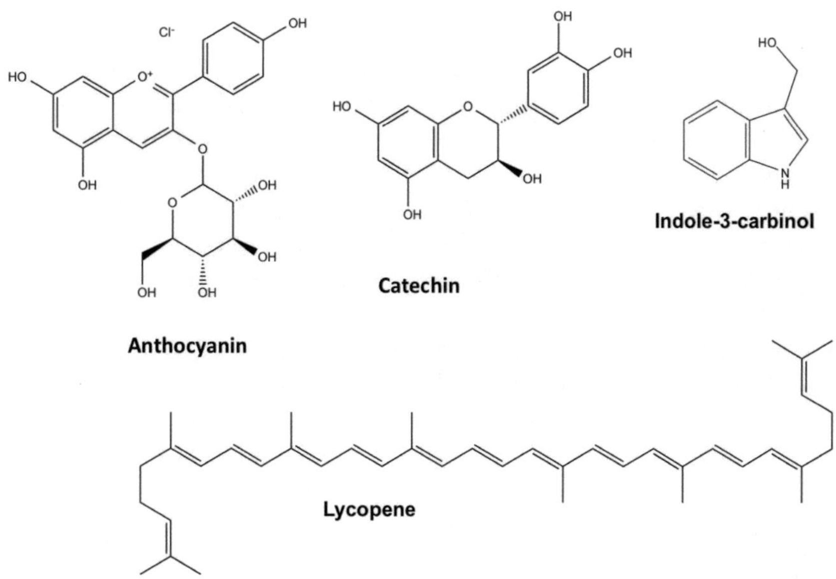

Figure 6. Pharmacological antioxidants of plant origins. Molecular structures were drawn with ChemDraw13 (Perkin Elmer).

Epigallocatechin gallate (EGCG) is the most abundant catechin found in green tea and curcumin-induced anticancer activity promoting cell cycle arrest, polyamine synthesis, and affecting transglutaminase (TG) activity along with regulation of signaling pathways mediated by NF-κB, AP-1, and MAPKs [94]. In a recent study, EGCG was shown to inhibit cell proliferation of cervical carcinoma Hela cells by promoting depolymerization of cellular microtubule and disrupting tubulin-microtubule equilibrium. Spectroscopic analysis revealed that EGCG bound to the α-subunit of tubulin at the interphase of α- and β-heterodimers preventing colchicine binding to the colchicine-binding site [95]. Also, in osteosarcoma cells, EGCG treatment induced cell cycle arrest, promoted apoptosis, and inhibited growth of transplanted tumors *in vivo* by regulating miR1/c-MET interaction [96] (**Figures 6** and **7**).

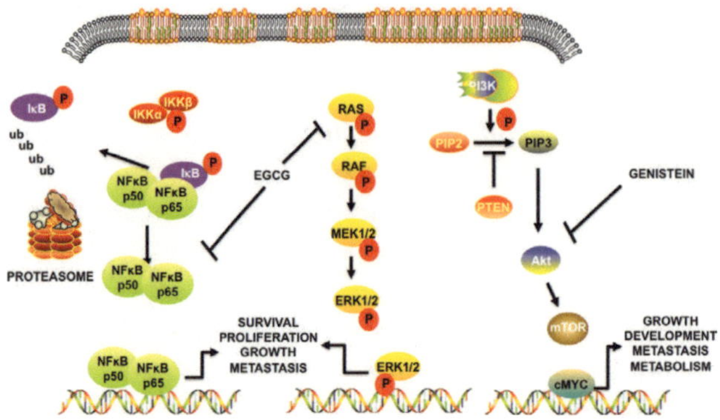

Figure 7. Molecular mechanisms involved in ROS-triggered survival. Scheme was drawn with ScienceSlides Suite 2105 (Visiscience).

Eugenol (4-allyl-2 methoxyphenol) is a naturally occurring phenolic compound that exhibits antioxidant properties. The antioxidant activity of eugenol was evaluated by the extent of protection offered against free radical-mediated lipid peroxidation using both in vitro and in vivo studies [97]. The chemopreventive and anticancer role of eugenol was evaluated on *N*-methyl-*N*′-nitro-*N*-nitrosoguanidine (MNNG)-induced gastric cancer in Wistar rats by analyzing the markers of apoptosis, invasion, and angiogenesis. Rats exposed to MNNG developed gastric cancer with upregulation of pro-invasive and angiogenic factors. Eugenol inhibited cell proliferation by suppression of NF-κB signaling. Apoptosis in these cells following eugenol treatment was mitochondrial pathway mediated that decreased the expression of Bcl-2, following release of cytochrome c and caspases activation. Anti-angiogenic and inhibition of invasion was evidenced by decreased expression of VEGF, its receptor VEGFR1 changes in the activities of MMPs and the expression levels of MMP-2 and MMP-9, VEGF, VEGFR1, tissue inhibitor of metalloproteinases (TIMP)-2 and reversion-inducing cysteine-rich protein with kazal motifs (RECK), a metastasis inhibitor [97].

Several studies aim toward proving the anticancer properties of flavonoids on an array of cancer cell types. Hirano and co-workers tested the anticancer activity of 28 flavonoids on human acute myeloid leukemia (AML) cell line HL-60. Eight of these flavonoids showed strong inhibition of cell proliferation with IC_{50} values in a nanomolar range [98]. In contingent to this finding, Kuntz et al. showed strong inhibition of proliferation induced by flavonoids on two colon cancer cell models with Caco-2 displaying features of small intestinal epithelial cells and

HT-29, resembling colonic cryptic cells [99]. Moreover, in vivo studies on mice strongly inhibited the growth and metastatic potential of melanoma cells B16-BL6 in response to flavonoid treatment [100].

Epigenetic modifications resulting in heritable changes into gene expression without changing the DNA sequence have been marked as key player in promoting cancer [101]. The most common types of epigenetic modifications that may contribute to tumor promotion are DNA methylation and histone acetylation or methylation. Antioxidant compounds mainly isoflavones, flavonols, and catechins have shown to modulate epigenetic features, thereby showing antitumor activity [102–104]. EGCG was shown to affect DNA methyltransferase by inhibiting DNMT and reactivating tumor suppressor genes RARα, p16, and O^6-methylguanine methyltransferase in esophageal cancer KYSE 510 cells [105]. Treatment with caffeic acid (3,4-dihydroxycinnamic acid) or chlorogenic acid [106] of hormone-dependent MCF-7 and hormone-independent MDA-MB-231 breast cancer cell lines partially inhibited the methylation of promoter region of the RARβ gene, thereby restoring its function [107]. Furthermore, studies also indicated that dietary antioxidants such as genistein, quercetin, parthenolide, and lycopene may affect DNA methylation status of different genes associated with cancer [108–111].

In addition to this, synergistic or additive effects of phytochemicals could be achieved when administered along with conventional chemotherapy or radiation therapy. This could be explained due to the fact that phytochemicals, which target different biochemical pathways, may enhance the efficacy of conventional therapies. Moreover, different studies have reported the synergistic cytotoxicity on different cancers when phytochemicals are administered together. Apple extracts and quercetin 3-β-D-glucoside combination showed synergistic antiproliferative effect on MCF-7 breast cancer cells [112]. Genistein a major phytoestrogen which has higher affinity for ERβ compared to ERα showed synergistic cytotoxicity in combination with indole-3-carbinol in HT-29 cells by simultaneously inhibiting Akt phosphorylation and progression of autophagic process [113]. Combination of δ-tocopherol and resveratrol showed strong inhibition of HMC-1 mastocytoma cell proliferation. The two compounds together strongly inhibited Ser473-phosphorylation of Akt, thereby reducing its activity compared to individual treatment [114]. Gagliano et al. suggested that the use of quercetin in combination with other antioxidants such as resveratrol or sulforaphane might be a novel approach for the treatment of human glioma, which has poor clinical prognosis in both adults and children [115].

Additionally, pharmacological implications of polyphenols have also been explored with respect to inhibition of cancer stem cells and self-renewal. It has been demonstrated that polyphenols can efficiently target pathways such as Wnt/β-catenin, Hedgehog, and Notch, which are critical for cancer stem, cells self-renewal [116]. Sulforaphane has been demonstrated to target cancer stem cells by modulating the pathways such as NF-κB, Hedgehog, and Wnt/β-catenin in different cancers such as breast, pancreas, and prostrate and has been proposed as an adjuvant of chemotherapy in different pre-clinical studies [117, 118]. As discussed earlier, cancer stem cells are characterized by a glycolytic metabolism with lower mitochondrial respiration compared to the tumor cells. Therefore, a proposed strategy to counteract CSCs population is to impair their metabolism by inhibiting glycolysis or by forcing CSCs into mitochondrial metabolism and oxidative phosphorylation. To this purpose, polyphenols have been implicated to regulate the cancer metabolism. For instance, EGCG in human breast cancer have been shown to target the 5′ adenosine monophosphate-activated protein kinase (AMPK) pathway, which is involved in maintaining cellular energy status, cell cycle, and protein synthesis [119] (**Figures 8** and **9**).

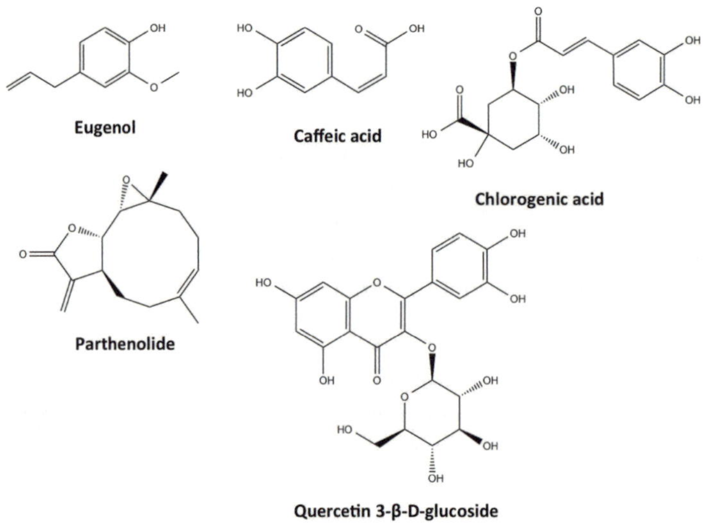

Figure 8. Pharmacological antioxidants of plant origins. Molecular structures were drawn with ChemDraw13 (Perkin Elmer).

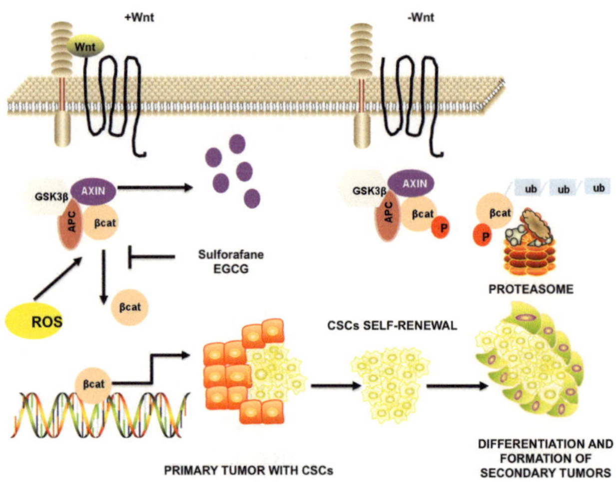

Figure 9. Molecular mechanisms involved in Wnt signaling. Scheme was drawn with ScienceSlides Suite 2105 (Visiscience).

http://dx.doi.org/10.5772/64183

8. Natural compounds as pharmacological pro-oxidants

As discussed earlier, cancer cells produce high levels of ROS that allow these cells to maintain a state of increased basal oxidative stress. The increased state of oxidative stress promotes survival but on the other hand makes the cancer cells vulnerable to further increase in ROS levels over a cancer-specific threshold. Accordingly, pro-oxidant agents and increased oxidative stress levels could then selectively target cancer cells. Different compounds of natural origins modulate the intracellular ROS levels and induce both chemopreventive and anticancer effect in different cancer types.

Polyphenolic extracts from artichokes (*Cynara cardunculus*) at high doses induce apoptosis and decrease the invasive potential of human metastatic breast cancer. Apoptosis was regulated in a caspase-independent manner. Additionally, sublethal concentrations of artichoke increased ROS and induced significant increase in senescence-associated β-galactosidase along with upregulation of tumor suppressor genes $p16^{INK4}$ and $p21^{Cip1//Waf1}$. Altogether, NAC attenuated the antiproliferative effect induced by artichoke extracts, which suggests that induction of premature senescence and apoptosis is regulated in a ROS-dependent manner [120].

20(S)-ginsenoside Rg3 [20(S)-Rg3], a chemical compound extracted from *Panax ginseng*, induced senescence in glioma cells at sublethal concentrations, which was abrogated by NAC treatment suggesting involvement of ROS. Moreover, depletion of Akt and inactivation of the p53/p21 pathway attenuated the compound-induced senescence. These results suggest that ROS is playing a role in activation of Akt and p53/p21, which leads to growth arrest in human glioma cancer [121].

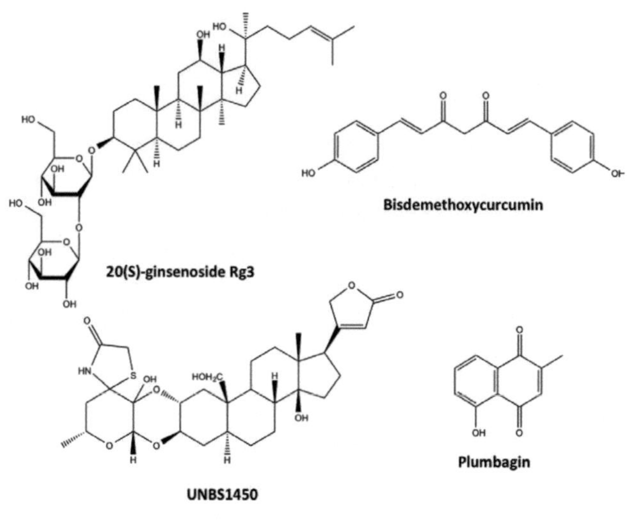

Figure 10. Molecular scaffolds involved ROS generation. Molecular structures were drawn with ChemDraw13 (Perkin Elmer).

Bisdemethoxycurcumin, a curcuminoid from turmeric, demonstrated potential chemotherapeutic activities by inhibiting proliferation and decreasing the cell viability of hormone-dependent breast cancer. Bisdemethoxycurcumin treatment leads to increased ROS production, which disrupted mitochondrial membrane potential assessed using mitochondrial potential sensor JC-1. Moreover, the compound induced increased expression of pro-apoptotic protein p53 and its downstream effector p21 along with cell cycle regulator p16 and its downstream regulator retinoblastoma protein (pRb). The results overall suggested bisdemethoxycurcumin-induced ROS accumulation, which leads to inhibition of hormone-dependent breast cancer [122].

We have previously reported that garlic-derived organosulfur compounds including diallyltetrasulfide induce growth arrest and apoptosis in colon cancer cells by disrupting the redox status in the cells. Drug-induced cell cycle arrest in G2/M phase followed by apoptosis was further associated with decreased Cdc25c expression, one of the key enzymes responsible for G2/M transition [32]. Moreover, we have also shown that plumbagin, a plant naphtoquinone, reduces cell viability and induces apoptosis in a series of hematopoietic cancer cell lines including HL-60, Jurkat, K562, Raji, and U937 with a most pronounced effect on AML U937 cells by 10-fold increase in ROS production. This was followed by decreased expression of anti-apoptotic proteins Mcl-1 and Bcl-2 along with activation of caspases-8, caspases-9, caspases-7, and caspases-3 [123]. Recently, we have also demonstrated ROS induction in neuroblastic and stromal neuroblastoma cells by hemisynthetic cardenolide UNBS1450. ROS induction was followed by autophagic response eventually leading to apoptosis or necroptosis. Time-dependent increase in ROS affected lysosomal integrity of the cells inducing lysosome-associated membrane protein (LAMP)-2 degradation leading to cathepsin B and L activation [124] (**Figure 10**).

9. Conclusion

Natural compounds or their derivatives comprise of more than 50% of cancer chemotherapeutic agents available in the clinics. Information encoded by the human genome project would definitely lead to identification of several gene products, which could potentially be targeted by novel anticancer drugs. Due to various advantages associated with the use of natural compounds such as high availability and reduced toxicity, it is likely that the natural products templates combined with chemistry will allow the generation of novel analogues with enhanced pharmacological benefits to enter clinics.

Malignant cells, which often exhibit increased ROS generation that is associated with tumor proliferation and drug resistance, highlight the crucial role of ROS stress in cancer. Therefore, targeting the redox-modulated biochemical properties of cancer cell may allow to develop a feasible therapeutic approach to overcome challenges associated with cancer treatment. Furthermore, not critically explored unique redox biology of cancer stem cells suggests the use of redox modulating strategies to eradicate these cells.

Acknowledgements

Aloran Mazumder and Marc Diederich are supported by RSL (Luxemburg) and by the Research Institute of Pharmaceutical Sciences, College of Pharmacy, Seoul National University, by the National Research Foundation grant funded by the MEST of Korea for Tumor Microenvironment GCRC 2012-0001184 and by Brain Korea (BK21) PLUS program.

Author details

Aloran Mazumder and Marc Diederich*

*Address all correspondence to: marcdiederich@snu.ac.kr

College of Pharmacy, Seoul National University, Seoul, Korea

References

[1] Mann J. Natural products in cancer chemotherapy: past, present and future. Nat Rev Cancer. 2002;2(2):143–8.

[2] Zubrod CG. Origins and development of chemotherapy research at the National-Cancer-Institute. Cancer Treat Rep. 1984;68(1):9–19.

[3] Kinghorn AD, Balandrin MF. Human medicinal agents from plants. American Chemical Society (ACS); Oxford University Press UK, 1993.

[4] Newman DJ, Cragg GM. Natural products as sources of new drugs over the 30 years from 1981 to 2010. J Nat Prod. 2012;75(3):311–35.

[5] Harvey AL, Edrada-Ebel R, Quinn RJ. The re-emergence of natural products for drug discovery in the genomics era. Nat Rev Drug Discov. 2015;14(2):111–29.

[6] Tsuda H, Ohshima Y, Nomoto H, Fujita K-I, Matsuda E, Iigo M, et al. Cancer prevention by natural compounds. Drug Metab Pharmacokinet. 2004;19(4):245–63.

[7] Cerella C, Teiten MH, Radogna F, Dicato M, Diederich M. From nature to bedside: pro-survival and cell death mechanisms as therapeutic targets in cancer treatment. Biotechnol Adv. 2014;32(6):1111–22.

[8] Morceau F, Chateauvieux S, Orsini M, Trecul A, Dicato M, Diederich M. Natural compounds and pharmaceuticals reprogram leukemia cell differentiation pathways. Biotechnol Adv. 2015;33(6 Pt 1):785–97.

[9] Schnekenburger M, Dicato M, Diederich M. Plant-derived epigenetic modulators for cancer treatment and prevention. Biotechnol Adv. 2014;32(6):1123–32.

[10] Schumacher M, Kelkel M, Dicato M, Diederich M. Gold from the sea: marine compounds as inhibitors of the hallmarks of cancer. Biotechnol Adv. 2011;29(5):531–47.

[11] Moriarty-Craige SE, Jones DP. Extracellular thiols and thiol/disulfide redox in metabolism. Annu Rev Nutr. 2004;24:481–509.

[12] Duvoix A, Schmitz M, Schnekenburger M, Dicato M, Morceau F, Galteau MM, et al. Transcriptional regulation of glutathione *S*-transferase P1-1 in human leukemia. BioFactors. 2003;17(1–4):131–8.

[13] Duvoix A, Schnekenburger M, Delhalle S, Blasius R, Borde-Chiche P, Morceau F, et al. Expression of glutathione *S*-transferase P1-1 in leukemic cells is regulated by inducible AP-1 binding. Cancer Lett. 2004;216(2):207–19.

[14] Schnekenburger M, Karius T, Diederich M. Regulation of epigenetic traits of the glutathione *S*-transferase P1 gene: from detoxification toward cancer prevention and diagnosis. Front Pharmacol. 2014;5:170.

[15] Brigelius-Flohe R. Tissue-specific functions of individual glutathione peroxidases. Free Radic Biol Med. 1999;27(9–10):951–65.

[16] Ursini F, Maiorino M, Brigelius-Flohe R, Aumann K, Roveri A, Schomburg D, et al. Diversity of glutathione peroxidases. Methods Enzymol. 1994;252:38–53.

[17] Townsend DM, Tew KD. The role of glutathione-*S*-transferase in anti-cancer drug resistance. Oncogene. 2003;22(47):7369–75.

[18] Sharma R, Yang Y, Sharma A, Awasthi S, Awasthi YC. Antioxidant role of glutathione *S*-transferases: protection against oxidant toxicity and regulation of stress-mediated apoptosis. Antioxid Redox Signal. 2004;6(2):289–300.

[19] Montero AJ, Jassem J. Cellular redox pathways as a therapeutic target in the treatment of cancer. Drugs. 2011;71(11):1385–96.

[20] Forman HJ, Torres M, Fukuto J. Redox signaling. Oxygen/nitrogen radicals: cell injury and disease. Springer Science + Business Media New York., 2002. p. 49–62.

[21] Duvoix A, Blasius R, Delhalle S, Schnekenburger M, Morceau F, Henry E, et al. Chemopreventive and therapeutic effects of curcumin. Cancer Lett. 2005;223(2): 181–90.

[22] Reuter S, Eifes S, Dicato M, Aggarwal BB, Diederich M. Modulation of anti-apoptotic and survival pathways by curcumin as a strategy to induce apoptosis in cancer cells. Biochem Pharmacol. 2008;76(11):1340–51.

[23] Teiten MH, Gaascht F, Eifes S, Dicato M, Diederich M. Chemopreventive potential of curcumin in prostate cancer. Genes Nutr. 2010;5(1):61–74.

[24] Teiten MH, Dicato M, Diederich M. Curcumin as a regulator of epigenetic events. Mol Nutr Food Res. 2013;57(9):1619–29.

[25] Kelkel M, Jacob C, Dicato M, Diederich M. Potential of the dietary antioxidants resveratrol and curcumin in prevention and treatment of hematologic malignancies. Molecules. 2010;15(10):7035–74.

[26] Teiten MH, Gaascht F, Dicato M, Diederich M. Targeting the wingless signaling pathway with natural compounds as chemopreventive or chemotherapeutic agents. Curr Pharm Biotechnol. 2012;13(1):245–54.

[27] Spagnuolo C, Cerella C, Russo M, Chateauvieux S, Diederich M, Russo GL. Quercetin downregulates Mcl-1 by acting on mRNA stability and protein degradation. Br J Cancer. 2011;105(2):221–30.

[28] Cerella C, Gaigneaux A, Dicato M, Diederich M. Antagonistic role of natural compounds in mTOR-mediated metabolic reprogramming. Cancer Lett. 2015;356(2 Pt A): 251–62.

[29] Cerella C, Dicato M, Jacob C, Diederich M. Chemical properties and mechanisms determining the anti-cancer action of garlic-derived organic sulfur compounds. Anticancer Agents Med Chem. 2011;11(3):267–71.

[30] Kelkel M, Cerella C, Mack F, Schneider T, Jacob C, Schumacher M, et al. ROS-independent JNK activation and multisite phosphorylation of Bcl-2 link diallyl tetrasulfide-induced mitotic arrest to apoptosis. Carcinogenesis. 2012;33(11):2162–71.

[31] Czepukojc B, Baltes AK, Cerella C, Kelkel M, Viswanathan UM, Salm F, et al. Synthetic polysulfane derivatives induce cell cycle arrest and apoptotic cell death in human hematopoietic cancer cells. Food Chem Toxicol. 2014;64:249–57.

[32] Busch C, Jacob C, Anwar A, Burkholz T, Aicha Ba L, Cerella C, et al. Diallylpolysulfides induce growth arrest and apoptosis. Int J Oncol. 2010;36(3):743–9.

[33] Viry E, Anwar A, Kirsch G, Jacob C, Diederich M, Bagrel D. Antiproliferative effect of natural tetrasulfides in human breast cancer cells is mediated through the inhibition of the cell division cycle 25 phosphatases. Int J Oncol. 2011;38(4):1103–11.

[34] Anwar A, Burkholz T, Scherer C, Abbas M, Lehr C-M, Diederich M, et al. Naturally occurring reactive sulfur species, their activity against Caco-2 cells, and possible modes of biochemical action. J Sulfur Chem. 2011;29(3–4):251–68.

[35] Storz P. Reactive oxygen species in tumor progression. Front Biosci. 2005;10(1–3):1881–96.

[36] Burdon RH, Gill V, Rice-Evans C. Oxidative stress and tumour cell proliferation. Free Radic Res Commun. 1990;11(1–3):65–76.

[37] Reddy KB, Glaros S. Inhibition of the MAP kinase activity suppresses estrogen-induced breast tumor growth both in vitro and in vivo. Int J Oncol. 2007;30(4):971–5.

[38] Parkash J, Felty Q, Roy D. Estrogen exerts a spatial and temporal influence on reactive oxygen species generation that precedes calcium uptake in high-capacity mitochondria: implications for rapid nongenomic signaling of cell growth. Biochemistry. 2006;45(9):2872–81.

[39] Li Q, Engelhardt JF. Interleukin-1β induction of NFkB is partially regulated by H2O2-mediated activation of NFkB-inducing kinase. J Biol Chem. 2006;281(3):1495–505.

[40] Manna SK, Zhang HJ, Yan T, Oberley LW, Aggarwal BB. Overexpression of manganese superoxide dismutase suppresses tumor necrosis factor-induced apoptosis and activation of nuclear transcription factor-kB and activated protein-1. J Biol Chem. 1998;273(21):13245–54.

[41] Felty Q, Singh KP, Roy D. Estrogen-induced G1/S transition of G0-arrested estrogen-dependent breast cancer cells is regulated by mitochondrial oxidant signaling. Oncogene. 2005;24(31):4883–93.

[42] Park S-A, Na H-K, Kim E-H, Cha Y-N, Surh Y-J. 4-Hydroxyestradiol induces anchorage-independent growth of human mammary epithelial cells via activation of IkB kinase: potential role of reactive oxygen species. Cancer Res. 2009;69(6):2416–24.

[43] Basseres DS, Baldwin AS. Nuclear factor-kappaB and inhibitor of kappaB kinase pathways in oncogenic initiation and progression. Oncogene. 2006;25(51):6817–30.

[44] Li N, Karin M. Is NF-kB the sensor of oxidative stress? FASEB J. 1999;13(10):1137–43.

[45] Chen CL, Lin CF, Chiang CW, Jan MS, Lin YS. Lithium inhibits ceramide- and etoposide-induced protein phosphatase 2A methylation, Bcl-2 dephosphorylation, caspase-2 activation, and apoptosis. Mol Pharmacol. 2006;70(2):510–7.

[46] Wang Y, Huang X, Cang H, Gao F, Yamamoto T, Osaki T, et al. The endogenous reactive oxygen species promote NF-k B activation by targeting on activation of NF-k B-inducing kinase in oral squamous carcinoma cells. Free Radical Res. 2007;41(9):963–71.

[47] Cristofanon S, Uguccioni F, Cerella C, Radogna F, Dicato M, Ghibelli L, et al. Intracellular prooxidant activity of melatonin induces a survival pathway involving NF-kappaB activation. Ann N Y Acad Sci. 2009;1171:472–8.

[48] Radogna F, Diederich M, Ghibelli L. Melatonin: a pleiotropic molecule regulating inflammation. Biochem Pharmacol. 2010;80(12):1844–52.

[49] Radogna F, Cristofanon S, Paternoster L, D'Alessio M, De Nicola M, Cerella C, et al. Melatonin antagonizes the intrinsic pathway of apoptosis via mitochondrial targeting of Bcl-2. J Pineal Res. 2008;44(3):316–25.

[50] Radogna F, Albertini MC, De Nicola M, Diederich M, Bejarano I, Ghibelli L. Melatonin promotes Bax sequestration to mitochondria reducing cell susceptibility to apoptosis via the lipoxygenase metabolite 5-hydroxyeicosatetraenoic acid. Mitochondrion. 2015;21:113–21.

[51] Cerella C, D'Alessio M, Cristofanon S, De Nicola M, Radogna F, Dicato M, et al. Subapoptogenic oxidative stress strongly increases the activity of the glycolytic key enzyme glyceraldehyde 3-phosphate dehydrogenase. Ann N Y Acad Sci. 2009;1171:583–90.

[52] Cristofanon S, Nuccitelli S, D'Alessio M, Radogna F, De Nicola M, Bergamaschi A, et al. Oxidative upregulation of Bcl-2 in healthy lymphocytes. Ann N Y Acad Sci. 2006;1091:1–9.

[53] Cristofanon S, Morceau F, Scovassi AI, Dicato M, Ghibelli L, Diederich M. Oxidative, multistep activation of the noncanonical NF-kappaB pathway via disulfide Bcl-3/p50 complex. FASEB J. 2009;23(1):45–57.

[54] Cristofanon S, Dicato M, Ghibelli L, Diederich M. Oxidative stress and apoptosis. Redox signaling and regulation in biology and medicine. Wiley-VCH Verlag GmbH & Co.11 KGaA Weinheim, 2009. p. 373–83.

[55] Brunet A, Bonni A, Zigmond MJ, Lin MZ, Juo P, Hu LS, et al. Akt promotes cell survival by phosphorylating and inhibiting a Forkhead transcription factor. Cell. 1999;96(6):857–68.

[56] Roberts P, Der C. Targeting the Raf-MEK-ERK mitogen-activated protein kinase cascade for the treatment of cancer. Oncogene. 2007;26(22):3291–310.

[57] Lander HM, Hajjar DP, Hempstead BL, Mirza UA, Chait BT, Campbell S, et al. A molecular redox switch on p21ras structural basis for the nitric oxide-p21ras interaction. J Biol Chem. 1997;272(7):4323–26.

[58] Chan DW, Liu VW, Tsao GS, Yao K-M, Furukawa T, Chan KK, et al. Loss of MKP3 mediated by oxidative stress enhances tumorigenicity and chemoresistance of ovarian cancer cells. Carcinogenesis. 2008;29(9):1742–50.

[59] McCubrey JA, Steelman LS, Chappell WH, Abrams SL, Wong EW, Chang F, et al. Roles of the Raf/MEK/ERK pathway in cell growth, malignant transformation and drug resistance. Biochimica et Biophysica Acta (BBA) MolCell Res. 2007;1773(8):1263–84.

[60] Liu L-Z, Hu X-W, Xia C, He J, Zhou Q, Shi X, et al. Reactive oxygen species regulate epidermal growth factor-induced vascular endothelial growth factor and hypoxia-inducible factor-1α expression through activation of AKT and P70S6K1 in human ovarian cancer cells. Free Radical Biol Med. 2006;41(10):1521–33.

[61] Mochizuki T, Furuta S, Mitsushita J, Shang W, Ito M, Yokoo Y, et al. Inhibition of NADPH oxidase 4 activates apoptosis via the AKT/apoptosis signal-regulating kinase 1 pathway in pancreatic cancer PANC-1 cells. Oncogene. 2006;25(26):3699–707.

[62] Burdick AD, Davis JW, 2nd, Liu KJ, Hudson LG, Shi H, Monske ML, et al. Benzo(a)pyrene quinones increase cell proliferation, generate reactive oxygen species, and transactivate the epidermal growth factor receptor in breast epithelial cells. Cancer Res. 2003;63(22):7825–33.

[63] Liou G-Y, Storz P. Reactive oxygen species in cancer. Free Radical Res. 2010;44(5):479–96.

[64] Broom OJ, Massoumi R, Sjolander A. Alpha2beta1 integrin signalling enhances cyclooxygenase-2 expression in intestinal epithelial cells. J Cell Physiol. 2006;209(3): 950–8.

[65] Pelicano H, Lu W, Zhou Y, Zhang W, Chen Z, Hu Y, et al. Mitochondrial dysfunction and reactive oxygen species imbalance promote breast cancer cell motility through a CXCL14-mediated mechanism. Cancer Res. 2009;69(6):2375–83.

[66] Hitchler MJ, Oberley LW, Domann FE. Epigenetic silencing of SOD2 by histone modifications in human breast cancer cells. Free Radical Biol Med. 2008;45(11):1573–80.

[67] Lewis A, Du J, Liu J, Ritchie JM, Oberley LW, Cullen JJ. Metastatic progression of pancreatic cancer: changes in antioxidant enzymes and cell growth. Clin Exp Metastasis. 2005;22(7):523–32.

[68] Heneberg P. Reactive nitrogen species and hydrogen sulfide as regulators of protein tyrosine phosphatase activity. Antioxidants Redox Signal. 2014;20(14):2191–209.

[69] Yano S, Arroyo N, Yano N. SHP2 binds catalase and acquires a hydrogen peroxide-resistant phosphatase activity via integrin-signaling. FEBS Lett. 2004;577(3):327–32.

[70] Werner E, Werb Z. Integrins engage mitochondrial function for signal transduction by a mechanism dependent on Rho GTPases. J Cell Biol. 2002;158(2):357–68.

[71] Lopez-Lazaro M. The warburg effect: why and how do cancer cells activate glycolysis in the presence of oxygen? Anti-Cancer Agents Med Chem (Formerly Current Medicinal Chemistry-Anti-Cancer Agents). 2008;8(3):305–12.

[72] Harris AL. Hypoxia—a key regulatory factor in tumour growth. Nat Rev Cancer. 2002;2(1):38–47.

[73] Spitz DR, Sim JE, Ridnour LA, Galoforo SS, Lee YJ. Glucose deprivation-induced oxidative stress in human tumor cells. A fundamental defect in metabolism? Ann N Y Acad Sci. 2000;899(1):349–62.

[74] Semenza GL, Roth PH, Fang H-M, Wang GL. Transcriptional regulation of genes encoding glycolytic enzymes by hypoxia-inducible factor 1. J Biol Chem. 1994;269(38): 23757–63.

[75] Xia C, Meng Q, Liu L-Z, Rojanasakul Y, Wang X-R, Jiang B-H. Reactive oxygen species regulate angiogenesis and tumor growth through vascular endothelial growth factor. Cancer Res. 2007;67(22):10823–30.

[76] Visvader JE, Lindeman GJ. Cancer stem cells in solid tumours: accumulating evidence and unresolved questions. Nat Rev Cancer. 2008;8(10):755–68.

[77] Tothova Z, Kollipara R, Huntly BJ, Lee BH, Castrillon DH, Cullen DE, et al. FoxOs are critical mediators of hematopoietic stem cell resistance to physiologic oxidative stress. Cell. 2007;128(2):325–39.

[78] Diehn M, Cho RW, Lobo NA, Kalisky T, Dorie MJ, Kulp AN, et al. Association of reactive oxygen species levels and radioresistance in cancer stem cells. Nature. 2009;458(7239): 780–3.

[79] Cadenas E. Mitochondrial free radical production and cell signaling. Mol Aspects Med. 2004;25(1):17–26.

[80] Szatrowski TP, Nathan CF. Production of large amounts of hydrogen peroxide by human tumor cells. Cancer Res. 1991;51(3):794–8.

[81] Vásquez-Vivar J, Martasek P, Hogg N, Masters BSS, Pritchard KA, Kalyanaraman B. Endothelial nitric oxide synthase-dependent superoxide generation from adriamycin. Biochemistry. 1997;36(38):11293–7.

[82] Chung YM, Bae YS, Lee SY. Molecular ordering of ROS production, mitochondrial changes, and caspase activation during sodium salicylate-induced apoptosis. Free Radical Biol Med. 2003;34(4):434–42.

[83] Gottlieb E, Vander Heiden MG, Thompson CB. Bcl-xL prevents the initial decrease in mitochondrial membrane potential and subsequent reactive oxygen species production during tumor necrosis factor alpha-induced apoptosis. Mol Cell Biol. 2000;20(15):5680–9.

[84] Saitoh M, Nishitoh H, Fujii M, Takeda K, Tobiume K, Sawada Y, et al. Mammalian thioredoxin is a direct inhibitor of apoptosis signal-regulating kinase (ASK) 1. EMBO J. 1998;17(9):2596–606.

[85] Schulze-Osthoff K, Beyaert R, Vandevoorde V, Haegeman G, Fiers W. Depletion of the mitochondrial electron transport abrogates the cytotoxic and gene-inductive effects of TNF. EMBO J. 1993;12(8):3095.

[86] Xu YC, Wu RF, Gu Y, Yang Y-S, Yang M-C, Nwariaku FE, et al. Involvement of TRAF4 in oxidative activation of c-Jun N-terminal kinase. J Biol Chem. 2002;277(31):28051–57.

[87] Perez-Mancera PA, Young AR, Narita M. Inside and out: the activities of senescence in cancer. Nat Rev Cancer. 2014;14(8):547–58.

[88] Imlay JA, Chin SM, Linn S. Toxic DNA damage by hydrogen peroxide through the Fenton reaction in vivo and in vitro. Science. 1988;240(4852):640–2.

[89] Levine RL. Carbonyl modified proteins in cellular regulation, aging, and disease 2, 3. Free Radical Biol Med. 2002;32(9):790–6.

[90] Squier TC, Bigelow DJ. Protein oxidation and age-dependent alterations in calcium homeostasis. Front Biosci. 2000;5:D504–26.

[91] Lauschke H, Tolba R, Burger B, Minor T, Hirner A. Lipid peroxidation as additional marker in patients with colorectal cancer. Results of a preliminary study. Eur Surg Res. 2002;34(5):346–50.

[92] Folmer F, Basavaraju U, Jaspars M, Hold G, El-Omar E, Dicato M, et al. Anticancer effects of bioactive berry compounds. Phytochem Rev. 2014;13(1):295–322.

[93] Kelkel M, Schumacher M, Dicato M, Diederich M. Antioxidant and anti-proliferative properties of lycopene. Free Radic Res. 2011;45(8):925–40.

[94] Lamoral-Theys D, Pottier L, Dufrasne F, Neve J, Dubois J, Kornienko A, et al. Natural polyphenols that display anticancer properties through inhibition of kinase activity. Curr Med Chem. 2010;17(9):812–25.

[95] Chakrabarty S, Ganguli A, Das A, Nag D, Chakrabarti G. Epigallocatechin-3-gallate shows anti-proliferative activity in HeLa cells targeting tubulin-microtubule equilibrium. Chem-Biol Interact. 2015;242:380–9.

[96] Zhu K, Wang W. Green tea polyphenol EGCG suppresses osteosarcoma cell growth through upregulating miR-1. Tumor Biol. 2015;37:1–10.

[97] Manikandan P, Murugan RS, Priyadarsini RV, Vinothini G, Nagini S. Eugenol induces apoptosis and inhibits invasion and angiogenesis in a rat model of gastric carcinogenesis induced by MNNG. Life Sci. 2010;86(25):936–41.

[98] Hirano T, Gotoh M, Oka K. Natural flavonoids and lignans are potent cytostatic agents against human leukemic HL-60 cells. Life Sci. 1994;55(13):1061–9.

[99] Kuntz S, Wenzel U, Daniel H. Comparative analysis of the effects of flavonoids on proliferation, cytotoxicity, and apoptosis in human colon cancer cell lines. Eur J Nutr. 1999;38(3):133–42.

[100] Caltagirone S, Rossi C, Poggi A, Ranelletti FO, Natali PG, Brunetti M, et al. Flavonoids apigenin and quercetin inhibit melanoma growth and metastatic potential. Int J Cancer. 2000;87(4):595–600.

[101] Rodriguez-Paredes M, Esteller M. Cancer epigenetics reaches mainstream oncology. Nat Med. 2011;17(3):330–9.

[102] Pudenz M, Roth K, Gerhauser C. Impact of Soy isoflavones on the epigenome in cancer prevention. Nutrients. 2014;6(10):4218–72.

[103] Gilbert ER, Liu D. Flavonoids influence epigenetic-modifying enzyme activity: structure – function relationships and the therapeutic potential for cancer. Curr Med Chem. 2010;17(17):1756–68.

[104] Henning SM, Wang P, Carpenter CL, Heber D. Epigenetic effects of green tea polyphenols in cancer. Epigenomics. 2013;5(6):729–41.

[105] Yang CS, Fang M, Lambert JD, Yan P, Huang TH. Reversal of hypermethylation and reactivation of genes by dietary polyphenolic compounds. Nutr Rev. 2008;66(Suppl. 1):S18–20.

[106] Gaascht F, Dicato M, Diederich M. Coffee provides a natural multitarget pharmacopeia against the hallmarks of cancer. Genes Nutr. 2015;10(6):51.

[107] Lee WJ, Zhu BT. Inhibition of DNA methylation by caffeic acid and chlorogenic acid, two common catechol-containing coffee polyphenols. Carcinogenesis. 2006;27(2):269–77.

[108] Xie Q, Bai Q, Zou LY, Zhang QY, Zhou Y, Chang H, et al. Genistein inhibits DNA methylation and increases expression of tumor suppressor genes in human breast cancer cells. Genes Chromosomes Cancer. 2014;53(5):422–31.

[109] Liu C-M, Ma J-Q, Xie W-R, Liu S-S, Feng Z-J, Zheng G-H, et al. Quercetin protects mouse liver against nickel-induced DNA methylation and inflammation associated with the Nrf2/HO-1 and p38/STAT1/NF-kB pathway. Food Chem Toxicol. 2015;82:19–26.

[110] Liu Z, Liu S, Xie Z, Pavlovicz RE, Wu J, Chen P, et al. Modulation of DNA methylation by a sesquiterpene lactone parthenolide. J Pharmacol Exp Ther. 2009;329(2):505–14.

[111] Fu LJ, Ding YB, Wu LX, Wen CJ, Qu Q, Zhang X, et al. The effects of lycopene on the methylation of the GSTP1 promoter and global methylation in prostatic cancer cell lines PC3 and LNCaP. Int J Endocrinol. 2014;2014:620165.

[112] Yang J, Liu RH. Synergistic effect of apple extracts and quercetin 3-β-D-glucoside combination on antiproliferative activity in MCF-7 human breast cancer cells in vitro. J Agric Food Chem. 2009;57(18):8581–6.

[113] Nakamura Y, Yogosawa S, Izutani Y, Watanabe H, Otsuji E, Sakai T. A combination of indol-3-carbinol and genistein synergistically induces apoptosis in human colon cancer HT-29 cells by inhibiting Akt phosphorylation and progression of autophagy. Mol Cancer. 2009;8(100):100.

[114] Reiter E, Azzi A, Zingg JM. Enhanced anti?proliferative effects of combinatorial treatment of δ?tocopherol and resveratrol in human HMC?1 cells. BioFactors. 2007;30(2):67–77.

[115] Gagliano N, Aldini G, Colombo G, Rossi R, Colombo R, Gioia M, et al. The potential of resveratrol against human gliomas. Anti-Cancer Drugs. 2010;21(2):140–50.

[116] Takahashi-Yanaga F, Kahn M. Targeting Wnt signaling: can we safely eradicate cancer stem cells? Clin Cancer Res. 2010;16(12):3153–62.

[117] Li Y, Yuan YY, Meeran SM, Tollefsbol TO. Synergistic epigenetic reactivation of estrogen receptor-alpha (ERalpha) by combined green tea polyphenol and histone deacetylase inhibitor in ERalpha-negative breast cancer cells. Mol Cancer. 2010;9:274.

[118] Rausch V, Liu L, Kallifatidis G, Baumann B, Mattern J, Gladkich J, et al. Synergistic activity of sorafenib and sulforaphane abolishes pancreatic cancer stem cell characteristics. Cancer Res. 2010;70(12):5004–13.

[119] Hadad SM, Fleming S, Thompson AM. Targeting AMPK: a new therapeutic opportunity in breast cancer. Crit Rev Oncol/Hematol. 2008;67(1):1–7.

[120] Mileo AM, Di Venere D, Abbruzzese C, Miccadei S. Long term exposure to polyphenols of artichoke (*Cynara scolymus* L.) exerts induction of senescence driven growth arrest in the MDA-MB231 human breast cancer cell line. Oxid Med Cell Longev. 2014;2014:1–17.

[121] Sin S, Kim SY, Kim SS. Chronic treatment with ginsenoside Rg3 induces Akt-dependent senescence in human glioma cells. Int J Oncol. 2012;41(5):1669–74.

[122] Li Y-B, Gao J-L, Zhong Z-F, Hoi P-M, Lee SM-Y, Wang Y-T. Bisdemethoxycurcumin suppresses MCF-7 cells proliferation by inducing ROS accumulation and modulating senescence-related pathways. Pharmacol Rep. 2013;65(3):700–9.

[123] Gaascht F, Teiten MH, Cerella C, Dicato M, Bagrel D, Diederich M. Plumbagin modulates leukemia cell redox status. Molecules. 2014;19(7):10011–32.

[124] Radogna F, Cerella C, Gaigneaux A, Christov C, Dicato M, Diederich M. Cell type-dependent ROS and mitophagy response leads to apoptosis or necroptosis in neuroblastoma. Oncogene. 2015.

Chapter 5

Oxidative Stress, Inflammation, and Formation of Beta-Amyloid 1-42 in Brain

Selva Rivas-Arancibia, Erika Rodriguez-Martinez,
Angélica Méndez-García,
Mariana Moctezuma-Salgado,
Paola Jiménez-Espíndola and Ulises López-Gonzales

Additional information is available at the end of the chapter

http://dx.doi.org/10.5772/64709

Abstract

Alzheimer's disease is characterized by the pathognomonic presence of intracellular neurofibrillary tangles containing hyperphosphorylated tau protein and extracellular senile plaques primarily formed by β-amyloid. Both the neurofibrillary tangles and the plaques formed by β-amyloid 1-42 are the final result of a chain of events that progressed along with the disease for a long time. Oxidative stress plays a fundamental role among those events as proven by the experiments carried out using animal models. This can be demonstrated since there are studies indicating that, although the formation of β-amyloid is inhibited through different mechanisms (using drugs or specific antibodies), cognitive deficit is not prevented. In this chapter, we will focus on reviewing the role the chronic state of oxidative stress plays in the development of Alzheimer's disease and how the loss of redox balance induces a vicious cycle that may change normal signaling. As a consequence, there are alterations in multiple metabolic pathways that end up in the formation of hyperphosphorylated tau and insoluble β-amyloid, leading to the advance of a progressive neurodegeneration process. This is characterized by neuronal dead, astrocytic changes, microglia activation, and the loss of brain repair.

Keywords: oxidative stress, Alzheimer's disease, β-amyloid 1-42, ozone, neurodegeneration

1. Introduction

Despite a great deal of studies and the efforts of researchers in the field, the physiopathology of Alzheimer's disease (AD) is not yet clear. There is neither an accurate early diagnosis nor an effective treatment that allows the patients to have better life expectancies [1]. Perhaps one of the most important problems to solve is understand that when the diagnosis is made, the symptoms and the signs of Alzheimer's disease are the result of a long chain of events that took place during an extended period of time and that such symptoms and signs change with time [2].

One can assume that intracellular signaling and metabolic changes found during the early stages of the disease are not the same as the ones found at more advanced stages. For this reason, recent postmortem studies fail to completely clarify the physiopathology of this disease.

2. Changes at cellular level caused by chronic oxidative stress

Acute oxidative stress is reversible and it is present in a number of physiological and pathological mechanisms that are reversible as well. These mechanisms play a defensive role in the organism during respiratory burst [3]. However, the chronic oxidative stress state is an epiphenomenon that affects the organism and the brain tissue at different levels. It is involved in the maintenance and advance of the chronic degenerative disease that is usually irreversible [4].

2.1. Cell signaling, redox balance, and oxidative stress state

It has been widely demonstrated that in redox balance, the rise in reactive species induces an increase in the production of antioxidant enzymes. In turn, the enzymes rapidly compensate the free radicals, allowing the system to return to redox balance [5]. During this state, free radicals also play a central role signaling the different intracellular cascades related to cell cycle and antioxidant response. The latter is associated to repair mechanisms and cell survival, regulation of inflammatory response, signaling of intracellular metabolic pathways, maintenance of energetic metabolism, and the efficient system of protein degradation by the proteasome [6].

In the brain, insulin signaling over its receptors is crucial to survival maintenance of neural metabolism. Similarly, the correct functioning of phosphorylation and dephosphorylation pathways that takes place during redox balance promotes an efficient functioning of the signaling pathways [7]. We must also include low-density lipoprotein (LDL) receptors, cholesterol, and receptors for advanced glycation end products [8–10].

Nevertheless, the loss of redox balance causes disturbances in the pathways mentioned above changing the signaling and the normal metabolism needed to maintain cell function.

2.2. Reactive oxygen species and antioxidant defenses

It has been reported that the excess of free radicals formed during normal metabolism is able to produce oxidation in proteins, DNA, and RNA. It also causes lipid peroxidation and sugar modification, thus inducing changes that lead to catastrophic neuronal death in the hippocampus, including neocortex regions [11]. Furthermore, free radicals are chemical species that have one or more unpaired electrons, which can act as acceptors of other electrons belonging to other molecules. As a result, they produce oxidation and cause a chain of molecular damage [12]. Free radicals come from sources that are endogenous (the own metabolism of the cell, mainly carried out during the respiratory chain in the internal membrane of the mitochondria) and exogenous (environmental pollution, tobacco, smoke, drugs, xenobiotics, or radiation) [13]. Despite the deleterious effects of oxidative stress, aerobic organisms have developed a wide variety of mechanisms to maintain genomic stability. These mechanisms include endogenous and exogenous antioxidants that can be divided into enzymatic and nonenzymatic antioxidants [14].

The enzymatic antioxidants are genetically codificated, for example, superoxide dismutase (SOD) cupper/zinc, manganese, glutathion peroxidase, glutathion reductase, and catalase [15]. The nonenzymatic antioxidants such as thioredoxin, vitamin C, vitamin A, and vitamin E have a strong role as scavengers [16].

2.3. Loss of redox balance and oxidative stress state

The free radicals are metabolized in the biological systems leading to the formation of reactive species that, depending on the radical (oxygen, nitrogen, iron, copper, etc.), receive their denomination. For example, the metabolism of the superoxide radical generates the reactive oxygen species (ROS), whereas the metabolism of the nitric oxide radical generates reactive nitrogen species (RNS) [17].

The increase of ROS together with the deficit of antioxidant systems causes a chronic oxidative stress state. It is interesting to point out that an acute increase of the ROS causes a stimulation of the antioxidant systems depending on the antioxidant capability of the organism; this is the basis of ozone therapy [18]. However, the production or the exposure chronic, whether by environmental pollutants or metabolic disorders, to low or moderate ROS concentrations in the organism induces a chronic oxidative stress state. Such state is found in several chronic degenerative diseases among which neurodegenerative diseases as Parkinson's and Alzheimer's are included [19].

The chronic oxidative stress state is an epiphenomenon that affects cell functions at different levels. They go from changes in signaling of the cell cycle [20], response to endogenous antioxidant systems [21], loss of repair and cell function mechanisms [22], and regulation of the dynamic of the cytoskeleton [23]. They also include protein misfolding and oxidation [24], alterations in function and signaling of the endoplasmic reticulum (ER) during protein synthesis and chaperone signaling [25], alteration and loss of cell receptor functionality [26, 27], and mitochondrial damage leading to a deficit of energy [28]. In addition, there is loss of the regulation and selectivity of the cell membrane [29], stimulation of phosphorylation pathways and inhibition of dephosphorylation pathways, which alter intracellular signaling [30, 31], and finally, the loss of regulation of inflammatory response [32], as is shown in **Figure 1**.

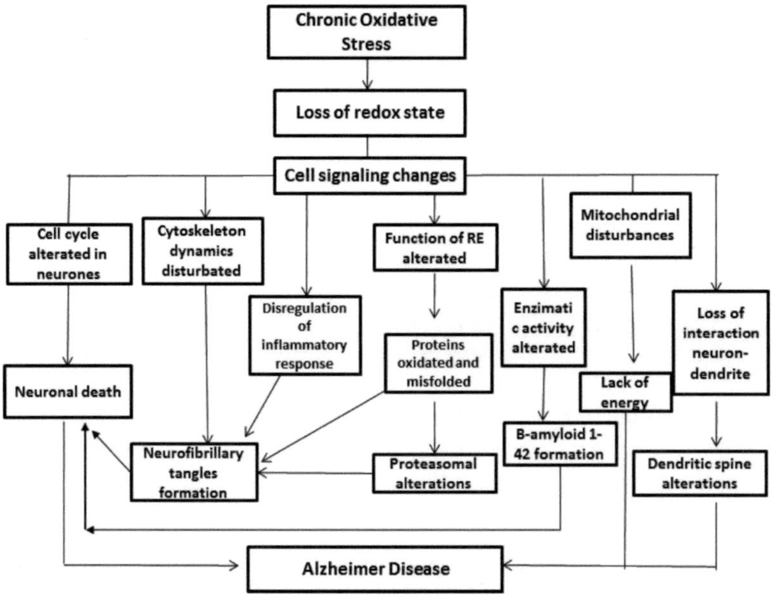

Figure 1. Effect of chronic oxidative stress on intracellular changes present during the development of Alzheimer's disease.

2.4. Cell cycle and oxidative stress

The presence of an oxidative stress state has been associated with an aberrant reentry into the cell cycle, a phenomenon associated with the death of terminally differentiated neurons. This mechanism has been observed in samples from Alzheimer's disease and Down syndrome patients [33, 34]. It has been proven that the increase in the cyclin D2 levels due to the loss of FoxO 1a downregulation on this cyclin may take part of the aberrant reentry into cell cycle. In consequence, the mature neurons do not divide activating cell death mechanisms by apoptosis where caspase-3 might play an important role [35].

2.5. Antioxidant enzyme regulation in an oxidative stress state

The increase of free radicals acts upon a series of pathways that lead to transcription of antioxidant enzymes. Transcription factors within these pathways allow the activation of antioxidant response elements (AREs) in the nucleus [36]. The AREs cause the raise in messenger RNA transcription for the increase in antioxidant enzyme synthesis. For instance, FoxO 3a activation stimulates the signaling pathway for the increase in the synthesis of superoxide dismutase enzymes, particularly the manganese superoxide dismutase, MnSOD [35]. The signaling pathway regulated by the transcription factor Nrf2 is also activated by the presence of ROS. Under oxidative stress conditions, Nrf2 transactivates the synthesis of hundreds of antioxidant genes such as HMOX-1, NQO-1, GCS, and GSTM1, among others [37]. In humans, the insufficient activation of this transcription factor has been related to chronic diseases as Parkinson's, Alzheimer's, and amyotrophic lateral sclerosis [38]. In brains of Alzheimer's patients, studies have also proven a reduction in the Nrf2 protein levels in hippocampus astrocytes. This is one of the key areas where ROS causes neurodegeneration in this disease [39]. In addition, some target genes of this transcription factor have been found to be reduced in the frontal cortex, as is the case of the protein p62 [40].

2.6. Regulation of the dynamic of the cytoskeleton and the effect of chronic oxidative stress

The neuronal cytoskeleton consists of microtubules, actin filaments, and neurofilaments (intermediate filaments). All these components are regulated through the changes in the levels of expression of the genes that code, posttranslational changes, and the set of proteins with which they interact. Oxidative stress affects the regulation mechanisms of the neuronal cytoskeleton when acting over its components. Because all the components are interconnected and regulate each other, the damage caused by oxidative stress affects the whole cytoskeleton network [41]. The microtubules are particularly susceptible to oxidative stress that causes its depolymerization [42]. Furthermore, oxidative stress affects the tubulin through aberrant posttranslational modifications [43]. For their part, actin filaments are less susceptible to the negative effects of oxidative stress because they use ROS for their reorganization [44]. Finally, neurofilaments are phosphorylated in the presence of reactive species, which causes the formation of protein aggregates as the ones found in neurodegenerative diseases like Alzheimer's [45].

2.7. Misfolding and protein oxidation by chronic oxidative stress

Oxidation can affect protein structure because the endoplasmic reticulum responds to oxidative stress by affecting chaperons and producing protein misfolding altering their spatial structure. This causes negative effects on the functionality of the proteins and makes them susceptible to aggregation, inducing to cell toxicity [46].

The disassembly in the ubiquitin-proteasome proteins is a protection mechanism to avoid the damages caused by oxidative stress [47]. A number of studies have reported that from the 26S proteasome complex, the 20S subunit is more resistant to the damage caused by ROS compared to the 19S subunit. It may bind and degrade misfolded oxidized proteins without the need of ubiquitination and ATP expenditure [48]. However, during a chronic oxidative stress state, proteasomal proteins are also modified by oxidation, thus altering their function and causing intracellular and extracellular protein accumulation [49].

2.8. Alterations in endoplasmic reticulum function and signaling by chronic oxidative stress

The endoplasmic reticulum is the organelle that within their functions include the calcium (Ca^{2+}) storage and protein folding with the participation of different enzymes and chaperones [50]. The redox state inside the ER lumen is highly oxidant and the changes caused by the presence of ROS affect the correct protein folding. It contributes to the breaking of the disulphide bonds by the binding of reactive species to thiol groups [51]. Misfolded proteins that are formed in the ER cause Ca^{2+} release in the cytoplasmic space. When the mitochondria capture excessive amounts of calcium, it loses the regulation of its membrane, creating a mitochondrial transition pore. This results in ATP deficit and ROS increase which induce, in turn, ER Ca^{2+} release; thus, a vicious cycle in the intracellular regulation of Ca^{2+} levels is created [52]. Studies performed with cerebral samples from Alzheimer's patients have demonstrated that the redox modifications caused by oxidative stress inhibit the function of chaperones and the correct folding proteins, causing protein misfolding and ER stress [53]. In Alzheimer's pathology, β-protein has been reported to induce stress in the ER and change the morphology of the ER and also of the mitochondria. This results in the loss of the mitochondrial membrane potential and the consequent production of ROS [54].

2.9. Mitochondrial damage by oxidative stress

The mitochondria play a number of cell functions, such as ATP synthesis, calcium homeostasis, and processes of cell survival and death. Additionally, this organelle is the main source of endogenous ROS; therefore, it is constantly exposed to oxidative stress [55]. Several metabolic and mitochondrial abnormalities have been found in hippocampal neurons of patients with Alzheimer's. Mitochondria of AD patients show a reduction in size, DNA alterations, and mitochondrial proteins in vacuoles, suggesting mitochondrial degradation by autophagy [56]. Studies have also observed deficiencies in the production of antioxidant enzymes that play a protective role protecting the mitochondria from the damage caused by ROS; for example, there are the cytochrome oxidase complex IV, MnSOD, and uncoupling proteins [57].

2.10. Loss of regulation of inflammatory response

The immune defense of the central nervous system (CNS) is composed of a number of small cells known as microglia, astrocytes, and an effective blood-brain barrier [58]. The presence of an oxidative stress state causes the activation of the microglia and the astrocytes. As a result, inflammatory and neurotoxic factors are released increasing the levels of oxidative stress and causing a chronic neuroinflammatory response. Depending on its duration, the response may cause damage in the brain tissue [59]. Neurodegenerative diseases are characterized by a chronic dysregulation of the inflammatory response that involves glial alteration. This produces alterations in the neuronal metabolism, neuronal survival, and repair that progress to neuronal death and memory disturbances [4].

2.11. Oxidative stress state and dendritic spines

The chronic oxidative stress state causes alterations in dendritic spines. These alterations consist of a reduction in the size of the spines as well as a decrease in their number. This phenomenon is present in neurodegenerative diseases and in chronic diseases as alcoholism [60, 61]. An explanation of this histologic alteration found in the hippocampus of the patients is the loss of the existing regulation in calcium metabolism during oxidative stress state. There is an increase of extracellular Ca^{2+} entry, which tries to be regulated by the cells; they send Ca^{2+} to the ER or the mitochondria to avoid the alteration Ca^{2+}-dependent cell functions [62].

http://dx.doi.org/10.5772/64709

In addition, some studies have proposed a neuronal defense mechanism in which the cell tries to decrease the membrane surface exposed to free radicals, with the final purpose to try to control the balance in the intraneuronal medium [63]. All these changes affect the number of synapses and the metabolic interaction between astrocytes and neurons.

2.12. Oxidative stress state and neuron-glia interaction

The signaling and metabolic changes that occur in the presence of oxidative stress affect the interaction between neurons and astrocytes, and cause the activation of the microglia, inducing and maintaining the loss of regulation of the inflammatory response [64]. Among these alterations, we find the loss of regulation in neurotransmitter metabolism as glutamate, dopamine, as well as alterations in the metabolism of antioxidant systems like glutathione [65, 66]. On the other hand, the changes in the expression of inducible nitric oxide synthase and in the extracellular Ca^{2+} levels cause the release of proinflammatory cytokines as interleukin (IL)-1, IL-3, IL-6, interferon (IFN)-α, IFN-β, and tumor necrosis factor (TNF)-α by the astrocytes (**Figure 2**). This promotes the maintenance of the inflammatory response and the stimulation of the glia, creating a vicious cycle consisting of oxidative stress, cytokine release, inflammatory response, and increase of oxidative stress [67].

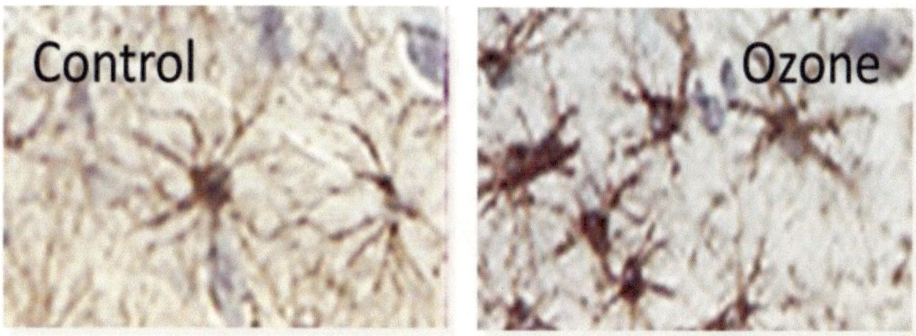

Figure 2. Microphotography that shows the chronic effect of oxidative stress in hippocampal astrocytes from rats exposed to low doses of ozone (40×). There are changes in the astrocytes in the samples from animals exposed to ozone.

2.13. Oxidative stress state and disturbance of the blood-brain barrier

The blood-brain barrier finely regulates the entry of substances into the brain. Among its functions is the capability of changing the affinity of the transporters according to the necessities of the nervous tissue [68]. This barrier is created by a close relationship between neurons, astrocytes, and endothelial cells; the microglia is involved as well [69]. The barrier creates a neurovascular unit that promotes neuronal homeostasis maintenance. Nevertheless, in neurodegenerative diseases and during inflammatory processes, this barrier is broken down and loses its selectivity [70]. We have proven that the blood-brain barrier is broken and there are changes in the morphology of the end feet of astrocytes in animal models of neurodegeneration caused by oxidative stress in the hippocampus of rats exposed to ozone [71]. Finally, this break is followed by endothelial cell edema, changes in the processes and in astrocytic feet, and an increase of the proinflammatory factors. It promotes the exacerbation of the neurodegenerative process [72]. Oligomer production of β-amyloid increases oxidative damage of the blood-brain barrier, attracting astrocytes, glia, and activated microglia [73].

3. Oxidative stress and Alzheimer's disease

3.1. APP processing and β-amyloid formation

The break of the amyloid precursor protein (APP) has two phases: a nonamyloidogenic pathway and an amyloidogenic pathway. The amino acid 83 is cleaved by the α-secretase on the carboxyl-terminal, producing a long amino N-terminal ectodomain (sAPPα). The result of this process is the formation of C83, which is retained by the membrane to be cleaved by gamma secretase, creating short p3 fragments. The break down by α-secretase occurs within the β-amyloid region, preventing the formation of β-amyloid [74].

On the other hand, the amyloidogenic pathway is an alternative APP breakdown which leads to the creation of β-amyloids. This pathway is created by the β-secretase cleaving in the amino acid 99, allowing sAPPβ release in the extracellular space [75]. In consequence, the breakdown of this fragment between the 38 and 43 residues by the γ-secretase releases an intact Aβ peptide [76]. The complete β-amyloid peptide is 40 residues long ($A\beta_{40}$) and 10% is a 42-residue variant ($A\beta_{42}$). This variant is more hydrophobic and easily induces the formation of fibrils. It is also the largest form of this peptides prevailing the β-amyloid plaques [77].

There is a variety of assembly forms in which the β-amyloid peptide can be found. This peptide can carry out different physiological or pathological functions depending on the assembly pathway [78]. The β-amyloid can be deposited in specific brain regions forming amyloid plaques [79, 80].

3.2. Oxidative stress and alteration of the enzymes involved in the processing of APP

Among the different hypotheses explaining the possible causes intervening in the development of the disease, the participation of oxidative stress is nowadays widely accepted. Results obtained in our laboratory show that oxidative stress in healthy animals is per se capable of producing hyperphosphorylated tau protein and the formation of isoforms of β-amyloids 1-42 in hippocampal neurons of rats chronically exposes to low doses of ozone [81] (**Figure 3**).

The formation of senile plaques is due to intracellular and extracellular accumulation of insoluble β-amyloids in the brain. The β-amyloid peptide is generated by APP cleavage where the enzymes α, β, and γ secretases are involved as previously indicated [82]. Both the enzymes of the amyloidogenic pathway as the enzymes of the nonamyloidogenic pathway are altered by a chronic oxidative stress state. Experiments performed in our laboratory demonstrate that chronic oxidative stress, caused by exposure to low doses of ozone, is capable of inhibiting the enzymes involved in the nonamyloidogenic pathway. It also increases the enzymes in the amyloidogenic pathway in the hippocampus of rats which were exposed to this gas for 4 hours during 60 and 90 days (**Figures 4** and **5**).

http://dx.doi.org/10.5772/64709

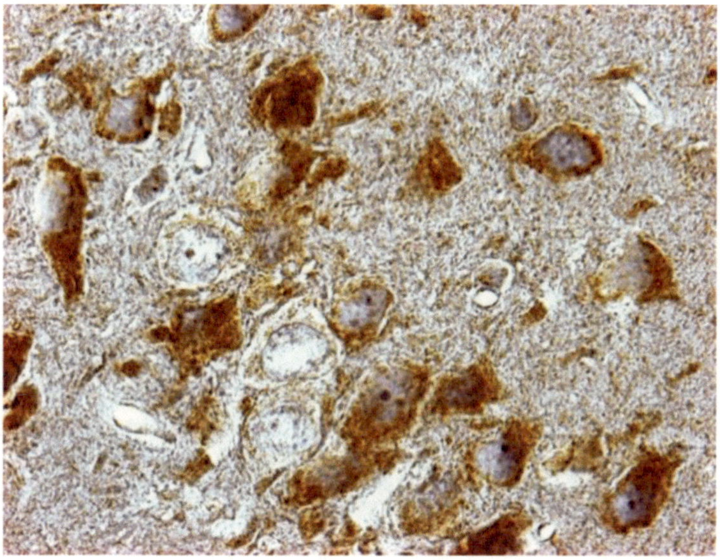

Figure 3. Micrography that shows the chronic effect of oxidative stress on the formation of β-amyloid 1-42 in rat hippocampus exposed to low doses of ozone for 90 days (100×). Note changes in intracellular accumulation of β-amyloid 1-42 in neurons of the dentate gyrus.

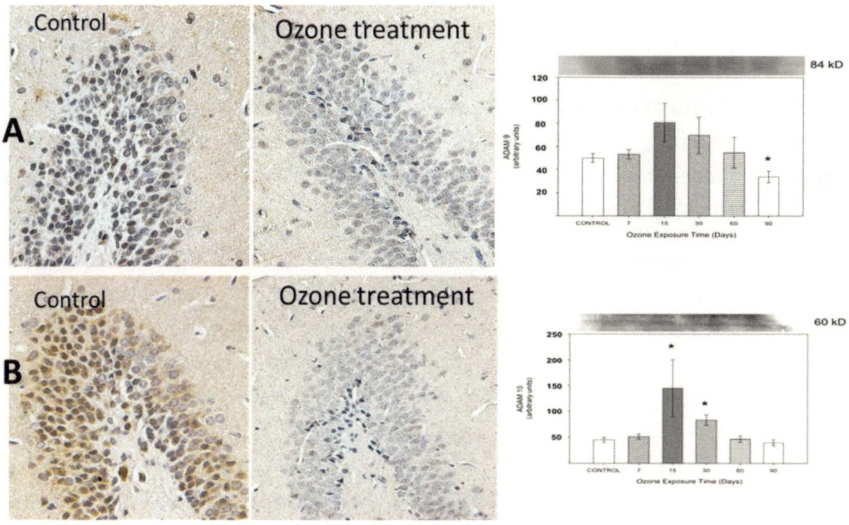

Figure 4. Micrography that shows the chronic effect of oxidative stress on the enzymes of the nonamyloidogenic pathway (A: ADAM 9; B: ADAM 10) in dentate gyrus of rat hippocampus exposed to low doses of ozone (40×). Note the decrease in immunoreactivity after 90 days of exposure to ozone compared to the control.

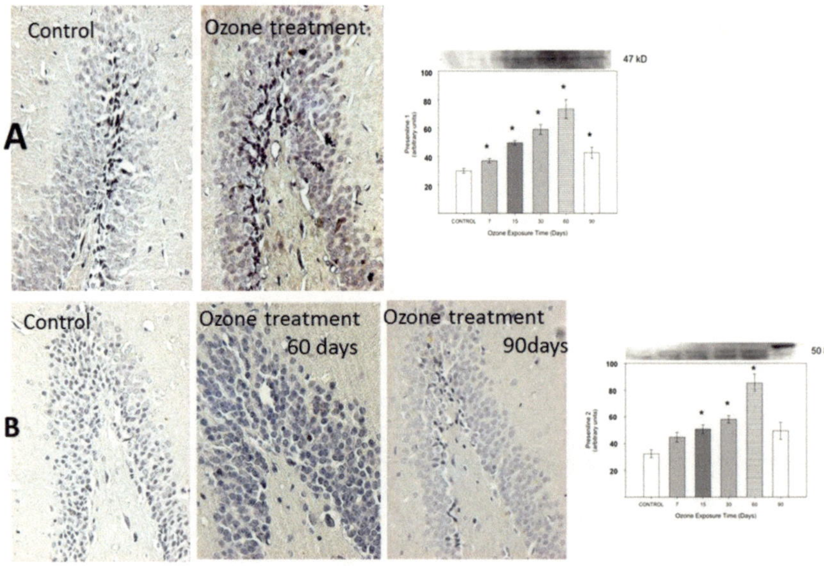

Figure 5. Micrography that shows the chronic effect of oxidative stress on the amyloidogenic pathway enzymes (A: presenilin 1; B: presenilin 2) in the dentate gyrus of rat hippocampus exposed to low doses of ozone (40×). Note the increase in immunoreactivity at 90 days for presenilin 1 and presenilin 2 to 60 days in the brains of animals exposed to ozone compared to the control.

The β-amyloid accumulation in specific compartments of the neuron causes an energy deficit and alterations in protein folding [83, 84]. For its part, the intracellular increase of these oligomers causes the inhibition of the proteasome activity, lowering the possibility of processing misfolded proteins and causing their accumulation buildup within the cell [85].

The β-amyloid accumulation attracts immune system cells such as astrocytes, activated microglia, and macrophages, among others. Glial cells maintain the loss of regulation of the inflammatory response, the inflammation, and the oxidative stress state, creating a vicious cycle that is maintained in time [86].

When the levels of the intracellular β-amyloid peptide decrease, the internalization of APP is induced. The internalization is mediated by the low density lipoprotein receptor-related protein 1B (LRP1B), one of the members of the LDL family. This receptor usually binds APP to the plasmatic membrane to prevent the internalization of the β-amyloid peptide, reducing its production [87]. The failure of these mechanisms by the effect of oxidative stress and the hyperphosphorylation of tau protein induced a disturbance in the formation of microtubules, producing neurofibrillary tangles [88]. Furthermore, tau protein associates with β-amyloids that might be involved in the internalization of the extracellular protein into the neurons. This produces and externalizes the insoluble isoform of β-amyloid [89]. During this phase, the synthesis of soluble β-amyloid is decreased while the synthesis of misfolded insoluble β-amyloids is increased. It forms part of the insoluble β-amyloid plaques [90].

Finally, our laboratory has developed a noninvasive model of oxidative stress using the exposure to low doses of ozone to that effect. Using this model, we have proven that oxidative stress per se is capable of producing progressive neurodegeneration in the hippocampus together with the formation of insoluble β-amyloid 1-42 and the accumulation of such peptides.

4. Conclusions

The loss of redox homeostasis accelerates ageing and plays a fundamental role in the pathogeny and development of Alzheimer's disease. It alters the cell signaling mechanisms of an important number of metabolic pathways, promotes epigenetic alterations, and alters the posttranslational mechanisms. Finally, the chronic alteration of the redox balance induces the misfolding of proteins by oxidative stress in ER, cholesterol oxidation, and alterations in insulin receptors that lead to changes in neuronal metabolism and survival.

We can infer that Alzheimer's disease is the final manifestation of a series of oxidative alterations of the metabolism. There is a slow involvement of different biomolecules during the development of the disease. The loss of redox balance plays a crucial role in the formation of hyperphosphorylated tau protein, insoluble β-amyloids, and the loss of regulation of the immune system.

Acknowledgements

This work was supported by CONACYT under grant 219703 to S. R-A.

Author details

Selva Rivas-Arancibia*, Erika Rodriguez-Martinez, Angélica Méndez-García, Mariana Moctezuma-Salgado, Paola Jiménez-Espíndola and Ulises López-Gonzales

*Address all correspondence to: srivas@unam.mx

Physiology Department, Faculty of Medicine, National Autonomous University of Mexico, Mexico City, Mexico

References

[1] Cacabelos R, Torrellas C, Carrera I, Cacabelos P, Corzo L, Fernández-Novoa L, Tellado I, Carril JC, Aliev G. Novel therapeutic strategies for dementia. CNS Neurol Disord Drug Targets. 2016;15(2):141–241. DOI: 10.2174/1871527315666160202121548

[2] Zafrilla P, Mulero J, Xandri JM, Santo E, Caravaca G, Morillas JM. Oxidative stress in Alzheimer patients in different stages of the disease. Curr Med Chem. 2006;13(9):1075–1083. DOI: 10.2174/092986706776360978

[3] Forman HJ, Torres M. Reactive oxygen species and cell signaling: respiratory burst in macrophage signaling. Am J Respir Crit Care Med. 2002;15:166(12 Pt 2):S4–S8. DOI: 10.1164/rccm.2206007

[4] Rivas-Arancibia S, Guevara-Guzmán R, López-Vidal Y, Rodríguez-Martínez E, Zanardo-Gomes M, Angoa-Pérez M, Raisman-Vozari R. Oxidative stress caused by ozone exposure induces loss of brain repair in the hippocampus of adult rats. Toxicol Sci. 2010;113(1):187–197. DOI: 10.1093/toxsci/kfp252

[5] Ursini F, Maiorino M, Forman HJ. Redox homeostasis: the golden mean of healthy living. Redox Biol. 2016;19(8):205–215. DOI: 10.1016/j.redox.2016.01.010

[6] Dröge W. Free radicals in the physiological control of cell function. Physiol Rev. 2002;82(1):47–95. DOI: 10.1152/physrev.00018.2001

[7] Kleinridders A, Ferris HA, Cai W, Kahn CR. Insulin action in brain regulates systemic metabolism and brain function. Diabetes. 2014;63(7):2232–2243. DOI: 10.2337/db14-0568

[8] Zhang J, Liu Q. Cholesterol metabolism and homeostasis in the brain. Protein Cell. 2015;6(4):254–264. DOI: 10.1007/s13238-014-0131-3

[9] Hayashi H, Campenot RB, Vance DE, Vance JE. Apolipoprotein E-containing lipoproteins protect neurons from apoptosis via a signaling pathway involving low-density lipoprotein receptor-related protein-1. J Neurosci. 2007;27(8):1933–1941. DOI:10.1523/JNEUROSCI.5471-06.2007

[10] Ott C, Jacobs K, Haucke E, Navarrete Santos A, Grune T, Simm A. Role of advanced glycation end products in cellular signaling. Redox Biol. 2014;2:411–429. DOI: 10.1016/j.redox.2013.12.016

[11] Zhao Y, Zhao B. Oxidative stress and the pathogenesis of Alzheimer's disease. Oxid Med Cell Longev. 2013;2013:316–523. DOI: 10.1155/2013/316523

[12] Fogarasi E, Croitoru MD, Fülöp I, Muntean DL. Is the oxidative stress really a disease? Acta Medica Marisiensis. 2016;62(1):112–120 DOI: 10.1515/amma-2015-0070

[13] Lobo V, Patil A, Phatak A, Chandra N. Free radicals, antioxidants and functional foods: impact on human health. Pharmacogn Rev. 2010;4(8):118–126. DOI: 10.4103/0973-7847.70902

[14] Valko M, Leibfritz D, Moncola J, Cronin M, Mazura M, Telser J. Free radicals and antioxidants in normal physiological functions and human disease. Int J Biochem Cell Biol. 2007;39(1):44–84. DOI:10.1016/j.biocel.2006.07.001

[15] Elias RJ, Kellerby SS, Decker EA. Antioxidant activity of proteins and peptides. Crit Rev Food Sci Nutr. 2008;48(5):430–441. DOI: 10.1080/10408390701425615

[16] Fang YZ, Yang S, Wu G. Free radicals, antioxidants, and nutrition. Nutrition. 2002 Oct; 18(10):872–879. DOI:10.1016/S0899-9007(02)00916-4

[17] Kehrer JP, Klotz LO. Free radicals and related reactive species as mediators of tissue injury and disease: implications for health. Crit Rev Toxicol. 2015;45(9):765–798. DOI: 10.3109/10408444.2015.1074159

[18] Smith AJ, Oertle J, Warren D, Prato D. Ozone therapy: a critical physiological and diverse clinical evaluation with regard to immune modulation, anti-infectious properties, anti-cancer potential, and impact on anti-oxidant enzymes. OJMIP. 2015;5:37–48. DOI: 10.4236/ojmip.2015.53004

[19] Taupin P. A dual activity of ROS and oxidative stress on adult neurogenesis and Alzheimer's disease. Cent Nerv Syst Agents Med Chem. 2010;10(1):16–21 1871-5249/10

[20] Klein JA, Ackerman SL. Oxidative stress, cell cycle, and neurodegeneration. J Clin Invest. 2003;111:785–793 DOI:10.1172/JCI200318182.

[21] Espinosa-Diez C, Miguel V, Mennerich D, Kietzmann T, Sánchez-Pérez P, Cadenas S, Lamas S. Antioxidant responses and cellular adjustments to oxidative stress. Redox Biol. 2015;6:183–197. DOI: 10.1016/j.redox.2015.07.008

[22] Barzilai A, Yamamoto KI. DNA damage responses to oxidative stress. DNA Repair. 2004;3(8–9):1109–1115. DOi:10.1016/j.dnarep.2004.03.002

[23] Wilson C, González-Billault C. Regulation of cytoskeletal dynamics by redox signaling and oxidative stress: implications for neuronal development and trafficking. Front Cell Neurosci. 2015;30(9):381. DOI: 10.3389/fncel.2015.00381

[24] Rao RV, Bredesen DE. Misfolded proteins, endoplasmic reticulum stress and neurodegeneration. Curr Opin Cell Biol. 2004;16(6):653–662. DOI:10.1016/j.ceb.2004.09.012

[25] Bhandary B, Marahatta A, Kim HR, Chae HJ. An involvement of oxidative stress in endoplasmic reticulum stress and its associated diseases, Int J Mol Sci. 2013;14:434–456. DOI:10.3390/ijms14010434

[26] Mančšek-Keber M, Frank-Bertoncelj M, Hafner-Bratkovič I, Smole A, Zorko M, Pirher N, Hayer S, Kralj-Iglič V, Rozman B, Ilc N, Horvat S, Jerala R. Toll-like receptor 4 senses oxidative stress mediated by the oxidation of phospholipids in extracellular vesicles. Sci Signal.2015;8(381):ra60. DOI: 10.1126/scisignal.2005860

[27] Guan ZZ. Cross-talk between oxidative stress and modifications of cholinergic and glutaminergic receptors in the pathogenesis of Alzheimer's disease. Acta Pharmacol Sin 2008;29 (7):773–780. DOI: 10.1111/j.1745-7254.2008.00819.x

[28] Salminen A, Ojala J, Kaarniranta K, Kauppinen A. Mitochondrial dysfunction and oxidative stress activate inflammasomes: impact on the aging process and

age-related diseases. Cell Mol Life Sci. 2012;69:2999–3013. DOI 10.1007/s00018-012-0962-0

[29] Tyurina YY, Shvedova AA, Kawai K, Tyurin VA, Kommineni C, Quinn PJ, Schor NF, Fabisiak JP, Kagan VE, Phospholipid signaling in apoptosis: peroxidation and externalization of phosphatidylserine. Toxicology. 2000;148:93–101. DOI:10.1016/S0300-483X(00)00199-2

[30] Soga M, Matsuzawa A, Ichijo H. Oxidative stress-induced diseases via the ASK1 signaling pathway. Int J Cell Biol. 2012;2012:439587. DOI: 10.1155/2012/439587

[31] Kim EK, Choi EJ. Pathological roles of MAPK signaling pathways in human diseases. Biochim Biophys Acta. 2010;1802(4):396–405. DOI: 10.1016/j.bbadis.2009.12.009

[32] di Penta A, Moreno B, Reix S, Fernandez-Diez B, Villanueva M, Errea O, Escala N, Vandenbroeck K, Comella JX, Villoslada P Oxidative stress and proinflammatory cytokines contribute to demyelination and axonal damage in a cerebellar culture model of neuroinflammation. PLoS One. 2013;8(2):e54722. DOI:10.1371/journal.pone.0054722. Epub 2013 Feb 19

[33] Wojsiat J, Prandelli C, Laskowska-Kaszub K, Martín-Requero A, Wojda U. Oxidative stress and aberrant cell cycle in Alzheimer's disease lymphocytes: diagnostic prospects. J Alzheimers Dis. 2015;46(2):329–350. DOI: 10.3233/JAD-141977

[34] Gimeno A, García-Giménez JL, Audí L, Toran N, Andaluz P, Dasí F, Viña J, Pallardó FV. Decreased cell proliferation and higher oxidative stress in fibroblasts from Down syndrome fetuses. Preliminary study. Biochim Biophys Acta. 2014;1842(1):116–125. DOI:10.1016/j.bbadis.2013.10.014

[35] Gómez-Crisóstomo NP, Rodríguez-Martínez E, Rivas-Arancibia S. Oxidative stress activates the transcription factors FoxO 1a and FoxO 3a in the hippocampus of rats exposed to low doses of ozone. Oxid Med Cell Longev. 2014;2014:805764. DOI: 10.1155/2014/805764

[36] Sandberg M1, Patil J1, D'Angelo B2, Weber SG3, Mallard C4. NRF2-regulation in brain health and disease: implication of cerebral inflammation Neuropharmacology. 2014;79:298–306. DOI:10.1016/j.neuropharm.2013.11.004..

[37] Lee JM, Li J, Johnson DA, Stein TD, Kraft AD, Calkins MJ, Jakel RJ, Johnson JA., Nrf2, a multi-organ protector? FASEB J. 2005;19(9):1061–1066. DOI: 10.1096/fj.04-2591hyp

[38] Calkins MJ, Johnson DA, Townsend JA, Vargas MR, Dowell JA, Williamson TP, Kraft AD, Lee JM, Li J, Johnson JA. The Nrf2/ARE pathway as a potential therapeutic target in neurodegenerative disease. Antioxid Redox Signal. 2009;11(3):497–508. DOI: 10.1089/ARS.2008.2242

[39] Ramsey CP, Glass CA, Montgomer MB, Lindl KA, Ritson GP, Chia LA, Hamilton RL, Chu CT, Jordan-Sciutto KL. Expression of Nrf2 in neurodegenerative diseases. J. Neuropathol Exp Neurol. 2007;66,75–85. DOI: 10.1097/nen.0b013e31802d6da9

[40] Komatsu M1, Kurokawa H, Waguri S, Taguchi K, Kobayashi A, Ichimura Y, Sou YS, Ueno I, Sakamoto A, Tong KI, Kim M, Nishito Y, Iemura S, Natsume T, Ueno T, Kominami E, Motohashi H, Tanaka K, Yamamoto M. The selective autophagy substrate p62 activates the stress responsive transcription factor Nrf2 through inactivation of Keap1. Nat Cell Biol. 2010;12(3):213–223. DOI: 10.1038/ncb2021

[41] Gardiner J, Overall R, Marc J. The nervous system cytoeskeleton under oxidative stress. Diseases. 2013;1:36–50. DOI:10.3390/diseases1010036

[42] Lee CF, Liu CY, Hsieh RH, Wei YH. Oxidative stress-induced depolymerization of microtubules and alteration of mitochondrial mass in human cells. Ann N Y Acad Sci. 2005;1042:246–254. DOI: 10.1196/annals.1338.027

[43] Parker AL, Kavallaris M, McCarroll JA. Front Microtubules and their role in cellular stress in cancer. Oncol. 2014;18:(4)153. DOI: 10.3389/fonc.2014.00153

[44] Farah ME, Sirotkin V, Haarer B, Kakhniashvili D, Amberg DC. Diverse protective roles of the actin cytoskeleton during oxidative stress. Cytoskeleton (Hoboken). 2011;68(6): 340–354. DOI: 10.1002/cm.20516

[45] Naini SM, Soussi-Yanicostas N. Tau hyperphosphorylation and oxidative stress, a critical vicious circle in neurodegenerative tauopathies? Oxid Med Cell Longev. 2015;2015:151979. DOI: 10.1155/2015/151979

[46] Rao RV, Ellerby HM, Bredesen DE. Coupling endoplasmic reticulum stress to the cell death program. Cell Death and Differentiation. 2004;11:372–380. DOI:10.1038/sj.cdd. 4401378

[47] Aiken CT, Kaake RM, Wang X Huang L. Oxidative stress-mediated regulation of proteasome complexes. Mol Cell Proteomics. 2011;10(5): R110.006924. DOI: 10.1074/ mcp.M110.006924

[48] Ben-Nissan G, Sharon M. Regulating the 20S proteasome ubiquitin-independent degradation pathway. Biomolecules. 2014;4(3):862–884 DOI: 10.3390/biom4030862

[49] Bader N1, Grune T. Protein oxidation and proteolysis. Biol Chem. 2006;387(10-11):1351–1355. DOI: 10.1515/BC.2006.169

[50] McLaughlin M, Vandenbroeck K. The endoplasmic reticulum protein folding factory and its chaperones: new targets for drug discovery? Br J Pharmacol. 2011;162(2):328–345. DOI: 10.1111/j.1476-5381.2010.01064.x

[51] Cremers CM, Jakob U. Oxidant sensing by reversible disulfide bond formation. J Biol Chem. 2013;288(37):26489–26496. DOI: 10.1074/jbc.R113.462929

[52] Calì T1, Ottolini D, Brini M. Mitochondrial Ca(2+) and neurodegeneration. Cell Calcium. 2012;52(1):73–85. DOI: 10.1016/j.ceca.2012.04.015

[53] Viana RJ, Nunes AF, Rodrigues CM. Endoplasmic reticulum enrollment in Alzheimer's disease. Mol Neurobiol. 2012;46(2):522–534. DOI: 10.1007/s12035-012-8301-x

[54] Ferreiro E, Baldeiras I, Ferreira IL, Costa RO, Rego AC, Pereira CF,Oliveira CR. Mitochondrial and endoplasmic reticulum associated oxidative stress in Alzheimer's disease: from pathogenesis to biomarkers. Int J Cell Biol. 2012;2012:735206. DOI: 10.1155/2012/735206

[55] Cadenas E, Davies K. Mitochondrial free radical generation, oxidative stress, and aging. Free Radic Biol Med. 2000;29(3-4):222–230. DOI:10.1016/S0891-5849(00)00317-8

[56] Lee J, Giordano S, Zhang J. Autophagy, mitochondria and oxidative stress: cross-talk and redox signaling. Biochem J. 2012;441:523–540 DOI:10.1042/BJ20111451

[57] Dumont M, Wille E., Stack C, Calingasan NY, Beal MF, Lin MT. Reduction of oxidative stress, amyloid deposition, and memory deficit by manganese superoxide dismutase overexpression in a transgenic mouse model of Alzheimer's disease. FASEB J. 2009;23:2459–2466. DOI: 10.1096/fj.09-132928

[58] Agostinho P, Cunha RA, Oliveira C. Neuroinflammation, oxidative stress and the pathogenesis of Alzheimer's disease. Curr Pharm Des. 2010;16(25):2766–2778. DOI: 10.2174/138161210793176572

[59] Cameron B, Landreth GE. Inflammation, microglia and Alzheimer's disease. Neurobiol Dis. 2010;37(3):503–509. DOI:10.1016/j.nbd.2009.10.006

[60] Knobloch M, Mansuy IM. Dendritic spine loss and synaptic alterations in Alzheimer's disease. Mol Neurobiol. 2008;37(1):73–82. DOI: 10.1007/s12035-008-8018-z

[61] Zhou FC1, Anthony B, Dunn KW, Lindquist WB, Xu ZC, Deng P. Chronic alcohol drinking alters neuronal dendritic spines in the brain reward center nucleus accumbens. Brain Res. 2007:1134(1):148–161. DOI:10.1016/j.brainres.2006.11.046

[62] Green KN, LaFerla FM. Linking calcium to Abeta and Alzheimer's disease. Neuron. 2008;59(2):190–194. DOI: 10.1016/j.neuron.2008.07.013

[63] Avila-Costa MR, Colín-Barenque L, Fortoul TI, Machado-Salas P, Espinosa-Villanueva J, Rugerio-Vargas C, Rivas-Arancibia S. Memory deterioration in an oxidative stress model and its correlation with cytological changes on rat hippocampus CA1. Neurosci Lett. 1999;30:270(2):107–179.

[64] Lopategui Cabezas I, Herrera Batista A, Pentón Rol G. The role of glial cells in Alzheimer disease: potential therapeutic implications. Neurologia. 2014;29(5):305–309. DOI: 10.1016/j.nrl.2012.10.006. Epub 2012 Dec 14.

[65] Francis PT. The interplay of neurotransmitters in Alzheimer's disease. CNS Spectr. 2005;10(11 Suppl 18):6–9. DOI: 10.1017/S1092852900014164

[66] Schulz JB1, Lindenau J, Seyfried J, Dichgans J Glutathione, oxidative stress and neurodegeneration. Eur J Biochem. 2000;267(16):4904–4911. DOI: 10.1046/j.1432-1327.2000.01595.x

[67] Sofroniew MV. Multiple roles for astrocytes as effectors of cytokines and inflammatory mediators. Neuroscientist. 2014;20(2):160–172. DOI: 10.1177/1073858413504466

[68] Zhou M, Xie, L,Fang CJ, Yang H, Wang YJ, Zhen XY, Yan CH, Wang Y, Zhao M, Peng S. Implications for blood-brain-barrier permeability, in vitro oxidative stress and neurotoxicity potential induced by mesoporous silica nanoparticles: effects of surface modification. RSC Adv. 2016;6:2800. DOI: 10.1039/c5ra17517h

[69] Abbott NJ, Patabendige AK, Dolman DE, Yusof SR, Begley DJ. Structure and function of the blood–brain barrier. Neurobiol Dis. 2010;37(1):13–25. DOI:10.1016/j.nbd.2009.07.030

[70] Zlokovic BV. The blood-brain barrier in health and chronic neurodegenerative disorders. Neuron. 2008;57(2):178–201. DOI:10.1016/j.neuron.2008.01.003

[71] Rivas-Arancibia S, Hernández-Zimbrón LF, Rodríguez-Martínez E, Borgonio-Pérez G, Velumani V, Durán-Bedolla J. Chronic exposure to low doses of ozone produces a state of oxidative stress and blood-brain barrier damage in the hippocampus of rat. ABB. 2013;4:24–29. DOI: 10.4236/abb.2013.411A2004

[72] Zlokovic BV. Blood brain barrier damage neuronal dysfunction, and degeneration. Journal of Alzheimer's Association. 2014;10(4):P285. DOI: http://dx.doi.org/10.1016/j.jalz.2014.04.472

[73] Qosa H, LeVine H, Keller JN, Kaddoumi A. Mixed oligomers and monomeric amyloid-β disrupts endothelial cells integrity and reduces monomeric amyloid-β transport across hCMEC/D3 cell line as an in vitro blood–brain barrier model. Biochim Biophys Acta. 2014;1842(9):1806–1815. DOI: 10.1016/j.bbadis.2014.06.029

[74] Bandyopadhyay S, Goldstein LE, Lahiri DK, Rogers JT. Role of the APP non-amyloidogenic signaling pathway and targeting α-secretase as an alternative drug target for treatment of Alzheimer's disease. Curr Med Chem. 2007;14(27):2848–2864. DOI: http://dx.doi.org/10.2174/092986707782360060

[75] Vassar R, Kovacs DM, Yan R, Wong PC. The β-secretase enzyme BACE in health and Alzheimer's disease: regulation, cell biology, function, and therapeutic potential. J Neurosci. 2009;29(41):12787–12794. DOI: 10.1523/JNEUROSCI.3657-09.2009

[76] Li H, Wolfe MS, Selkoe DJ. Toward structural elucidation of the γ-secretase complex. Structure. 2009;17(3):326–334. DOI:10.1016/j.str.2009.01.007

[77] Schmidt M, Sachsea C, Richterd W, Xua C, Fandrichb M, Grigorieffa N. Comparison of Alzheimer Aβ(1–40) and Aβ(1–42) amyloid fibrils reveals similar protofilament structures. Proc Natl Acad Sci U S A. 2009;106(47):19813–19818. DOI: 10.1073/pnas.0905007106

[78] Sadigh-Eteghad S, Sabermarouf B, Majdi A, Talebi M, Farhoudi M, Mahmoudi J. Amyloid-beta: a crucial factor in Alzheimer's disease. Med Princ Pract. 2015;24(1):1–10. DOI: 10.1159/000369101

[79] LaFerla FM, Green KN, Oddo S Intracellular amyloid-beta in Alzheimer's disease. Nat Rev Neurosci. 2007;8(7):499–509. DOI:10.1038/nrn2168

[80] Sam Gandy The role of cerebral amyloid β accumulation in common forms of Alzheimer disease. J Clin Invest. 2005;115(5):1121–1129. DOI:10.1172/JCI200525100

[81] Hernández-Zimbrón LF, Rivas-Arancibia S. Oxidative stress caused by ozone exposure induces β-amyloid 1-42 overproduction and mitochondrial accumulation by activating the amyloidogenic pathway. Neuroscience. 2015;304:340–348. DOI: 10.1016/j.neuroscience.2015.07.011

[82] Zhang YW, Thompson R, Zhang H, Huaxi X. APP processing in Alzheimer's disease. Mol Brain. 2011;4:3. DOI: 10.1186/1756-6606-4-3

[83] Spuch C, Ortolano S, Navarro C. New insights in the amyloid-beta interaction with mitochondria. J Aging Res. 2012;2012:324968. DOI: 10.1155/2012/324968

[84] Vattemi G, Engel WK, McFerrin J, Askanas V. Endoplasmic reticulum stress and unfolded protein response in inclusion body myositis muscle. Am J Pathol. 2004;164(1): 1–7. DOI:10.1016/S0002-9440(10)63089-1

[85] Gruschus JM. Do amyloid oligomers act as traps for misfolded proteins? A hypothesis. Amyloid. 2008;15(3):160–165. DOI: 10.1080/13506120802193746

[86] Sondag CM, Dhawan G, Combs CK. Beta amyloid oligomers and fibrils stimulate differential activation of primary microglia. J Neuroinflammation. 2009;6:1. DOI: 10.1186/1742-2094-6-1

[87] Ramanathan A, Nelson AR, Sagare AP, Zlokovic BV. Impaired vascular-mediated clearance of brain amyloid beta in Alzheimer's disease: the role, regulation and restoration of LRP1. Front Aging Neurosci. 2015;7:136. DOI: 10.3389/fnagi.2015.00136

[88] Qi H, Prabakaran S, Cantrelle FC, Chambraud BE, Gunawardena J, Lippens G, Landrieu I. Characterization of neuronal tau protein as a target of extracellular-signal-regulated kinase. J Biol Chem. 2016;1;291(14):7742-53. DOI: 10.1074/jbc.M115.700914

[89] Mucke L, Selkoe DJ. Neurotoxicity of amyloid β-protein: synaptic and network dysfunction. Cold Spring Harb Perspect Med. 2012;2(7):a006338. DOI: 10.1101/cshperspect.a006338.

[90] Haass C, Selkoe DJ. Soluble protein oligomers in neurodegeneration: lessons from the Alzheimer's amyloid beta-peptide. Nat Rev Mol Cell Biol. 2007;8(2):101–112. DOI: 10.1038/nrm2101

Chapter 6

Biomarkers in ROS and Role of Isoprostanes in Oxidative Stress

Mini Chandra, Manikandan Panchatcharam and
Sumitra Miriyala

Additional information is available at the end of the chapter

http://dx.doi.org/10.5772/64706

Abstract

Biomarkers of reactive oxygen species serve as indicators of oxidative stress in the pathology of cardiovascular diseases. This chapter presents an overview of the various biomarkers available to quantify oxidative stress to advance the understanding of the pathophysiology of cardiovascular diseases as well as to serve as an adjunct in their diagnosis and prognosis. The plasma levels of reactive oxygen species themselves are unstable and unreliable markers of oxidative stress. The commonly used stable biomarkers are derivatives of oxygen radicals such as products of lipid peroxidation and protein oxidation, with isoprostanes and malondialdehyde (MDA) being the most widely used biomarkers due to higher specificity and ease of measurement. Recently, micro-RNA is emerging as stable and specific biomarkers for detection of heart failure. Other biomarkers have a role in certain conditions; for example, advanced oxidation protein products indicate acute inflammation, whereas advanced glycation end products serve as indicators of chronic disease.

Keywords: biomarkers, reactive oxygen species, isoprostanes, lipid peroxidation, cardiovascular diseases

1. Introduction

Reactive oxygen species (ROS) are formed as by-products of cellular activity or cellular metabolism or cellular respiration. They have useful function-serving roles in cell signaling, cell differentiation, cell immunity, etc., when present in low concentrations, all of which are important in maintaining the body's physiological functions known as redox signaling [1].

Their concentration is controlled by the various antioxidants produced in the body such as superoxide dismutases, catalase, and glutathione peroxidase, with the goal to keep ROS concentration low [2]. Oxidative stress is a condition resulting from excessive reactive oxygen species due to either increased production or inadequacy of antioxidants to eliminate them. This increase in ROS results in damage to the cell which includes oxidizing lipids, nucleic acids, and proteins, thus leading to a change or loss in their function and ultimately causes cell death by apoptosis or necrosis. Due to this effect on the cells, oxidative stress has been implicated in aging [3] as well as many diseases including but not limited to cardiovascular disease [4], neurodegenerative diseases [5, 6], cancer [7], and diabetes [8].

Biomarkers are measurable characteristics of a biological condition; in this case, biomarkers of ROS serve as indicators of oxidative stress and how it influences a given disease. Hallmarks of a good biomarker are sensitivity, specificity, ease of obtaining and measuring samples, and cost-effectiveness. The quantification of oxidative stress with biomarkers is important not only in understanding the pathophysiology of cardiovascular disease but also in the diagnosis, prognosis as well as in designing new therapeutic measures for individual intervention. Oxidative stress plays a major role in the pathology of cardiovascular disease. In the heart, oxidative stress results in the inhibition of Na+-K- pump [9]. The mitochondrial electron transport chain and enzymes xanthine oxidase and nicotinamide-adenine dinucleotide phosphate (NADPH) oxidase are the main producers of ROS. Risk factors and conditions which predispose to a cardiovascular event such as smoking, hypertension, atherosclerosis, hypercholesterolemia, diabetes, and obesity increase the effect of these enzymes which results in an increased production of ROS [10, 11].

2. ROS as biomarkers

ROS themselves act as biomarkers, their plasma levels being indicators of ROS production. A method known as the reactive oxygen metabolites (ROM) kit is used to measure total oxidative stress and measures superoxides (02-) and hydroxyl radical (HO) as well as hypochlorous acid (HOCl) and hydrogen peroxide (H_2O_2) [12] among others. This kit measures reactive oxidants in biological fluids and has been used to assess oxidative stress in animals such as in a study on ewes done by Rizzo et al. [13]. Cytochrome C reduction has been used in many studies to measure the production of superoxide (O_2^-) in the atrium [14], mouse aorta [15], and vessels [16]. Chemiluminescent probes which release photon when in contact with ROS can be detected and used for various ROS measurements with the lucigenin-enhanced chemiluminescence being the most commonly used to understand the way superoxide and diseases related to the cardiovascular system are affected in tissues [10]. Electron spin resonance detects free radical by the presence of its unpaired electron. Reactive radicals are detected by addition of probes [10]. As of 2003, the spin traps were not fit to be used in humans due to the potential for toxicity, but they can be used on tissues and body fluids; for example, PBN was used to show free radicals in coronary sinus blood during bypass surgery [17]. Aromatic traps for free radicals such as salicylate have been used in studies to detect superoxide in myocardial infarction [18]. High levels of dityrosine, an oxidation product of ROS, have been used to demonstrate the role of oxidative damage in atherosclerotic plaques [19]. Even though each reactive oxidant can be measured individually, they have drawbacks of being too costly and time-consuming. Their property of being inherently unstable with short half-lives of merely seconds, both of which combined with the antioxidants in the circulation, results in very low intracellular concentration of ROS thus making them unreliable markers of ROS.

The derivatives of oxygen radicals such as products of lipid peroxidation and protein oxidation on the other hand are stable and thus are more commonly used to measure the presence of ROS. The serum derivatives are new biomarkers of ROS which are mainly indicators of hydroperoxide levels produced by lipid peroxidation and have been shown to be high in atrial fibrillation [20]. The diacron reactive oxygen metabolites (dROM) test is an inexpensive analysis which measures ROS in both serum and plasma.

3. Peroxidation of lipids biomarkers

Lipids, especially polyunsaturated lipids, are more susceptible to oxidative damage due to the presence of many double bonds in their molecular structure [21], and thus, the indicators of lipid peroxidation are important indicators of free radicals. The presence of biomarkers in cardiovascular disease confirms the hypothesis that lipid peroxidation contributes to the development of cardiovascular diseases. There are many biomarkers of lipid peroxidation—MDA and isoprostanes being the most widely used. Others are lipid hydroperoxides, oxysterols, and oxidation resistance assays.

4. Isoprostanes

More accurate biomarkers of lipid peroxidation are isoprostanes along with its metabolites as stated in a study done by the National Institute of Health (NIH) [22]. In 1990, Roberts and Morrow discovered F2-isoprostane formed by the peroxidation of arachidonic acid [23] which is polyunsaturated fatty acid found in the cell membrane phospholipids and is one of the many targets of ROS. They are specific indicators of lipid peroxidation both *in vitro* and *in vivo* [24] and are stable compounds which are formed in large quantities *in vivo* following oxidative damage such as with CCl4 which is a producer of free radicals [25] as well as having detectable amounts present even in non-injured tissue making them reliable as a biomarker of ROS [26]. Isoprostanes are excellent biomarkers and have numerous advantages over other biomarkers of oxidative stress; they are chemically stable markers and are formed *in vivo*. They are specific to lipid peroxidation and are not affected by the dietary lipid content [27]. Since they are detectable in biological fluids, they have the significant advantage over other oxidative stress markers due to the ease of measuring them since they can be measured by noninvasive methods extracellularly in the urine, plasma, and tissue [27, 28]. High levels of F2-isoprostanes are found in many human diseases such as coronary heart disease [29], obesity, cancer, and even genetic disorders [30]. They are shown to be increased in risk factors such as smoking, obesity, hypercholesterolemia, and myocardial ischemia reperfusion [31–33] as well as in atherosclerosis [34]. They are also observed in bypass [35] and angioplasty. The extent of lipid peroxidation can be measured by calculating the level of F2-IsoPs which is esterified in phospholipids due to them being initially formed esterified and subsequently gain their free form [27]. In humans, the two major metabolites of isoprostane which are detectable in the urine are 2,3-dinor-15-F2t-IsoP and 2,3 dinor-5,6-dihydro-15-F2t-IsoP [36]. Elevated levels of 8-isoprostane in the plasma and urine are also observed in cardiovascular disease [37]. There are many other derivatives identified [38]. The method for detecting isoprostanes is gas chromatography-mass spectrometry (GC-MS) and liquid chromatography-mass spectrometry (LC-MS), but drawbacks in using mass spectrometry is the expense and time required for measurement [22]. ELISA-based isoprostane detection is currently most reliable indicator of lipid oxidation [39]. There are commercially available kits to measure them using the sandwich ELISA method where the isoprostanes in biological samples compete with isoprostane conjugated with an enzyme to bind to an isoprostane-specific antibody present in the micro-plate. The activity of the enzyme results in increased intensity of color development with increased amount of conjugated isoprostane bound. Isoprostanes are biomarkers of choice, but since the results obtained by these two methods do not corroborate, the result of the immune assays is yet to be given clinical validation [40]. There have been studies showing the variation in isoprostane levels according to the time of day, and thus, this needs to be taken into account when further research is conducted [41, 42].

5. MDA

Malondialdehyde (MDA) is a ketoaldehyde which is produced as an end product of polyunsaturated fatty acid and is found in increased concentration in tissue injury. It forms a red pigmentation when it reacts with thiobarbituric acid. This thiobarbituric acid-reactive substance (TBARS) assay can be used to measure lipid peroxidation using spectrophotometry. In relation to cardiovascular disease, elevated levels of MDA are associated with smoking [43]. They are seen to be elevated with the progression of atherosclerosis [44] and are predictors of future cardiovascular events in patients with coronary artery disease [45]. Limitations of this method include low specificity since TBARS includes many other products of lipid peroxidation other than MDA [46], tendency for inaccurate results due to the varying results generated with different assay conditions used as well as the production of artifacts due to the fact that the MDA measured is mostly generated *in vitro* [47] with most of the MDA formed due to the high temperature used in the procedure [48]. Now, high-pressure liquid chromatography (HPLC) is preferred over TBARS due to higher specificity [49]. Commercially available ELISA kits are also available for MDA detection which show better specificity [50].

6. Isolevuglandins

Isolevuglandins (IsoLGs) are also produced due to oxidation of arachidonic acid, but unlike isoprostanes, they are highly reactive and react with primary amines for example phosphatidylethanolamine to form lactam and hydroxylactam. The unreacted isolevuglandins are not detected in the tissues or cells. They have been implicated in many disease processes such as atherosclerosis and neurodegenerative diseases [51]. Though methods such as mass spectrometry and immunohistochemical studies have shown increased levels of IsoLG, there is still not enough evidence connecting them with severity of a disease or of their use in predicting the onset of disease. Further studies need to be conducted to determine the utility of IsoLG as clinical biomarkers.

7. Oxidation of proteins biomarkers

7.1. Myeloperoxidase (MPO)

MPO is an enzyme found in inflammatory cells such as macrophages and neutrophils. It generates ROS by the conversion of hydrogen peroxide to hydroxy radical (OH), nitric oxide (ONOO-NO2), and hypochlorous acid (HOCl) and is a proinflammatory agent responsible for the oxidation of low-density lipoprotein (LDL) [52]. It is found in abundance in the atherosclerosis plaques [53] and coronary artery disease where it can serve as an inflammatory marker for both the risk of CAD and its existence [54]. MPO concentration is measured in biological samples by ELISA which is commercially available. Its function is measured by spectrophotometry by peroxidase activity assays such as measuring the formation of guaiacol oxidation products [55]. Its levels in the serum can predict risk for acute coronary syndromes [56], for risk of cardiovascular event in patients with chest pain [57] and increased risk of coronary artery disease in seemingly healthy population [58]. It is prone to varying and unreliable results due to the fact that the values are altered during the process of collection and handling as seen in a study done in 2008 by Shih et al. where it was determined that the concentration of MPO varied depending on the collection tube used and the presence of heparin in the patient serum [59]. A concern in the measurement of MPO is the artificial release of MPO from the neutrophils leading to false results showing an increase in MPO. In their study, Shih et al. used nine different types of tubes containing EDTA, citrate plasma, and heparin samples and serum samples. The level of MPO varied in all these tubes, with EDTA and citrate samples showing the lowest concentration and heparin and serum samples showing 10 and 100% higher values, respectively. This suggests that the serum levels of MPO are higher due to their release from leukocytes during coagulation. It has previously been shown by Li et al. that heparin leads to release of MPO from neutrophils during neutrophil activation [60].

8. Growth differentiation factor-15

It is a cytokine expressed in many cells including cardiomyocytes [61]. It increases in many cardiovascular diseases such as atherosclerosis [62] and heart failure [63]. It has been studied with respect to the progress and outcome of disease since it has a protective role in the heart

[64] such as against ischemia reperfusion injury [61] and acute myocardial infarction [65] making it a useful biomarker in clinical settings though more research still needs to be conducted.

9. Oxidized low-density lipoprotein (OxLDL)

The use of OxLDL as a biomarker of oxidative stress in cardiovascular diseases has been reported due to its ability to promote lipid deposition. The oxidation of LDL is linked to the pathology of atherosclerosis by immunohistochemical staining apolipoprotein B-100 [66]. It is thought to be formed by activated platelets [67]. High-density lipoproteins (HDL) lead to decreased activation of platelets since it competes with them to bind to oxidized LDL protecting against the development of atherosclerosis [68]. Circulating OxLDL is already proven to be able to predict the presence of atherosclerosis [69] and coronary artery disease [70]. OxLDL is detected by immune assays in plasma. According to Trpkovic et al., there are currently three ELISA assays namely 4E6, E06, and DLH3 developed to detect OxLDL in the blood [71]. Out of these, 4E6 binds to LDL but also detects native LDL and the other two, DLH3 which measures LDL and E06 are used for oxidized phosphatidylcholine [72]. A drawback of E06 method is its non-specificity to oxidized lipids. In 2001, Holvoet et al. measured circulating LDL levels by ELISA using monoclonal antibody 4E6 which detected higher number of circulating OxLDL in patients with coronary artery disease [73].

10. Allantoin

Over the years, allantoin has emerged as a reliable biomarker of oxidative damage both *in vivo* and *in vitro.* It is formed by the ROS-induced oxidation of uric acid [74], where uric acid is converted to allantoin due to overproduction of ROS [75]. In relation to cardiovascular diseases, increased levels of allantoin in the plasma have been shown in people with type 2 diabetes [75] as well as in heavy smokers [76] both of which are risk factors for developing cardiovascular disease. It has been shown to be increased in the plasma in oxidative stress-related chronic heart failure [77]. The use of allantoin as a widely applied biomarker is limited due to the difficulty of measuring allantoin in the body fluids [78]. The most specific and sensitive method for its measurement is liquid chromatography [79].

11. Protein carbonyls

Oxidation of protein amino acid residues leads to the formation of protein carbonyls by different means such as deamination of glutamic acid and lysine or due to the resulting breakage of protein backbone [80]. They are stable compounds formed early and are usually higher in concentration due to their multiple sources, making them good biomarkers due to the ease of detection as well as no need of expensive equipment. It is a commonly used protein oxidation marker, and there are various assays for its detection. They have been shown to increase with age implicating them in the process of aging [81]. They have even been reported in the human heart following coronary surgery [82]. Assay has been done to observe them in dilated cardiomyopathy [83]. In 1990, Levine et al. were the first ones to determine various methods to measure carbonyls in oxidized protein [84].

A highly sensitive assay is protein carbonyl content (PCC) which has various modifications but in all of them 2,4-dinitrophenylhydrazine (DNPH) reacts with the protein carbonyls and forms its 2,4-dinitrophenyl (DNP) hydrazone which is stable and can then be optically measured by immunohistochemistry or by radioactive counting [85]. Spectrophotometric assay can be employed due the ability of this hydrazone product to absorb ultraviolet light which when coupled with high-performance liquid chromatography, in short HPLC, makes the measurement more specific and sensitive [86]. One sensitive method is to detect carbonyls by first labeling them with tritiated sodium borohydride then separating with SDS-PAGE [87] or by reducing with tritiated sodium borohydride in solution [88]. An important limitation of carbonyl measurement is that there are different protocols used by researchers leading to variable levels of carbonyls in tissues.

12. Advanced oxidation protein products (AOPPS)

Advanced oxidation protein products (AOPPs) are the end products of free radical affected proteins. They have been shown to be linked to many human diseases such as diabetes mellitus [89], coronary artery disease [90], and chronic renal disease [91] among others, and since they have been shown to produce oxidative stress in inflammatory conditions [92], they serve to indicate acute inflammation.

13. Advanced glycation end products (AGES)

They are molecules which are formed as a result of the reaction between reducing sugars and amino groups. Their concentration tends to increase in conditions of oxidative stress. The two main advanced glycation end products are pentosidine and carboxymethyl valine which result from a process known as glycoxidation where the amino acids lysine and arginine react with carbohydrates as well as the oxidizing effect of ROS on polyunsaturated fatty acids. A precursor of carboxymethyl valine known as glyoxal is formed when RNase incubates with arachidonate [93]. The presence of AGES has been shown in diseases such as diabetes mellitus and obesity among others [94]. They also have a role in diabetic heart failure as shown by Brouwers et al., where they overexpressed glyoxalase-I, a glycation precursor detoxifying enzyme in order to reduce AGES, and found that it leads to prevention of diabetes-induced oxidative damage in the heart [95]. They are detected after derivatization with 2, 4-dinitrophenylhydrazine (DNP). The hydrazone formed is then detected using a spectrophotometer or by using anti-DNP antibodies with along with ELISA [96] or by high-performance liquid chromatography (HPLC) or by Western blot or immunohistocytochemistry

[97]. Out of these methods, HPLC is more specific and can measure carboxymethyl lysine CML [98] and pentosidine [99]. They mainly serve as indicators of chronic diseases [100].

14. Glutathione and glutathione disulfide

Reduced glutathione (GSH) is present in large quantities in the cells and acts as an inhibitor of lipid peroxidase. Glutathione disulfide (GSSG) is the oxidized form of glutathione. Protein glutathionylation regulates cardiovascular function [101]. Its values have been shown to increase in ischemia reperfusion injury [102], atherosclerosis [103], and cardiac hypertrophy [104]. In patients with atherosclerosis obliterans, increased glutathionylation is shown to be related to the progression of the disease proving to be a biomarker at early stage [105]. The ratio of GSH and GSSG is used as an indicator of ROS due to the fact that there occurs a decrease in GSH and increase in GSSG concentration in oxidative stress [106]. There are a number of methods to detect protein s-glutathionylation. Quantifying the total amount of s-glutathionylated proteins is by measuring fluorescence [107]. Labeling glutathione is a method for glutathionylation analysis such as 35s radiolabeling [108], though it is not very sensitive and can only be used in cell culture; furthermore, it cannot detect proteins which have already undergone glutathionylation. Biotinylated glutathione either reduced or oxidized is superior to the 35s labeling methods, it detects only glutathionylated proteins thus is specific plus it can be analyzed by multiple methods such as fluorescence microscopy [109] or immunoblotting using biotin antibodies [110]. One drawback of this method is that the presence of biotin tag on glutathione may have an effect on the protein function. Anti-glutathione antibodies allow the detection of glutathionylated proteins in physiological conditions. Studies done with antibodies are by using mouse monoclonal antibodies [111–113]. Drawback of antibody method is the lack of specificity, and it can only detect a few proteins in total extract [109] limiting its utility in detecting glutathionylated proteins on a large scale. Recently, the use of liquid chromatography-couple mass spectrometry using whole proteins is found to be a good method to identify proteins in larger numbers [114].

Recently, the role of micro-RNA (miRNA) in the generation of ROS and its consequences such as inflammation, angiogenesis, cell proliferation, and apoptosis has been a subject of research. They are found intracellularly and outside cells in body fluids [115]. They are stable and specific such as miR-499 miRNA for the heart. Another advantage of miRNA as a biomarker is that they are not affected by posttranslational modifications. They can also be easily assessed by methods like polymerase chain reaction (PCR) and microarrays. PCR is an expensive method which detects small quantities of miRNA, but the results are affected by the primer used. Microarray measurements require the development of probes and can thus be useful in that many RNAs can be detected at the same time [116]. Other less used methods are direct sequencing by next-generation sequencing [117], which eliminates the influence of primers as in the case of PCR but is still not used widely because of expense. Stem loop probe ligation [118] and Northern blotting are other methods which may be used to measure concentration of miRNA. The miRNA found most abundantly in the heart is mR-1 which is heart specific and can be used as a sensitive and specific marker for diagnosis of acute myocardial infarction [119, 120].

Elevated miRNAs specifically miR423-5p has also been observed in heart failure patients making them important clinical biomarkers in the diagnosis of heart failure [121]. Although miRNA measurement has shown promise, there are still various issues that need to be addressed. The concentration of miRNA in body fluids is low making its isolation rather difficult. The values obtained also tend to be different in different body fluids which need to be normalized. Therefore, it is necessary to develop a method to obtain accurate results with miRNA measurement across the various samples [116]. The product of DNA damage, 8 dydroxy-2'-deoxyguanosine urinary levels, seems to be elevated in dilated cardiomyopathy [122]. It is also evidently a predictor of future events following myocardial infarction [123]. Other specific biomarkers have also been studied but are not yet studied as extensively as the above biomarkers. Ascorbic acid is an endogenous antioxidant which has been linked to unstable coronary syndrome where it is thought to have an effect on the lesion [124]. Glutathione peroxidase-I is evidently decreased in coronary artery disease patients [125] which is an antioxidant enzyme. Low levels of bilirubin have been linked to cigarette smoking and increased levels of triglycerides and cholesterol making it a potential biomarker of cardiovascular disease [126]. Oxidative bilirubin metabolites called biopyrrins are elevated in the urine in patients with heart failure [127] and are thought to be predictors of future cardiac events in acute myocardial infarction [128].

Several biomarkers of oxidative stress have been studied over the years in an effort to understand the mechanism of cardiovascular generation with the intention to use the information by targeting oxidative stress with cardio-protective drugs. Further research into understanding the mechanism of ROS generation and their role in therapeutic intervention will be beneficial for the management of cardiovascular diseases.

Author details

Mini Chandra, Manikandan Panchatcharam and Sumitra Miriyala*

*Address all correspondence to: smiriy@lsuhsc.edu

Department of Cellular Biology and Anatomy, Louisiana Health Sciences-Shreveport, Shreveport, LA, USA

References

[1] Schieber, M. and N.S. Chandel, ROS function in redox signaling and oxidative stress. Curr Biol, 2014. 24(10): p. R453–62.

[2] Miller, J.K., E. Brzezinska-Slebodzinska, and F.C. Madsen, Oxidative stress, antioxidants, and animal function. J Dairy Sci, 1993. 76(9): p. 2812–23.

[3] Finkel, T. and N.J. Holbrook, Oxidants, oxidative stress and the biology of ageing. Nature, 2000. 408(6809): p. 239–47.

[4] Griendling, K.K. and G.A. FitzGerald, Oxidative stress and cardiovascular injury: Part I: basic mechanisms and in vivo monitoring of ROS. Circulation, 2003. 108(16): p. 1912–6.

[5] Halliwell, B., Role of free radicals in the neurodegenerative diseases: therapeutic implications for antioxidant treatment. Drugs Aging, 2001. 18(9): p. 685–716.

[6] Butterfield, D.A., Amyloid beta-peptide (1-42)-induced oxidative stress and neurotoxicity: implications for neurodegeneration in Alzheimer's disease brain. A review. Free Radic Res, 2002. 36(12): p. 1307–13.

[7] Klaunig, J.E. and L.M. Kamendulis, The role of oxidative stress in carcinogenesis. Annu Rev Pharmacol Toxicol, 2004. 44: p. 239–67.

[8] Maritim, A.C., R.A. Sanders, and J.B. Watkins, 3rd, Diabetes, oxidative stress, and antioxidants: a review. J Biochem Mol Toxicol, 2003. 17(1): p. 24–38.

[9] Figtree, G.A., et al., Oxidative regulation of the Na(+)–K(+) pump in the cardiovascular system. Free Radic Biol Med, 2012. 53(12): p. 2263–8.

[10] Dikalov, S., K.K. Griendling, and D.G. Harrison, Measurement of reactive oxygen species in cardiovascular studies. Hypertension, 2007. 49(4): p. 717–27.

[11] Touyz, R.M. and A.M. Briones, Reactive oxygen species and vascular biology: implications in human hypertension. Hypertens Res, 2011. 34(1): p. 5–14.

[12] Reilly, P.M., H.J. Schiller, and G.B. Bulkley, Pharmacologic approach to tissue injury mediated by free radicals and other reactive oxygen metabolites. Am J Surg, 1991. 161(4): p. 488–503.

[13] Rizzo, A., et al., First demonstration of an increased serum level of reactive oxygen species during the peripartal period in the ewes. Immunopharmacol Immunotoxicol, 2008. 30(4): p. 741–6.

[14] Dudley, S.C., Jr., et al., Atrial fibrillation increases production of superoxide by the left atrium and left atrial appendage: role of the NADPH and xanthine oxidases. Circulation, 2005. 112(9): p. 1266–73.

[15] Landmesser, U., et al., Oxidation of tetrahydrobiopterin leads to uncoupling of endothelial cell nitric oxide synthase in hypertension. J Clin Invest, 2003. 111(8): p. 1201–9.

http://dx.doi.org/10.5772/64706

[16] Guzik, T.J., et al., Mechanisms of increased vascular superoxide production in human diabetes mellitus: role of NAD(P)H oxidase and endothelial nitric oxide synthase. Circulation, 2002. 105(14): p. 1656–62.

[17] Clermont, G., et al., Systemic free radical activation is a major event involved in myocardial oxidative stress related to cardiopulmonary bypass. Anesthesiology, 2002. 96(1): p. 80–7.

[18] Tubaro, M., et al., Demonstration of the formation of hydroxyl radicals in acute myocardial infarction in man using salicylate as probe. Cardiology, 1992. 80(3–4): p. 246–51.

[19] Fu, S., et al., Evidence for roles of radicals in protein oxidation in advanced human atherosclerotic plaque. Biochem J, 1998. 333(Pt 3): p. 519–25.

[20] Shimano, M., et al., Reactive oxidative metabolites are associated with atrial conduction disturbance in patients with atrial fibrillation. Heart Rhythm, 2009. 6(7): p. 935–40.

[21] Porter, N.A., S.E. Caldwell, and K.A. Mills, Mechanisms of free radical oxidation of unsaturated lipids. Lipids, 1995. 30(4): p. 277–90.

[22] Milne, G.L., et al., Quantification of F2-isoprostanes as a biomarker of oxidative stress. Nat Protoc, 2007. 2(1): p. 221–6.

[23] Morrow, J.D., et al., A series of prostaglandin F2-like compounds are produced in vivo in humans by a non-cyclooxygenase, free radical-catalyzed mechanism. Proc Natl Acad Sci USA, 1990. 87(23): p. 9383–7.

[24] Fam, S.S. and J.D. Morrow, The isoprostanes: unique products of arachidonic acid oxidation—a review. Curr Med Chem, 2003. 10(17): p. 1723–40.

[25] Morrow, J.D., et al., Formation of novel non-cyclooxygenase-derived prostanoids (F2-isoprostanes) in carbon tetrachloride hepatotoxicity. An animal model of lipid peroxidation. J Clin Invest, 1992. 90(6): p. 2502–7.

[26] Iuliano, L., et al., Angioplasty increases coronary sinus F2-isoprostane formation: evidence for in vivo oxidative stress during PTCA. J Am Coll Cardiol, 2001. 37(1): p. 76–80.

[27] Roberts, L.J. and J.D. Morrow, Measurement of F(2)-isoprostanes as an index of oxidative stress in vivo. Free Radic Biol Med, 2000. 28(4): p. 505–13.

[28] Cracowski, J.L., T. Durand, and G. Bessard, Isoprostanes as a biomarker of lipid peroxidation in humans: physiology, pharmacology and clinical implications. Trends Pharmacol Sci, 2002. 23(8): p. 360–6.

[29] Davies, S.S. and L.J. Roberts, 2nd, F2-isoprostanes as an indicator and risk factor for coronary heart disease. Free Radic Biol Med, 2011. 50(5): p. 559–66.

[30] Milne, G.L., Q. Dai, and L.J. Roberts, 2nd, The isoprostanes—25 years later. Biochim Biophys Acta, 2015. 1851(4): p. 433–45.

[31] Delanty, N., et al., 8-epi PGF2 alpha generation during coronary reperfusion. A potential quantitative marker of oxidant stress in vivo. Circulation, 1997. 95(11): p. 2492–9.

[32] Keaney, J.F., Jr., et al., Obesity and systemic oxidative stress: clinical correlates of oxidative stress in the Framingham Study. Arterioscler Thromb Vasc Biol, 2003. 23(3): p. 434–9.

[33] De Caterina, R., et al., Low-density lipoprotein level reduction by the 3-hydroxy-3-methylglutaryl coenzyme-A inhibitor simvastatin is accompanied by a related reduction of F2-isoprostane formation in hypercholesterolemic subjects: no further effect of vitamin E. Circulation, 2002. 106(20): p. 2543–9.

[34] Gniwotta, C., et al., Prostaglandin F2-like compounds, F2-isoprostanes, are present in increased amounts in human atherosclerotic lesions. Arterioscler Thromb Vasc Biol, 1997. 17(11): p. 3236–41.

[35] Ulus, A.T., et al., Cardiopulmonary bypass as a cause of free radical-induced oxidative stress and enhanced blood-borne isoprostanes in humans. Free Radic Biol Med, 2003. 34(7): p. 911–7.

[36] Roberts, L.J., 2nd, et al., Identification of the major urinary metabolite of the F2-isoprostane 8-iso-prostaglandin F2alpha in humans. J Biol Chem, 1996. 271(34): p. 20617–20.

[37] Aviram, M., Review of human studies on oxidative damage and antioxidant protection related to cardiovascular diseases. Free Radic Res, 2000. 33(Suppl): p. S85–97.

[38] Chiabrando, C., et al., Identification of metabolites from type III F2-isoprostane diastereoisomers by mass spectrometry. J Lipid Res, 2002. 43(3): p. 495–509.

[39] Milne, G.L., E.S. Musiek, and J.D. Morrow, F2-isoprostanes as markers of oxidative stress in vivo: an overview. Biomarkers, 2005. 10(Suppl 1): p. S10–23.

[40] Smith, K.A., et al., A comparison of methods for the measurement of 8-isoPGF(2alpha): a marker of oxidative stress. Ann Clin Biochem, 2011. 48(Pt 2): p. 147–54.

[41] Kanabrocki, E.L., et al., Circadian variation in oxidative stress markers in healthy and type II diabetic men. Chronobiol Int, 2002. 19(2): p. 423–39.

[42] Helmersson, J. and S. Basu, F(2)-isoprostane and prostaglandin F(2 alpha)metabolite excretion rate and day to day variation in healthy humans. Prostaglandins Leukot Essent Fatty Acids, 2001. 65(2): p. 99–102.

[43] Miller, E.R., 3rd, et al., Association between cigarette smoking and lipid peroxidation in a controlled feeding study. Circulation, 1997. 96(4): p. 1097–101.

[44] Salonen, J.T., et al., Lipoprotein oxidation and progression of carotid atherosclerosis. Circulation, 1997. 95(4): p. 840–5.

[45] Walter, M.F., et al., Serum levels of thiobarbituric acid reactive substances predict cardiovascular events in patients with stable coronary artery disease: a longitudinal analysis of the PREVENT study. J Am Coll Cardiol, 2004. 44(10): p. 1996–2002.

[46] Meagher, E.A. and G.A. FitzGerald, Indices of lipid peroxidation in vivo: strengths and limitations. Free Radic Biol Med, 2000. 28(12): p. 1745–50.

[47] Halliwell, B. and S. Chirico, Lipid peroxidation: its mechanism, measurement, and significance. Am J Clin Nutr, 1993. 57(5 Suppl): p. 715S–724S; discussion 724S–725S.

[48] Moore, K. and L.J. Roberts, 2nd, Measurement of lipid peroxidation. Free Radic Res, 1998. 28(6): p. 659–71.

[49] Lykkesfeldt, J., Determination of malondialdehyde as dithiobarbituric acid adduct in biological samples by HPLC with fluorescence detection: comparison with ultraviolet-visible spectrophotometry. Clin Chem, 2001. 47(9): p. 1725–7.

[50] Bevan, R.J., et al., Validation of a novel ELISA for measurement of MDA-LDL in human plasma. Free Radic Biol Med, 2003. 35(5): p. 517–27.

[51] Salomon, R.G. and W. Bi, Isolevuglandin adducts in disease. Antioxid Redox Signal, 2015. 22(18): p. 1703–18.

[52] Hazen, S.L. and J.W. Heinecke, 3-Chlorotyrosine, a specific marker of myeloperoxidase-catalyzed oxidation, is markedly elevated in low density lipoprotein isolated from human atherosclerotic intima. J Clin Invest, 1997. 99(9): p. 2075–81.

[53] Daugherty, A., et al., Myeloperoxidase, a catalyst for lipoprotein oxidation, is expressed in human atherosclerotic lesions. J Clin Invest, 1994. 94(1): p. 437–44.

[54] Zhang, R., et al., Association between myeloperoxidase levels and risk of coronary artery disease. JAMA, 2001. 286(17): p. 2136–42.

[55] Capeillere-Blandin, C., Oxidation of guaiacol by myeloperoxidase: a two-electron-oxidized guaiacol transient species as a mediator of NADPH oxidation. Biochem J, 1998. 336(Pt 2): p. 395–404.

[56] Baldus, S., et al., Myeloperoxidase serum levels predict risk in patients with acute coronary syndromes. Circulation, 2003. 108(12): p. 1440–5.

[57] Brennan, M.L., et al., Prognostic value of myeloperoxidase in patients with chest pain. N Engl J Med, 2003. 349(17): p. 1595–604.

[58] Meuwese, M.C., et al., Serum myeloperoxidase levels are associated with the future risk of coronary artery disease in apparently healthy individuals: the EPIC-Norfolk Prospective Population Study. J Am Coll Cardiol, 2007. 50(2): p. 159–65.

[59] Shih, J., et al., Effect of collection tube type and preanalytical handling on myeloperoxidase concentrations. Clin Chem, 2008. 54(6): p. 1076–9.

[60] Li, G., et al., Effects of unfractionated heparin and glycoprotein IIb/IIIa antagonists versus bivalirdin on myeloperoxidase release from neutrophils. Arterioscler Thromb Vasc Biol, 2007. 27(8): p. 1850–6.

[61] Kempf, T., et al., The transforming growth factor-beta superfamily member growth-differentiation factor-15 protects the heart from ischemia/reperfusion injury. Circ Res, 2006. 98(3): p. 351–60.

[62] Schlittenhardt, D., et al., Involvement of growth differentiation factor-15/macrophage inhibitory cytokine-1 (GDF-15/MIC-1) in oxLDL-induced apoptosis of human macrophages in vitro and in arteriosclerotic lesions. Cell Tissue Res, 2004. 318(2): p. 325–33.

[63] Lindahl, B., The story of growth differentiation factor 15: another piece of the puzzle. Clin Chem, 2013. 59(11): p. 1550–2.

[64] Ago, T. and J. Sadoshima, GDF15, a cardioprotective TGF-beta superfamily protein. Circ Res, 2006. 98(3): p. 294–7.

[65] Khan, S.Q., et al., Growth differentiation factor-15 as a prognostic marker in patients with acute myocardial infarction. Eur Heart J, 2009. 30(9): p. 1057–65.

[66] Yla-Herttuala, S., et al., Evidence for the presence of oxidatively modified low density lipoprotein in atherosclerotic lesions of rabbit and man. J Clin Invest, 1989. 84(4): p. 1086–95.

[67] Massberg, S., et al., Platelet adhesion via glycoprotein IIb integrin is critical for atheroprogression and focal cerebral ischemia: an in vivo study in mice lacking glycoprotein IIb. Circulation, 2005. 112(8): p. 1180–8.

[68] Badrnya, S., A. Assinger, and I. Volf, Native high density lipoproteins (HDL) interfere with platelet activation induced by oxidized low density lipoproteins (OxLDL). Int J Mol Sci, 2013. 14(5): p. 10107–21.

[69] Hulthe, J. and B. Fagerberg, Circulating oxidized LDL is associated with subclinical atherosclerosis development and inflammatory cytokines (AIR Study). Arterioscler Thromb Vasc Biol, 2002. 22(7): p. 1162–7.

[70] Meisinger, C., et al., Plasma oxidized low-density lipoprotein, a strong predictor for acute coronary heart disease events in apparently healthy, middle-aged men from the general population. Circulation, 2005. 112(5): p. 651–7.

[71] Trpkovic, A., et al., Oxidized low-density lipoprotein as a biomarker of cardiovascular diseases. Crit Rev Clin Lab Sci, 2015. 52(2): p. 70–85.

[72] Itabe, H., et al., Oxidized phosphatidylcholines that modify proteins. Analysis by monoclonal antibody against oxidized low density lipoprotein. J Biol Chem, 1996. 271(52): p. 33208–17.

[73] Holvoet, P., et al., Circulating oxidized LDL is a useful marker for identifying patients with coronary artery disease. Arterioscler Thromb Vasc Biol, 2001. 21(5): p. 844–8.

[74] Grootveld, M. and B. Halliwell, Measurement of allantoin and uric acid in human body fluids. A potential index of free-radical reactions in vivo? Biochem J, 1987. 243(3): p. 803–8.

[75] Kand'ar, R., P. Zakova, and V. Muzakova, Monitoring of antioxidant properties of uric acid in humans for a consideration measuring of levels of allantoin in plasma by liquid chromatography. Clin Chim Acta, 2006. 365(1–2): p. 249–56.

[76] Seet, R.C., et al., Biomarkers of oxidative damage in cigarette smokers: which biomarkers might reflect acute versus chronic oxidative stress? Free Radic Biol Med, 2011. 50(12): p. 1787–93.

[77] Doehner, W., et al., Effects of xanthine oxidase inhibition with allopurinol on endothelial function and peripheral blood flow in hyperuricemic patients with chronic heart failure: results from 2 placebo-controlled studies. Circulation, 2002. 105(22): p. 2619–24.

[78] Berthemy, A., et al., Quantitative determination of an extremely polar compound allantoin in human urine by LC-MS/MS based on the separation on a polymeric amino column. J Pharm Biomed Anal, 1999. 19(3–4): p. 429–34.

[79] Turner, R., L.K. Stamp, and A.J. Kettle, Detection of allantoin in clinical samples using hydrophilic liquid chromatography with stable isotope dilution negative ion tandem mass spectrometry. J Chromatogr B Analyt Technol Biomed Life Sci, 2012. 891–892: p. 85–9.

[80] Dalle-Donne, I., et al., Protein carbonyl groups as biomarkers of oxidative stress. Clin Chim Acta, 2003. 329(1–2): p. 23–38.

[81] Mutlu-Turkoglu, U., et al., Age-related increases in plasma malondialdehyde and protein carbonyl levels and lymphocyte DNA damage in elderly subjects. Clin Biochem, 2003. 36(5): p. 397–400.

[82] Pantke, U., et al., Oxidized proteins as a marker of oxidative stress during coronary heart surgery. Free Radic Biol Med, 1999. 27(9–10): p. 1080–6.

[83] Lynch, T.L.t., et al., Oxidative stress in dilated cardiomyopathy caused by MYBPC3 mutation. Oxid Med Cell Longev, 2015. 2015: p. 424751.

[84] Levine, R.L., et al., Determination of carbonyl content in oxidatively modified proteins. Methods Enzymol, 1990. 186: p. 464–78.

[85] Chevion, M., E. Berenshtein, and E.R. Stadtman, Human studies related to protein oxidation: protein carbonyl content as a marker of damage. Free Radic Res, 2000. 33(Suppl): p. S99–108.

[86] Levine, R.L., et al., Carbonyl assays for determination of oxidatively modified proteins. Methods Enzymol, 1994. 233: p. 346–57.

[87] Yan, L.J. and R.S. Sohal, Gel electrophoretic quantitation of protein carbonyls derivatized with tritiated sodium borohydride. Anal Biochem, 1998. 265(1): p. 176–82.

[88] Lenz, A.G., et al., Determination of carbonyl groups in oxidatively modified proteins by reduction with tritiated sodium borohydride. Anal Biochem, 1989. 177(2): p. 419–25.

[89] Kalousova, M., J. Skrha, and T. Zima, Advanced glycation end-products and advanced oxidation protein products in patients with diabetes mellitus. Physiol Res, 2002. 51(6): p. 597–604.

[90] Kaneda, H., et al., Increased level of advanced oxidation protein products in patients with coronary artery disease. Atherosclerosis, 2002. 162(1): p. 221–5.

[91] Witko-Sarsat, V., et al., Advanced oxidation protein products as novel mediators of inflammation and monocyte activation in chronic renal failure. J Immunol, 1998. 161(5): p. 2524–32.

[92] Witko-Sarsat, V., et al., Advanced oxidation protein products as a novel molecular basis of oxidative stress in uraemia. Nephrol Dial Transplant, 1999. 14(Suppl 1): p. 76–8.

[93] Fu, M.X., et al., The advanced glycation end product, Nepsilon-(carboxymethyl)lysine, is a product of both lipid peroxidation and glycoxidation reactions. J Biol Chem, 1996. 271(17): p. 9982–6.

[94] Brix, J.M., et al., The soluble form of the receptor of advanced glycation endproducts increases after bariatric surgery in morbid obesity. Int J Obes (Lond), 2012. 36(11): p. 1412–7.

[95] Brouwers, O., et al., Mild oxidative damage in the diabetic rat heart is attenuated by glyoxalase-1 overexpression. Int J Mol Sci, 2013. 14(8): p. 15724–39.

[96] Buss, H., et al., Protein carbonyl measurement by a sensitive ELISA method. Free Radic Biol Med, 1997. 23(3): p. 361–6.

[97] Keller, R.J., et al., Immunochemical detection of oxidized proteins. Chem Res Toxicol, 1993. 6(4): p. 430–3.

[98] Friess, U., et al., Liquid chromatography-based determination of urinary free and total N(epsilon)-(carboxymethyl)lysine excretion in normal and diabetic subjects. J Chromatogr B Analyt Technol Biomed Life Sci, 2003. 794(2): p. 273–80.

[99] Takahashi, M., et al., Direct quantification of pentosidine in urine and serum by HPLC with column switching. Clin Chem, 1996. 42(9): p. 1439–44.

[100] Kalousova, M., et al., Advanced glycoxidation end products in chronic diseases-clinical chemistry and genetic background. Mutat Res, 2005. 579(1–2): p. 37–46.

[101] Mieyal, J.J., et al., Molecular mechanisms and clinical implications of reversible protein S-glutathionylation. Antioxid Redox Signal, 2008. 10(11): p. 1941–88.

[102] Eaton, P., et al., Glyceraldehyde phosphate dehydrogenase oxidation during cardiac ischemia and reperfusion. J Mol Cell Cardiol, 2002. 34(11): p. 1549–60.

[103] Okuda, M., et al., Expression of glutaredoxin in human coronary arteries: its potential role in antioxidant protection against atherosclerosis. Arterioscler Thromb Vasc Biol, 2001. 21(9): p. 1483–7.

[104] Pimentel, D.R., et al., Strain-stimulated hypertrophy in cardiac myocytes is mediated by reactive oxygen species-dependent Ras S-glutathiolation. J Mol Cell Cardiol, 2006. 41(4): p. 613–22.

[105] Nonaka, K., et al., Serum levels of S-glutathionylated proteins as a risk-marker for arteriosclerosis obliterans. Circ J, 2007. 71(1): p. 100–5.

[106] Jones, D.P., Redox potential of GSH/GSSG couple: assay and biological significance. Methods Enzymol, 2002. 348: p. 93–112.

[107] Townsend, D.M., et al., Novel role for glutathione S-transferase pi. Regulator of protein S-Glutathionylation following oxidative and nitrosative stress. J Biol Chem, 2009. 284(1): p. 436–45.

[108] Lind, C., et al., Studies on the mechanism of oxidative modification of human glyceraldehyde-3-phosphate dehydrogenase by glutathione: catalysis by glutaredoxin. Biochem Biophys Res Commun, 1998. 247(2): p. 481–6.

[109] Brennan, J.P., et al., The utility of N,N-biotinyl glutathione disulfide in the study of protein S-glutathiolation. Mol Cell Proteomics, 2006. 5(2): p. 215–25.

[110] Reynaert, N.L., et al., Dynamic redox control of NF-kappaB through glutaredoxin-regulated S-glutathionylation of inhibitory kappaB kinase beta. Proc Natl Acad Sci USA, 2006. 103(35): p. 13086–91.

[111] Passarelli, C., et al., Susceptibility of isolated myofibrils to in vitro glutathionylation: potential relevance to muscle functions. Cytoskeleton (Hoboken), 2010. 67(2): p. 81–9.

[112] Passarelli, C., et al., Myosin as a potential redox-sensor: an in vitro study. J Muscle Res Cell Motil, 2008. 29(2–5): p. 119–26.

[113] West, M.B., et al., Protein glutathiolation by nitric oxide: an intracellular mechanism regulating redox protein modification. FASEB J, 2006. 20(10): p. 1715–7.

[114] Pastore, A. and F. Piemonte, Protein glutathionylation in cardiovascular diseases. Int J Mol Sci, 2013. 14(10): p. 20845–76.

[115] Hanson, E.K., H. Lubenow, and J. Ballantyne, Identification of forensically relevant body fluids using a panel of differentially expressed microRNAs. Anal Biochem, 2009. 387(2): p. 303–14.

[116] Etheridge, A., et al., Extracellular microRNA: a new source of biomarkers. Mutat Res, 2011. 717(1–2): p. 85–90.

[117] Thomas, M.F. and K.M. Ansel, Construction of small RNA cDNA libraries for deep sequencing. Methods Mol Biol, 2010. 667: p. 93–111.

[118] Li, J., et al., Real-time polymerase chain reaction microRNA detection based on enzymatic stem-loop probes ligation. Anal Chem, 2009. 81(13): p. 5446–51.

[119] Cheng, Y., et al., A translational study of circulating cell-free microRNA-1 in acute myocardial infarction. Clin Sci (Lond), 2010. 119(2): p. 87–95.

[120] Ai, J., et al., Circulating microRNA-1 as a potential novel biomarker for acute myocardial infarction. Biochem Biophys Res Commun, 2010. 391(1): p. 73–7.

[121] Tijsen, A.J., et al., MiR423-5p as a circulating biomarker for heart failure. Circ Res, 2010. 106(6): p. 1035–9.

[122] Kono, Y., et al., Elevated levels of oxidative DNA damage in serum and myocardium of patients with heart failure. Circ J, 2006. 70(8): p. 1001–5.

[123] Nagayoshi, Y., et al., Urinary 8-hydroxy-2'-deoxyguanosine levels increase after reperfusion in acute myocardial infarction and may predict subsequent cardiac events. Am J Cardiol, 2005. 95(4): p. 514–7.

[124] Vita, J.A., et al., Low plasma ascorbic acid independently predicts the presence of an unstable coronary syndrome. J Am Coll Cardiol, 1998. 31(5): p. 980–6.

[125] Blankenberg, S., et al., Glutathione peroxidase 1 activity and cardiovascular events in patients with coronary artery disease. N Engl J Med, 2003. 349(17): p. 1605–13.

[126] Madhavan, M., et al., Serum bilirubin distribution and its relation to cardiovascular risk in children and young adults. Atherosclerosis, 1997. 131(1): p. 107–13.

[127] Hokamaki, J., et al., Urinary biopyrrins levels are elevated in relation to severity of heart failure. J Am Coll Cardiol, 2004. 43(10): p. 1880–5.

[128] Shimomura, H., et al., Comparison of urinary biopyrrin levels in acute myocardial infarction (after reperfusion therapy) versus stable angina pectoris and their usefulness in predicting subsequent cardiac events. Am J Cardiol, 2002. 90(2): p. 108–11.

Chapter 7

Redoxomics and Oxidative Stress: From the Basic Research to the Clinical Practice

Simona Tafuri, Natascia Cocchia, Francesco Landolfi,
Eugenio Luigi Iorio and Francesca Ciani

Additional information is available at the end of the chapter

http://dx.doi.org/10.5772/64577

Abstract

Potentially oxidant chemical species, which include not only free radicals but also other oxidizing chemical species such as reactive oxygen species (ROS), for example, hydroxyl radical and hydrogen peroxide, and nitrogen reactive species (RNS), for example, nitric oxide, play a relevant role in all biological processes and especially in cell defenses and molecular signaling. Their action is finely modulated by the antioxidant network that is composed either by endogenous or exogenous compounds (e.g., enzymes, peptides, lipids, and vitamins). An impaired modulation of oxidant species can lead to the so-called oxidative stress that is now considered an emerging health risk factor in almost all living organisms including plants, animals, and humans. Indeed, oxidative stress is related to a reduced lifespan and many diseases (e.g., cardiovascular diseases, neurodegenerative disorders, and metabolic diseases) both in humans and in animals. Unfortunately, oxidative stress does not show any clinical picture, but it can be detected only by means of specific laboratory tests. The recent recognition of a specific "redox code" and the definition of a redoxomics as a new "omics" are now enlarging the horizon of the traditional oxidative stress field leading to the definition of the so-called electrophilic stress. The aim of this chapter is to review the basic principles of redox reaction starting from the concept of free radicals and antioxidant in order to define the "electrophilic stress" as an emerging health risk factor for early aging and almost 1000 illness from infectious diseases to cancer. A paragraph is dedicated to the tests to measure oxidative stress in clinical practice either in humans or in animals in order to prevent, to treat and to monitor electrophilic-related diseases.

Keywords: ROS, RNS, antioxidants, redoxomics

1. Reactive species, free radicals, and oxidative processes

Free radicals play a fundamental role in the metabolic activity and function of different organs. Interactions between prooxidants (free radicals) and antioxidants lead to the maintenance of the intracellular homeostasis. A state of oxidative stress begins when there is an imbalance between the prooxidants and antioxidants, in favor of free radicals. Oxidative stress is a health risk factor involved in aging and in several diseases, in humans and/or in animals. In normal conditions, paired electrons create stable bonds in biomolecules; a free radical is defined as any independent species that contains one or more unpaired electrons in external orbital. Free radicals have a greater or lesser reactivity for the spontaneous tendency to exist as molecules with all electrons arranged in couples; this state is equivalent to the chemical stability.

The radicals do not show the same reactivity. Their increase of charge and the volumetric ratio is directly proportional to their reactivity. They will only reach their stability stripping electrons to other chemical species with which they are in contact and oxidize them [1].

Free radicals are classified according to the nature of atom that owns the orbital with unpaired electron. Reactive species include either radical or nonradical chemical species with oxidant potential. There are, therefore, free radicals centered on oxygen, carbon, nitrogen, or chlorine, and so on. Free radicals and other reactive species act as signaling molecules. Reactive species modulate transcription and epigenetics.

Free radicals/reactive species can be produced either by a "nonenzymatic" or an "enzymatic" way (**Figure 1**).

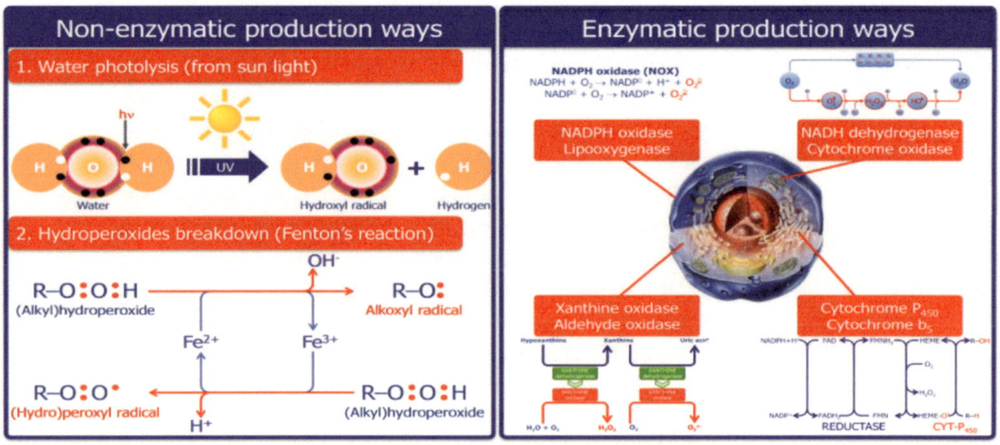

Figure 1. The "origin" of free radicals and other reactive species in living organisms.

The cell is the first target of oxidative damage. The destructive action of free radicals on cells is addressed mainly through the following reactions: membrane lipid peroxidation, oxidative modification of proteins and amino acids, nucleic acids' damage, and sugar oxidation (**Figure 2**).

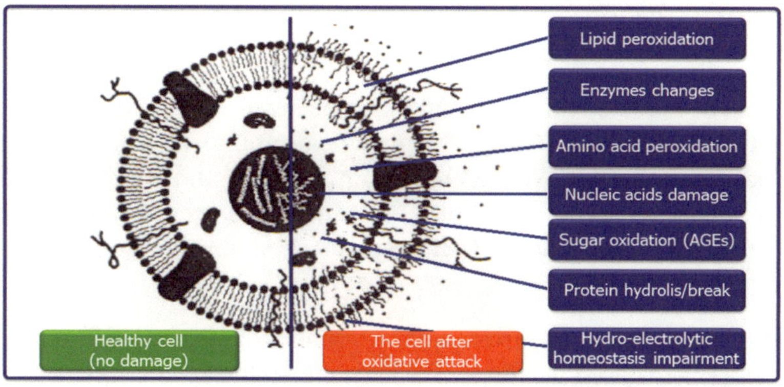

Figure 2. The cell: the first target of oxidative damage. Reactive species can hit not only lipids but also proteins and nucleic acids.

The damage, initially cellular, if prolonged through time, spreads to the tissues, organs and then it becomes a systemic damage. Oxidative stress is responsible, then, of cardiovascular diseases, dementia, Parkinson, early senescence, inflammation, cancers, and other diseases (**Figure 3**).

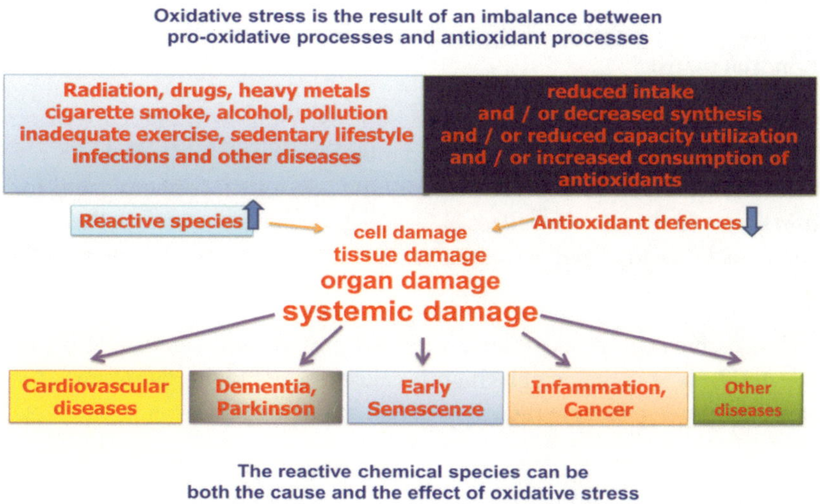

Figure 3. Consequences of the imbalance between pro-oxidants and antioxidants.

2. The antioxidants and biochemical classification

Antioxidants are substances that, when they are present at a low concentration compared to those of an oxidizable substrate, retard or prevent the oxidation of the same substrate. The keyword "oxidized substrate" includes every kind of molecule that is located *in vivo*.

In nature, there are no universal best antioxidants, but there are different antioxidants that are required to protect several molecules *in vivo* [2].

Antioxidants can be classified into enzymatic and nonenzymatic. The enzymatic antioxidants include glutathione reductase (GSH), superoxide dismutase (SOD), and catalase (CAT). Among the nonenzymatic antioxidants are vitamins (C, E, and B), carotenoids, carnitine, cysteine, some metals, taurine, and albumin [3]. Reductase and peroxidase glutathione are the main reducing endogenous agents and act as scavenger antioxidants especially in the epididymis and testes [4].

SOD is an enzyme that catalyzes the dismutation reactions of the superoxide anion (O_2^-). It can be found in intra- and extracellular forms. The intracellular forms are copper-zinc SOD present in the cytoplasm and contain copper and zinc in the active site (Cu, ZnSOD, SOD1); and manganese SOD localized mainly in the mitochondrial matrix and contains manganese in the active site (MnSOD, SOD2). Instead, SOD extracellular form (EC-SOD, SOD3), working into the extracellular space, is correlated to the polysaccharides of surface or in a free form [5].

CAT catalyzes the conversion of H_2O_2 to O_2 and H_2O and presents a heme system with a central iron atom. It acts mainly in endoplasmic reticulum, peroxisomes, mitochondria, and the cytosol of many cell types [6].

Glutathione peroxidase (GPX) catalyzes the reduction of H_2O_2 and organic peroxides [5].GPX contains selenium in the form of selenocysteine in its active site. It is located in the sperm in the mitochondrial matrix.

The nonenzymatic exogen antioxidants are vitamins. Vitamin E encompasses a group of potent, lipid-soluble, chain-breaking antioxidants. Structural analyses have revealed that molecules having vitamin E antioxidant activity include four tocopherols and four tocotrienols. Vitamin E (α-tocopherol) neutralizes H_2O_2 and quenches free radicals, therefore, stopping chain reactions that develop lipid peroxides and protecting the membrane from the oxidative damage.

Vitamin C (L-ascorbic acid or ascorbate), a pivotal nutrient for organisms, is present in the extracellular fluid. It is a principal chain-breaking antioxidant neutralizing superoxide, hydroxyl, and hydrogen peroxide radicals. Also, it has an important action to recycle vitamin E [7].

A class of natural pigments, carotenoids, is synthesized from plants and microorganisms, but not animals. They, present as microcomponents in fruits and vegetables, are responsible for their colors (yellow, orange, and red). Carotenoids are held liable for the beneficial effects of fruits and vegetables to prevent illnesses such as cardiovascular disease, cancer, and different chronic disease [7].

Cysteines, intracellular GSH precursors, enhancement the quantity of GSH synthesized, which avoids oxidative damage to the cell membrane and DNA.

In addition, albumin, taurine/hypotaurine, inositol and any metal are other minor antioxidants which help to reduce oxidative stress.

One of the plasma proteins, the albumin, reacts with peroxyl radicals and prevents the chain reactions that produce ROS (Reactive Oxygen Species) formation.

Taurine, nonenzymatic antioxidant, scavenges ROS, inositol enhances GSH activity.

Selenium is an important component in the regular development and maturation of cells and contributes to the protection of DNA and cell membranes, particularly when used as an adjunct to vitamin E.

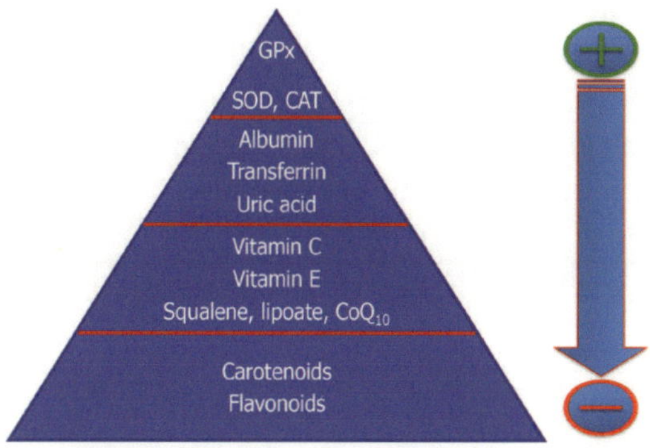

Figure 4. The antioxidant pyramid. Vertical stratification (power hierarchy).

Zinc acts as a chelator and binds ROS [8]. Chrome, another essential micronutrient, is a component of enzymes involved in carbohydrate metabolism. Its supplementation reduces fat deposition in rats, preventing obesity, initial phase of inflammation and oxidative stress [9].

Figure 4 shows the power hierarchy of antioxidant pyramid. Endogenous enzyme antioxidants have a higher antioxidant capacity and are located at the top of the pyramid.

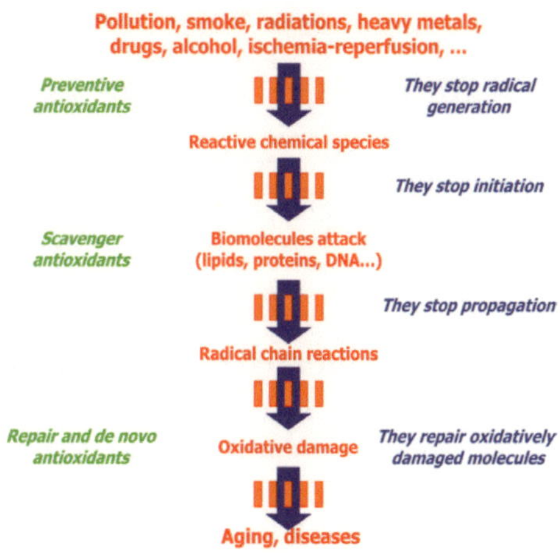

Figure 5. Antioxidant defense mechanisms.

The mechanisms of antioxidant action are shown in **Figure 5**. According to their function, they can be classified into preventive, scavenger, and repair antioxidants. Preventive antioxidants stop radical generation; scavenger antioxidants stop initiation and propagation; and repair and *de novo* antioxidants repair oxidated damaged molecules.

Polyphenols are abundant micronutrients in our diet, and there is evidence for their role in the prevention of degenerative diseases. Their bioavailability differs greatly among the polyphenol groups, depending on their composition, dietary sources, forms, and their containing so that the most abundant polyphenols in our diet are not necessarily those leading to the highest concentrations of active metabolites in target tissues. The plasma concentrations of total metabolites range from 0 to 4 mol/L with an intake of 50-mg aglycone equivalents. Among the polyphenols, isoflavones and gallic acid are the ones that are absorbed most by humans following, with different kinetics, flavonoids, catechins, and quercetin glycosides. Less absorbed polyphenols are proanthocyanidins, catechins galloylated tea, and anthocyanins. The data for other polyphenols remain poorly understood. Other studies would be necessary for the investigations on the health effects of polyphenols (**Figure 6**) [10].

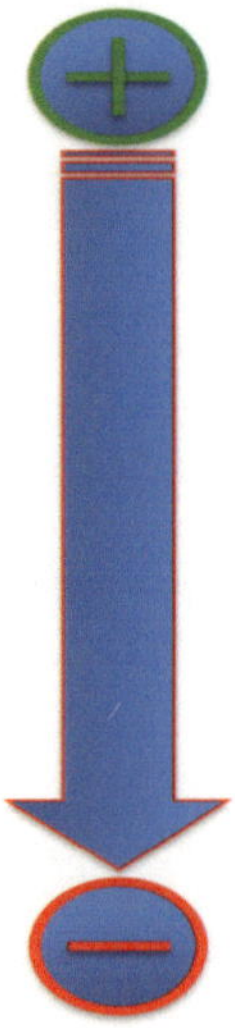

Classes of compounds	Active principles
Hydroxybenzoic acids	Gallic acid
Hydroxycinamic acids	Ferulic acid
Isoflavones	Daidzeidin, glycetin
Catechines	Epicatechin, epigallocatechin
Flavanones	Naringin, esperidin
Flavanols	Quercetin, rutin
Proanthocyanidines	Dimeric, trimeric
Anthocyanidines	Cyanidin, malvidin

Figure 6. Antioxidant: polyphenol classes.

3. Oxidative stress: from the biochemistry to the clinics

Oxidative stress is a particular kind of chemical stress, which is induced—locally and/or systemically—by an excess of potentially oxidant reactive species, mostly centered on the oxygen (reactive oxygen species, ROS). It can be due to an increased production of reactive species and/or to a reduced efficiency of antioxidant defense system. The effects of oxidative stress can range from the impairment of cell signaling to the apoptosis or necrosis.

The systematic assessment in biological samples of primary oxidizing chemical species, such as free radicals and their derivatives, such as hydroperoxides, as well as the dosage of antioxidant compounds and/or antioxidant activities (selenium and/or glutathione peroxidase), are not a "ring terminal" in the diagnostic chain of the information flows in biological systems (DNA > RNA > protein > metabolites > oxidants), but should make a "central place" compared to genomics, transcriptomics, proteomics, and metabolomics [11]. Precisely for this reason it has been newly introduced the new concept of "redoxomics" [12], a word previously used to detect only a few oxidized byproducts in the area of proteomics [13].

Redoxomics is a new field of "applied biochemistry" and "molecular diagnostic" with the following objectives: to examine the structure, the physiological role, and the deploying of oxidant and antioxidant systems into a living organism; to identify the mutual interactions of oxidant and antioxidant systems in a biological system (e.g., cell, tissue, organ, apparatus, and whole organism) in a defined phase of its development, under basic conditions as well as after stimulation potentially stressful; to assess the implications of these results from the point of view of epidemiology, pathophysiology, clinic, pharmacology, and so on [14].

The aspiring objective of redoxomics (as well as for another "-omics" in other areas) is "mapping" dynamically—through all the analytical and sophisticated techniques, from electron spin resonance to imaging—the whole oxidative-antioxidant repertoire [15].

This "integrated" approach allows us to track any qualitative/quantitative changes of oxidative balance and can support clinicians to give an optimum and "customized" solution for fixing any anomalies of redox status related to human diseases, in particular, in the area of aesthetic and antiaging medicine [16].

4. The breakdown of oxidant/antioxidant balance

The biological concept of stress: the word "stress", as it is currently in use, was first coined by Hans Selye (1907–1982) in 1936, he defined "stress" as "the nonspecific response of the body to any demand for change."

Selye had observed in many experiments that laboratory animals underwent sharp stimuli but different physical and emotional harmful (e.g., high beam, loud noise, extreme heat or cold, and constant frustration) all shown the identical pathologic changes of gastric ulcers narrowing of the lymphoid tissue and widening of the adrenal glands. Following they showed that persistent stress could be the cause of the development of different diseases in these animals similar to those observed in humans, like heart attacks, strokes, kidney diseases, and rheumatoid arthritis. The Selye's concept and dynamics of stress overlaps with that of oxidative stress (**Figure 7**) [17]. Most of oxidative stress-related diseases are related to life style [13].

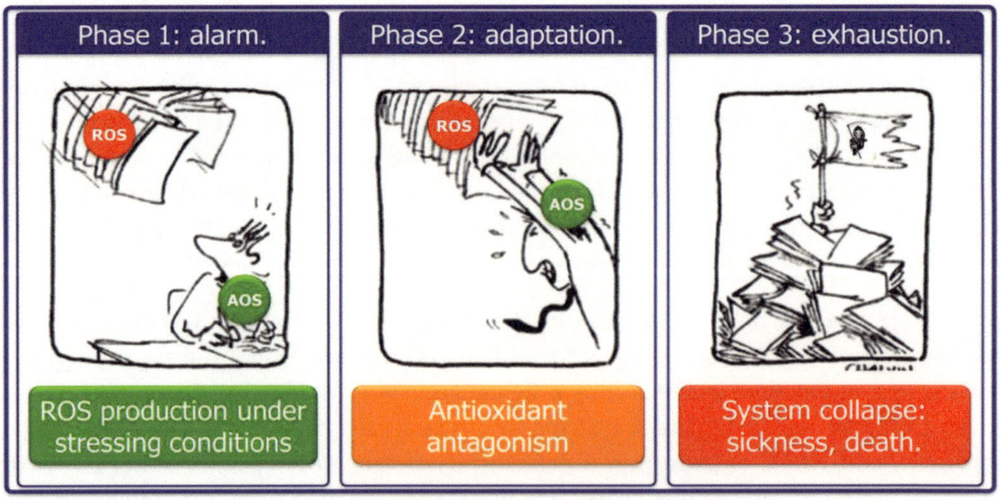

Figure 7. Classical stress and oxidative stress: two overlapping concepts.

Oxidative distress from oxidative eustress can happen for several reasons: formation of reactive species from stimulated polymorphonuclear leukocytes that can hit not only bacteria but also tissues; an overload of oxygen (e.g., by strong aerobic exercise) into the mitochondria and consequent increase ROS production; detoxification from acetaminophen (paracetamol) into the microsomes may increase ROS liver production; reperfusion after ischemia may lead to reactive oxygen species production due to xanthine oxidase activation.

In any case, an amount of oxidants is synthesized and by the old Greek language, *oxys* means *acids*, it is possible to establish a new paradigma: oxidative stress + acidosis = electrophilic stress.

5. Measurement of oxidative stress

The focus is now put on oxidative stress biomarkers that are objectively measured and assessed as markers of normal biological processes, pathogenic processes, or pharmacological responses to therapy performed. A biomarker, to be used as a predictor of illness, must first be endorsed. The validation criteria are intrinsic qualities like the specificity, sensitivity, the degree of inter- and intraindividual variability, and understanding of factors that can change.

In particular, features of the sample and analytical procedures are significant, therefore, noninvasiveness of the sampling, biomarker stability, sensitivity, specificity, velocity and simplicity of the analytical method are important. Below, the most commonly used biomarkers for the evaluation of oxidative/nitrosative damage are listed.

Oxidative stress depends on an imbalance that is created between the production of ROS (pro-oxidants) and the action of the antioxidants. Direct assays, which measure the oxidation of the cell membrane of many cell types, are available.

http://dx.doi.org/10.5772/64577

The most widespread assay assesses the concentration of malondialdehyde (MDA), one of the end products of lipid peroxidation [18, 19]. The increased levels of MDA may be related, for example, to the decrease of sperm parameters. To quantify the damage of sperm DNA, another assay is also used; it measures the concentration of a specific product of oxidative DNA damage, 8-oxo-7,8, dihydro 2′deoxyguanosine (8-OHdG). This product is particularly employed as a specific marker of oxidative damage to sperm DNA [20].

The assay of the indirect chemiluminescence is one of the most popular methods for the determination of ROS in the spermatic semen. Luminol (5-amino-2,3, dihydro 1,4, phthalazinedione) and lucigen are substances used to determine the redox activity in the cells [20]. Lucigen quantizes only extracellular superoxide radicals, while the luminol is able to determine the extracellular and intracellular levels of ROS.

In order to use the nitrobluetetrazolium assay an optical microscope is needed: it allows us to determine the differentiation of ROS in different cell types. This reagent, nitrobluetetrazolium, reacts with superoxide radicals, for example, in spermatozoa and in leukocytes, changing to diformazan, a blue pigment. The concentration of diformazan is directly proportional to the intracellular concentration of ROS [21].

To assess serum total oxidant and antioxidant levels, commercially available d-ROMs and anti-ROM (Reactive Oxygen Metabolites) tests (Diacron International, Grosseto, Italy) are utilized. These tests are performed using Free Carpe Diem, a dedicated spectrophotometer (Diacron International, Grosseto, Italy).

Oxidative status is evaluated by measuring hydroperoxides in the serum using d-ROMs' test. The d-ROMs test measures the oxidant ability of a serum sample toward a particular substance (modified aromatic amine) used as an indicator (chromogen, N,N-diethyl-para-phenylendiamine) (DEPPD). The phenomenon is associated with the progressive and gradual color change to pink reaction mixture (serum + chromogen), which was initially colorless. In the d-ROMs test, the metabolites of reactive oxygen species (ROMs), particularly hydroperoxides (ROOH), of a biological sample, in the presence of iron, issued by the serum proteins by an acid buffer, can produce alkoxyl and peroxyl radicals, in accordance with Fenton's reaction.

Such radicals are able to oxidize an alkyl-substituted aromatic amine that is solubilized in a chromogenic mixture, thus producing a pink-colored derivative which is photometrically quantified at 505 nm [22]. The intensity of developed color is directly proportional to the concentration of ROMs, according to the Lambert–Beer's law and is expressed as Carratelli units (1 CARR U = 0.08 mg hydrogen peroxide/dl). The method is linear up to 1000 CARR U.

The measurement of antioxidant capacity in serum samples can be performed by the anti-ROM test. The anti-ROM test measures the antioxidant capacity of serum in terms of iron-reducing capacity; in fact, it is based on the ability of serum antioxidants to reduce ferric iron to ferrous iron, which reacting with $\alpha\alpha$-dipyridyl, gives rise to a reddish purple. The intensity of color increases in proportion to the amount of iron reduced by antioxidants present in the sample.

In the BAP (Biological Antioxidant Potential) test, adding a sample of plasma to a dye solution, obtained as a mixture of ferric chloride with a derived thiocyanate solution, a discoloration is caused. The intensity of this discoloration is determined photometrically by using a wavelength of 505 nm and it results proportional to the ability of plasma to reduce ferric ions [23]. The results obtained are evaluated as μmol/L or reduced ferric ions.

The antioxidant levels can be evaluated in the semen too, both with a chemiluminescence and through a colorimetric assay. The antioxidant amounts are determined by the addition of a well-known concentration of ROS to semen, developing the chemiluminescent signal or the color changes. The antioxidants present in the sperm behave toward ROS as a scavenger, so it is possible to measure the residual levels of ROS. Then, the intensity of the developed signal is inversely proportional to the total antioxidant activity of the sample [24].

The total oxidant capacity/potential of a blood plasma/serum sample can be evaluated by exploiting the ability of N,N-diethyl-paraphenylendiamine to give electrons (oxidation) after the reaction with a biological sample. The newly generated radical cation can be detected—thus providing a suitable measure of oxidant capacity—either by evaluating the absorbance change at 505 nm (the solution becomes pink to red, depending on the concentration) or the specific spin resonance signal [22].

6. The oxidative stress evaluation in clinical practice

Oxidative stress does not show any clinical picture; thus, the study of basic mechanisms of oxidative stress can lead to the identification of suitable biomarkers. Searching for the "ideal" biomarker of oxidative stress is not an easy matter; it should be validated by means of the golden standard technique (e.g., electron spin resonance); acceptably high levels of sensitivity, specificity, and precision; chemically stable over the time; able to measure suitably oxidative stress level; able to provide reliable information even in an early stage of the disease; able to anticipate the progression of disease during a systemic monitoring; modifiable with adequate sensitivity after medical/surgery/antioxidant treatments; minimally invasive, highly compliant, fast; and optimal cost/benefit ratio. Unfortunately, an accomplished biomarker of oxidative stress with all these features is not yet available.

The blood plasma/serum of apparently healthy people (and that one of many animal species) is able to oxidize the DEPPD (as described above) in a precise range of absorbance change as a function of either genetic or environment factors (age, gender, race, physiological conditions like pregnancy, and so on) and according to a Gauss-like curve of distribution (**Figure 8**) [25].

Primary mechanism	Primary cell site involved	Main biochemical mechanisms	Main reactive species involved	Causes and clinical correlations
Reactive changes of cell surface	Plasmamembrane	Activation of NADPH oxidase	Superoxide anion	Inflammatory diseases
		Activation of arachidonic acid metabolism	Hydroperoxides Superoxide anion	Infectious diseases
Impaired cell respiration	Mitochondria	Metabolic activation	Superoxide anion Hydrogen peroxide Hydroxyl radical	Caloric excess Strong erobic activity Thyroid hyperactivity
		Mithocondrial dysfunction	Superoxide anion Hydrogen peroxide	Nervous system and muscle genetic disorders
Pharmaco-metabolic induction	Endoplasmic reticulum/ microsomes	Activation of cytochrome P_{450} and b_5	Variable	Alcohol abuse Drugs, xenobiotics
Abnormal changes of intracellular pO_2	Citosol	Activation of xanthine oxidase	Superoxide anion Hydrogen peroxide Hydroxyl radical	Ischemia/reperfusion diseases (e. g. infarction)
Multiple	Variable	Variable	Variable	Cigarette smoke,toxicities, radiations, metabolism

Figure 8. Causes, mechanisms, and clinical pictures of oxidative stress.

The blood plasma/serum of apparently healthy people, which are exposed to factors that are classically able to induce a condition of oxidative stress, shows a total oxidant capacity constantly and significantly higher than that found in apparently healthy nonexposed peoples, and patients suffering from diseases classically related to oxidative stress show significantly higher levels of blood plasma/serum total oxidant capacity compared to those found in apparently healthy controls (**Figure 9**).

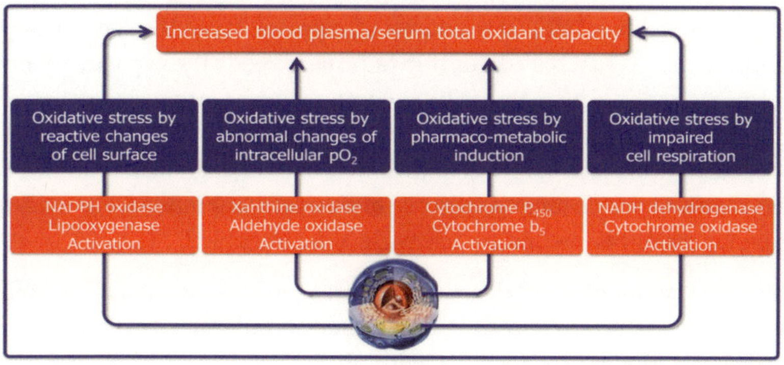

Figure 9. Oxidative stress-related diseases. Pathophysiological and clinical pictures.

Some studies have shown that between the work done on standing and chronic venous insufficiency of the lower limbs, there is a statistically significant correlation. This correlation has been associated with an oxidative stress in an advanced stage that, according to several studies, would represent a risk factor for cardiovascular systemic disorders; in fact, standing workers exhibit significantly higher mean levels of ROS after work [26].

It is known that elevated levels of blood reactive oxygen species are correlated with the severity of periodontitis. An improvement of clinical parameters in chronic periodontitis patients, through a nonsurgical periodontal treatment, is able to determine a decrease in blood reactive oxygen species [27].

Moreover, free radicals' cigarette smoke is a complex chemical system and there are many potential pathways for these species to interact with one another and with biopolymers in a smoker's lung. There is ample evidence that the free radical system plays a significant role in cigarette smoke toxicology. It is becoming increasingly strong and necessary to try to place some possibilities in perspective [28, 29].

Chronic alcohol abuse appears to be linked to increased serum levels of reactive oxygen species, such as hydroperoxides, with a normal antioxidant capacity. The study performed by Trotti et al. [30] suggested that both alterations in the redox balance and a thrombophilic condition can be observed in heavy drinkers without severe liver diseases, such as cirrhosis, hepatitis, and hepatitis C virus (HCV).

Oxidative stress by impaired cell respiration increased oxidant capacity in strenuous exercise. Physical activity increases the free radicals in several ways, such as oxidative phosphorylation enhances in answer to exercise; therefore, there is a simultaneous production of free radicals. Catecholamines, issued when exercising, can produce free radicals. The free radicals that enhance with exercise are produced by the metabolism of prostanoids, by xanthine oxidase, NADPH (Nicotinamide Adenine dinucleotide Phosphate-Oxidase) oxidase, and other secondary sources, for example, by macrophages hired to fix the injured tissue that can produce free radicals [31].

Antioxidant supplements are sold and used by athletes to counteroxidative stress due to strenuous exercise. It is not yet clear if strenuous exercise increases the need for supplementary antioxidants in the diet. When the rise of free radicals exceeds the capacity of antioxidants to neutralize them, the radicals have the cellular components as targets in particular lipids. The lipid attack starts a chain reaction known as lipid peroxidation, which results in formation of a high number of radicals and reactive species that can damage other cellular components. The organism is able to bear a limited increase of free radicals; indeed, the evidence suggests that an ROS enhancement is needed for a muscle adjustment [32, 33].

In a study of Chen and Kotani [34], oxidative stress in premenopausal women with oral contraceptive therapy, which is now commonly used in millions of women worldwide, was investigated. This treatment is associated with an increased risk of deep vein thrombosis, venous thromboembolism, and stroke, so it is critically important to evaluate risks and benefits of therapies. The results of the study show that use of oral contraceptive therapy may increase oxidative stress levels, independently on traditional cardiovascular risk factors, in premenopausal women, providing new perspectives to the prevention of vascular complications in these subjects.

The cells normally generate reactive oxygen species (ROS) during energy metabolism for the respiratory chain. ROS at low or moderate concentrations have important physiological roles. However, an excessive enhancement of ROS in conditions of oxidative stress may be very harmful. The central nervous system (CNS) is helpless to oxidative stress for its high oxygen consume, for the weak antioxidant systems and terminal differentiation of neurons. Therefore, oxidative stress causes several neurodegenerative illnesses. Also, chemotherapy can cause serious side effects on the CNS and peripheral nervous system (PNS) in treated cancer patients, and then several studies show the involvement of ROS in the neurotoxicity induced by drugs. For this reason, the growth of neuroprotective drugs such as antioxidants can be considered a beneficial strategy for clinical treatment [35].

The worldwide incidence of diabetes mellitus (DM) has recently increased rapidly due to lifestyle changes, with DM projected to affect over 300 million people in the last years. DM is related to several complications and poor quality of life of the affected patients; this also leads to an increase in health spending. DM can lead not only to microangiopathy (related to major complications of diabetes, such as diabetic retinopathy, nephropathy, and neuropathy) but can also be considered a major risk factor for macroangiopathy, like coronary heart and cerebrovascular diseases. Moreover, oxidative stress can be an important factor for the development and progression of diabetic complications, related to insulin resistance and reduced insulin secretion with consequent development of DM. Therefore, the oxidative stress in DM is an important factor involved in the development of diabetic complications and in that of the same DM [36].

Numerous studies have shown that the transition metals could be affected in the pathogenesis of various neurodegenerative diseases for their ability to produce oxidative stress. Alzheimer's disease is the most common cause of dementia in older people. The metals, such as iron and copper, which can catalyze the Fenton's reaction by reactive oxygen species, are highly concentrated within the neuritic plaques that represent the features of the Alzheimer's disease brain.

A large body of experimental and *postmortem* findings indicates that Alzheimer's disease is associated with increased oxidative stress levels in the brain. Despite the current limitations of oxidative stress assessment in living subjects, recent data suggest that oxidative challenge might increase early both in the central nervous system and peripheral fluids [37].

7. Antioxidants and disease prevention

Numerous studies show that diets high in fruits and vegetables are protective against cardiovascular diseases (CVD), several kinds of cancer, and other chronic diseases. However, although a broad consensus, it is still unclear what their mechanism(s) of action enable the protection against certain diseases. The antioxidant hypothesis connects the high content of antioxidant molecules found in plant foods and their health benefits by a direct impact on the decrease of oxidative stress.

Some clinical studies have shown contrasting results: some showing protective effects, while others do not. Antioxidants do not act just in isolation or in synergistic interactions; it should be taken into account that in part they are involved in the antioxidant regeneration. The data emerged from these studies are that dietary and endogenous antioxidants, with various activities and features, act synergistically contributing to the overall effect of protective plant foods.

The efficacy of the nonenzymatic antioxidant barrier can be evaluated by determining the total antioxidant capacity (TAC), termed as moles of oxidizing neutralized by 1 L of the sample tested. TAC treats the cumulative action of all antioxidants in the matrix, thus providing an integrated parameter instead of the simple sum for measurable antioxidants, giving a view balance among antioxidant molecules. Some experiments have shown that plasma TAC of patients with various chronic diseases such as diabetes, AIDS, ulcerative colitis, Crohn's disease, meningitis, cardiovascular diseases, colorectal, lung and breast cancer, is much lower than in healthy controls, suggesting impairment of antioxidant barrier in the development of these pathologies.

In order to optimize the intake of dietary antioxidants, particular attention should be paid to the possibility that the interaction between foods consumed in a meal might affect the *in vivo* efficiency of dietary antioxidants [38].

Lycopenes, which represent more than 80% of the total tomato carotenoids, can reduce the risk of cardiovascular disease by inhibiting cholesterol synthesis, reducing the expression of cell surface adhesion molecules and the binding of monocytes to endothelial cells, and modulating LDL (low-density lipoprotein) susceptibility to oxidation. *In vitro* studies demonstrated that the highest beneficial effects as a cancer preventive of lycopene in the diet occur when it is associated with other compounds. A recent study suggests that α-tocopherol or whole tomato lipophilic extracts (containing more than 80% lycopene along with other compounds) potentiate the effects of lycopene during oxidative stress [39].

Neurons are particularly prone to oxidative stress. Particularly, ROS were shown implicated in the pathology of a number of neurological disorders. The brain, mostly neuronal plasma-membranes, houses large concentrations of polyunsaturated fatty acids, which may undergo lipid peroxidation in such an oxygen-rich environment. Brain catecholamines easily undergo auto-oxidation phenomena, thus generating reactive oxygen species. Furthermore, brain contains conspicuous amount of iron (a powerful catalyst of free radical generation), although in an inactive form (chelated). Physiologically, brain exhibits low antioxidant defenses (vitamin C, vitamin E, glutathione, and superoxide dismutase); moreover, reduced levels of antioxidants such as vitamins E and C have been reported in many neurological conditions. It was demonstrated that vitamin E supplementation in deficient individuals is able to either prevent or at least halt the progression of many neurological features. However, supplementation of vitamin E in patients suffering from Parkinson's disease had no apparent benefits [40].

The study has compared the activity and bioavailability of some antioxidants, which have been used in doses very close to those of an average daily meal. Three different formulations (F1, F2, and F3) were tried. Each one was prepared both in fluid and dry formulations and given to the same group of subjects for 1 week. The antioxidants provided in combination with a dosage near to one RDA (Recommended Daily Allowance) decreased oxidative stress, and the fluid formulation was found to be more active and bioavailable than the dry one. The antioxidants present in F1 are those with affinity for membranes (vitamin A, vitamin E, and carotene), minerals (selenium and zinc), components of antioxidant enzymes, and L-cysteine, which is needed for the synthesis of glutathione peroxidase. In F2, the antioxidants comprise circulating substances (vitamin C, bioflavonoids, and vitamin B-6) and a cytosol antioxidant (coenzyme Q10). In this study, F1 was significantly more active than F2, and F3 enhances the F1 activity without a true synergism. Nevertheless, especially in healthy subjects, the existence of a "roof" effect of antioxidants cannot be ruled. The antioxidant activity can be much more evident in subjects with a chronic oxidative stress. A group of antioxidants in low doses decreased oxidative stress as highlighted by the values expressed as U CARR. Since oxidative stress is important for the prevention and/or treatment of an illness, the dROMs' test appears to be a suitable instrument with which to identify the type and dose of antioxidants [41].

Ascorbic acid (ascorbate or vitamin C) has a controversial history in cancer treatment. Pharmacologic concentrations of ascorbate, only achievable by intravenous (i.v.) administration, produce H_2O_2, causing cancer and cell death *in vitro* [42]. Parenteral administration of ascorbate in pharmacologic doses produces millimolar concentrations in blood and extracellular fluid, with preferential generation of Asc•, the product of a loss of one electron from ascorbate, and H_2O_2 in extracellular fluid but not blood. When ascorbate is given parenterally, Asc• is detected preferentially in extracellular fluid compared with blood. Asc• generation in extracellular fluid depended on the ascorbate dose and the resulting concentrations. These findings are all consistent with the hypothesis that pharmacologic ascorbate concentrations *in vivo* serve as a prodrug for selective delivery of H_2O_2 to the extracellular space. In humans, these experiments are based on principles of tight control of ascorbate. After oral ingestion, control of intracellular and extracellular ascorbate concentrations is mediated by three mechanisms: intestinal absorption, tissue transport, and renal reabsorption. These three mechanisms work in coordination with each other, ensuring that ascorbate is tightly controlled. Parenteral administration bypasses tight control, which is restored as kidneys excrete ascorbate. The results demonstrate an explanation on why tight control happens. If the tight control is exceeded, H_2O_2 is formed into the extracellular space. When tight control is reset, the production of H_2O_2 stops. If there was no tight control, the formation of H_2O_2 and exposure to it could be steady, with disagreeable impact on division and cell growth. Tight control prevents continued exposure of tissues to high concentrations of H_2O_2. Bypassing provisionally the tight control with the ascorbate parenteral administration, H_2O_2 is able to form for only a fair period of time, decreasing the damage, and gives a drug for therapeutic of i.v. use of ascorbate [43].

Also, endothelium performs an important role in the regulation of vascular tone, platelet activity, leukocyte adhesion, and thrombosis, and is also implicated in the development of atherosclerosis. In patients with determined coronary heart disease or coronary risk factor, endothelial dysfunction was observed. Treatment with lipid lowering drugs, ACE (Angiotensin Converting Enzyme inhibitor) inhibitors, physical activity, and antioxidant agents has shown an improvement in endothelial function in the coronary and peripheral vessels. Vitamin C is a very efficient antioxidant, and is a scavenger of several reactive oxygen species, such as superoxide anion and peroxynitrite. Several researches have demonstrated that the beneficial effect of vitamin C (24 mg/min) on endothelial dysfunction in subjects with risk factors or coronary artery disorders is specific, because it was observed neither in healthy control subjects nor on the endothelium-independent vasodilation induced by nitroglycerin or SNP (Sodium Nitroprusside) [44].

8. Conclusions

An unhealthy diet, alcohol abuse, chronic intake of drugs, cigarette smoking, inadequate exercise, and environmental pollution are just some causes of a particular form of "stress" which experts have called "oxidative stress" [45]. It is very different and definitely more dangerous than the more common "emotional distress" that affects every day much of the population in Western countries with high economic level [46]. Oxidative stress is a form of "chemical stress" induced by the presence, in our organism, of high quantities of harmful substances acting as oxidants, whose members are the most dangerous oxygen free radicals [47].

Oxidative stress is considered responsible for premature and many diseases ranging from hypertension to atherosclerosis, infarction to stroke, from Parkinson's to Alzheimer's disease, from colitis to pancreatitis, from obesity to diabetes, from chronic bronchitis to rheumatoid arthritis, from AIDS to several forms of cancer [48, 49]. Oxidative stress is much more sneaky, because it gives rise to characteristic symptoms, or to a particular clinical picture, because its causes are to be found in "invisible" entities, such as free radicals [50]. Therefore, the clinician could not suspect the existence; oxidative stress does not provide any evidence to suggest a more detailed diagnosis, when performing simple laboratory tests allow to understand immediately the problem, avoiding the patient a series of consequences such compromise the duration and/or the quality of life in the short or medium term. It is not currently provided for the execution of any preliminary laboratory tests, although available for clinical routine, to show—by means of the quantification in the blood of suitable biochemical markers—the objective need for such formulations. While it is now known that a cholesterol-lowering drug is taken only after a test that has documented a high blood level of cholesterol, it is now an increasingly widespread tendency to assume antioxidants even without the documentation in the blood, an increase in the level of free radicals and/or a reduction of its "physiological" antioxidant defenses. It is not yet a good practice to perform a preliminary evaluation of the laboratory of oxidative stress.

However, the scientific evidence supports that only adequate assessment biochemistry may allow the identification and the definition of a state of oxidative stress and make monitoring of a possible antioxidant therapy. Because of these specific tests for the evaluation and determination of free radicals and antioxidant defenses, it makes the initial diagnosis of oxidative stress extremely accurate and reliable, whether the two opposite components, either pro- or antioxidant, are measured separately [51]. It is possible to determine in real time whether oxidative stress is due to an increased production and/or a reduced ability to eliminate free radicals. It would be appropriate to undergo the oxidative stress evaluation, even in good health and, more so, when exposed to pro-oxidant

http://dx.doi.org/10.5772/64577

factors (e.g., incorrect lifestyles, excessive aerobic exercise, and pollutants in the workplace) or when affected from chronic degenerative diseases (e.g., diabetes, atherosclerosis, cancer, dementia, and rheumatoid arthritis) or, eventually, when performed specific treatments (e.g., dialysis, by-pass, organ transplant, radiotherapy, and chemotherapy) [52, 53]. For this evaluation it will be possible to use specific therapies and to monitor the real efficacy of antioxidants, too often assumed without a preliminary test able to demonstrate its necessity. The same "prescription" of supplements, finally, will lean—in this sensitive field—on a more solid and leave the empirical phase in which it often finds itself.

The evaluation of a real state of oxidative stress may be covered in the predictive medicine area. Predictive medicine is the emerging field of medicine that entails predicting the probability of disease and taking proactive steps to either prevent the disease altogether or significantly decrease its impact upon the patient (such as by preventing mortality or limiting morbidity). The aim of predictive medicine is to predict the likelihood of disease so that healthcare providers and the patients will have an active role in changing the way of life and increase the medical surveillance, such as complete biannual skin examinations by a dermatologist or internist if their patient is found to have an increased risk of melanoma; an ECG and cardiac examination by a cardiologist if a patient has an increased risk of cardiac arrhythmia or alternating magnetic resonance imaging (MRI); or mammograms if a patient has an increased risk of breast cancer. Predictive medicine is useful for both healthy individuals (predictive health) and those with illnesses (predictive medicine); its aim is to provide information on the possibility of having a disease and to predict the progression and treatment for a specific disease. Aside from genetic testing, predictive medicine utilizes a wide variety of tools to predict health and disease, including assessments of exercise, nutrition, spirituality, quality of life, and oxidative stress.

Author details

Simona Tafuri[1], Natascia Cocchia[1], Francesco Landolfi[2], Eugenio Luigi Iorio[3] and Francesca Ciani[1*]

*Address all correspondence to: ciani@unina.it

1 Department of Veterinary Medicine and Animal Productions, University of Naples Federico II, Naples, Italy

2 ASL Na 3 Sud, Castellammare di Stabia, Naples, Italy

3 International Observatory of Oxidative Stress, Salerno, Italy

References

[1] Banfi G., Iorio E.L., Corsi M.M. Oxidative stress, free radicals and bone remodeling. Clin Chem Lab Med. 2008; 46(11); 1550–1555. doi: 10.1515/CCLM.2008.302.

[2] Halliwell B. Antioxidants and human disease: a general introduction. Nutr Rev. 1997; 55; S44–S49.

[3] Bansal A.K., Bilaspuri G.S. Impacts of oxidative stress and antioxidants on semen functions. Vet Med Int. 2010; 2011; 1–7. doi: 10.4061/2011/686137.

[4] Mora-Esteves C., Shin D. Nutrient supplementation: improving male fertility fourfold. Semin Reprodt Med. 2013; 31; 293–300.

[5] Galecka E., Jacewicz R., Mrowicka M., Florkowski A. Galecki P. Antioxidative enzymes —structure, properties, functions. Polski Merkuriusz Lekarski. 2008; 25; 266–268.

[6] Scibior D, Czeczot H. Catalase: structure, properties, functions. Postepy Hig Med Dosw (Online). 2006; 60; 170–180.

[7] Lampiao F. Free radicals generation in an *in vitro* fertilization setting and how to minimize them. World J Obstet Gynecol. 2012; 1; 29–34.

[8] Sies H. Strategies of antioxidant defense. Eur J Biochem. 1993; 21; 213–219.

[9] Park S., Park N.Y., Valacchi G., Lim Y. Calorie restriction with a high-fat diet effectively attenuated inflammatory response and oxidative stress-related markers in obese tissues of the high diet fed rats. Mediat Inflammation. 2012; 2012; 1–11. doi: 10.1155/2012/984643.

[10] Manach C., Williamson G., Morand C., Scalbert A., Rémésy C. Bioavailability and bioefficacy of polyphenols in humans. I. Review of 97 bioavailability studies. Am J Clin Nutr. 2005; 81(Suppl); 230S–242S.

[11] Iorio E-L., Ferreri C. Lipidomics [original title "Lipidomica"]. In: Italian Treatise of Laboratory Medicine [original title "Trattato Italiano di Medicina di Laboratorio"]. Angelo Burlina (Ed)., Piccin, Padua (Italy). 2009; pp. 341–360.

[12] Iorio E.L., Marin M.G. Redoxomics. An integrated and practical approach to genomics, metabolomics and lipidomics to manage oxidative stress. Gen-T. 2008; 2; 67.

[13] Dalle-Donne I., Scaloni A., Butterfield D.A. Redox Proteomics: from Protein Modifications to Cellular Dysfunction and Diseases. Wiley Press, New York. 2006.

[14] Iorio E.L. New perspectives in oxidative stress research: the Redoxomics. Proceedings International Conference on Advances in Free Radicals Research, Natural Products, Antioxidants and Radioprotectors in Health—Ninth Annual Meeting of the Society of Free Radical Research India. January 11–13, 2010. Hyderabad (India). 2010; pp. 26–27.

[15] Iorio E.L. The novel field of Redoxomics. Proceedings BIT Life Sciences' 3rd Annual PepCon-2010. March 21–23, 2010. Beijing (China). 2010; p. 283.

[16] Iorio E.L., Balestrieri M.L.. The oxidative stress [original title "Lo stress ossidativo"]. In: Italian Treatise of Laboratory Medicine [original title "Trattato Italiano di Medicina di Laboratorio"]. Angelo Burlina (Ed.), Piccin, Padua (Italy). 2009; pp. 533–549.

[17] Szabo S., Tache Y., Somogyi A. The legacy of Hans Selye and the origins of stress research: a retrospective 75 years after his landmark. Brief "Letter" to the Editor of Nature. Stress. 2012; 15(5); 472–478.

[18] Shang X.J., Li K., Ye Z.Q., Chen Y.G., Yu X., Huang Y.F. Analysis of lipid peroxidative levels in seminal plasma of infertile men by high performance liquid chromatography. Arc Androl. 2004; 50; 411–416.

[19] Aitken R.J., Harkiss D., Buckingham D. Leukocytic infiltration into the human ejaculate and its association with semen quality, oxidative stress, and sperm function. J Reprod Fert. 1993; 98; 257–265.

[20] Loft S., Kold-Jensen T., Hjollund N.H. Oxidative DNA damage in human sperm influences time to pregnancy. Human Reprod. 2003; 18; 1265–1272.

[21] Agarwal A., Makker K., Sharma R. Clinical relevance of oxidative stress in male factor infertility: an update. Am J Reprod Immunol. 2008; 59; 2–11.

[22] Alberti A., Bolognini L., Macciantelli D., Carratelli M. The radical cation of N,N-diethyl-para-phenylendiamine: a possible indicator of oxidative stress in biological samples. Res Chem Intermed. 2000; 26(3); 253–267.

[23] Benzie I.F.F., Strain J.J. The ferric redicing ability of plasma (FRAP) as a measure of "antioxidant power": the FRAP assay. Anal Biochem. 1996; 239; 70–76.

[24] Said T.M., Kattal N., Sharma R.K. Enhanced chemiluminescence assay vs colorimetric assay for measurement of the total antioxidant capacity of human seminal plasma. J Androlol. 2003; 24; 676–680.

[25] Pasquini A., Luchetti E., Marchetti V., CardiniG., Iorio E.L. Analytical performances of d-ROMs test and BAP test in canine plasma. Definition of the normal range in healthy Labrador dogs. Vet Res Commun. 2008; 32; 137–143. doi 10.1007/s11259-007-9014-x.

[26] Flore R., Gerardino L., Santoliquido A., Pola R., Flex A., Di Campli C., Pola P., Tondi P. Enhanced oxidative stress in workers with a standing occupation. Occup Environ Med. 2004; 61; 548–550. doi: 10.1136/oem.2003.008805.

[27] Tamaki N., Tomofuji T., Ekuni D., Yamanaka R., Yamamoto T, Morita M. Short-term effects of non-surgical periodontal treatment on plasma level of reactive oxygen metabolites in patients with chronic periodontitis. J Periodontol. 2009; 80(6); 901–906. doi: 10.1902/jop.2009.080640.

[28] Church D.F., Pryor W.A. Free radical chemistry of cigarette smoke and its toxicological implications. Environ Health Perspect. 1985; 64; 111–126.

[29] Dal Negro R.W., Visconti M., Micheletto C., Tognella S. Changes in blood ROS, e-NO, and some pro-inflammatory mediators in bronchial secretions following erdosteine or placebo: a controlled study in current smokers with mild COPD. Pulm Pharm Ther. 2008; 21¸304–308.

[30] Trotti R., Carratelli M., Barbieri M., Micieli G., Bosone D., Rondanelli M., Bo P. Oxidative stress and a thrombophilic condition in alcoholics without severe liver disease. Haematologica. 2001; 86; 85–91.

[31] Jackson M.J. Handbook of Oxidants and Antioxidants in Exercise. In: Hanninen O., Packer L., Sen C.K. (Eds.), Elsevier, Amsterdam. 2000; pp. 57–68.

[32] Jackson, M.J. Free radicals in skin and muscle: damaging agents or signals for adaptation? Proc Nutr Soc 1999; 58(3); 673–676.

[33] Iorio E.L. d-ROMs test in sport. Cosmetic News. 2004; 157; 272–275.

[34] Chen J.-T., Kotani K. Oral contraceptive therapy increases oxidative stress in pre menopausal women. Int J Prev Med. 2012; 3(12); 893–896.

[35] Li J., Wuliji O., Li W., Jiang Z-G., Ghanbari H.A. Oxidative stress and neurodegenerative disorders. Int J Mol Sci. 2013;14(12):24438–24475. doi: 10.3390/ijms141224438.

[36] Kayama Y., Raaz U., Jagger A., Adam M., Schellinger I.N., Sakamoto M., Suzuki H., Toyama K., Spin J.M., Tsao P.S. Diabetic cardiovascular disease induced by oxidative stress. Int J Mol Sci. 2015; 16(10); 25234–63. doi: 10.3390/ijms161025234.

[37] Squitti R. Metals in Alzheimer's disease: a systemic perspective. Front Biosci (Landmark Ed). 2012; 17; 451–72.

[38] Serafini M., The role of antioxidants in disease prevention. Medicine. 2006; 34; 512 533.

[39] Balestrieri M.L., De Prisco R., Nicolaus B., Pari P., Schiano Moriello V., Strazzullo G., Iorio E.L, Servillo L., Balestrieri C. Lycopene in association with a-tocopherol or tomato lipophilic extracts enhances acyl-platelet-activating factor biosynthesis in endothelial cells during oxidative stress. Free Radical Biol Med. 2004; 36(8); 1058–1067.

[40] Uttara B., Singh A.V., Zamboni P., Mahajan R.T. Oxidative stress and neurodegenerative diseases: a review of upstream and downstream antioxidant therapeutic options. Curr Neuropharmacol. 2009; 7(1); 65–74.

[41] Cornelli U., Terranova R., Luca S., Cornelli M., Alberti A. Bioavailability and antioxidant activity of some food supplements in men and women using the D-Roms test as a marker of oxidative stress. J Nutr. 2001; 131(12); 3208–3211.

[42] Chen Q., Espey M.G., Sun A.Y., Pooput C., Kenneth C.P., Kirk L., Murali L.K., Krishna M.C., Khosh D.B., Drisko J., Levine M. Pharmacologic doses of ascorbate act as a

prooxidant and decrease growth of aggressive tumor xenografts in mice. PNAS. 2008; 105(32); 11105–11109.

[43] Chen Q., Espey M.G., Andrew Y. Sun A.Y., Lee J-H., Krishna M.C., Shacter E., Choyke P.L., Pooput C., Kirk K.L., Buettner G.R., Levine M. Ascorbate in pharmacologic concentrations selectively generates ascorbate radical and hydrogen peroxide in extracellular fluid *in vivo*. PNAS. 2007; 104 (21); 8749–8754.

[44] Heitzer T., Schlinzig T., Krohn K., Meinertz T., Münzel T. Endothelial dysfunction, oxidative stress, and risk of cardiovascular events in patients with coronary artery disease. Circulation. 2001; 104(22); 2673–2678.

[45] Iorio E.L. Oxidative stress as a risk factor for health. The role of the environmental factors. Proceedings Days Medical-Surgical Romane "Environment: health or disease". October 31, 2003. Rome. 2003.

[46] Cornelli U., Cornelli M., Terranova R., Luca S., Belcaro G. Importance of oxidative stress as a risk factor for morbidity. The Med Biol .2000; 1; 13–18.

[47] Halliwell B. Free radicals, antioxidants, and human disease: curiosity, cause, or consequence? Lancet. 1994; 344; 721–724.

[48] Iorio E.L. The global assessment of oxidative stress. The Clinical Pathologist. 2003; 5/6; 155–159.

[49] Carratelli M., Iorio E.L., Bianchi L. Methods of oxidative stress measurement.. ADI 2 Magazine. 2006; 4(10); 405–414.

[50] Ridker P.M., Brown N.J., Vaughan D.E., et al. Established and emerging plasma biomarkers in the prediction of first atherothrombotic events. Circulation. 2004; 109 (Suppl. IV); IV-6–IV-19.

[51] Iorio E.L., Cinquanta L., Pisano R. A diagnostic algorithm to manage oxidative stress. Austral J Cosmet Surg. 2006; 2 (1); 26–30.

[52] Carratelli M., Iorio E.L. Potential usefulness of oxidative stress in nutrition and food supplementation. Proceedings IV Greek Congress on Free Radicals and Oxidative Stress. October, 7–10, 2004. Larissa, Greece. 2004; 15.

[53] Iorio E.L. d-ROMs test in sport. Cosmetic News. 2004; 157; 272–275.

Chapter 8

The Role of *Attractin* in Neurodegeneration Caused by Oxidative Stress

Ayuka Ehara, Shin-ichi Sakakibara and Shuichi Ueda

Additional information is available at the end of the chapter

http://dx.doi.org/10.5772/63330

Abstract

Oxidative stress is linked to dopaminergic (DA) neurodegeneration in Parkinson's disease. Our laboratory reported slowly progressive DA neurodegeneration in the zitter (*zi*) rat, which is *Attractin* (*Atrn*) deficient. However, little is known about the function of *Atrn* in the central nervous system (CNS). Thus, we investigated whether DA neurodegeneration in the *zi* rat was induced by oxidative stress, and how *Atrn* affects oxidative stress. First, we summarize our previous *in vivo* data, which revealed suppression of DA neurodegeneration using antioxidants (vitamin E and melatonin) in *zi* rats. Second, our current *ex vivo* and *in vitro* studies are introduced. Using primary neuronal cultures of *zi* mesencephalon as a model of *Atrn*-deficient neurons or *Atrn*-GFP-overexpressing HEK293 cells, accumulation of reactive oxygen species (ROS) in mitochondria and cell viability was examined under oxidative stress. *Atrn*-deficient neurons accumulated excess ROS in mitochondria, resulting in neurodegeneration, whereas *Atrn*-overexpressing cells showed suppression of ROS accumulation under oxidative stress. These results showed that *Atrn* plays a suppressive role against ROS and that the loss of *Atrn* function induced excess ROS accumulation and led to DA neurodegeneration. This is the first report to show that *Atrn* directly modulates mitochondrial ROS accumulation in the CNS.

Keywords: dopaminergic neurodegeneration, *Attractin*, reactive oxygen species, Parkinson's disease, oxidative stress

1. Introduction

Oxidative stress is considered to be the cause of several neurological diseases. In particular, dopaminergic (DA) neurons are vulnerable to oxidative stress, which is normally generated by dopamine metabolism [1, 2]. The progressive DA neurodegeneration that occurs with age in Parkinson's disease (PD) is caused by increased oxidative stress. The neurotoxins 1-methyl-4-phenyl-1,2,3,6-tetrahydropyridine and6-hydroxydopamine induce free radicals (H_2O_2, O_2^-,and OH) that destroy DA neurons [3, 4] and are used to produce acute animal models of PD. Recently, we reported slowly progressive DA neurodegeneration, which is similar to the symptoms of humans with PD, in a mutant rat, the *zitter* (*zi*) rat [5].

The *zi* rat, which occurred in a colony of Sprague-Dawley (SD) rats, is a spontaneous autosomal recessive mutant rat with body tremors. The gene symbol of the mutation is designated *zi* (zitter means shake and tremble in German). The rats develop the tremor at around 15 days of age and progressive flaccid paresis of hind limbs at 6 months of age. The behavioral defects are associated with progressive hypomyelination and vacuolation in the central nervous system (CNS) [6]. *Zi* is homozygous for an 8-bp deletion in intron 12 of *Attractin* (*Atrn*) [7]. *Atrn* is involved in regulating physiological processes such as initial immune cell clustering during an inflammatory response, melanocortin signaling pathways that regulate energy homeostasis, pigmentation, and normal myelination in the CNS. *Atrn* encodes a protein that is secreted or transmembrane form as a result of alternative splicing of the same mRNA. Both forms of the protein have several domains in common such as epidermal growth factor-related domains, a CUB domain, and a C-type lectin. The transmembrane form, which has a transmembrane domain, has a long N-terminal extracellular domain. Rats and humans express both secreted and transmembrane proteins. However, mice express only the transmembrane protein. The *zi* rat expresses neither the secreted nor the transmembrane form of Atrn proteins. The abnormalities in the CNS of *zi* rats are mainly caused by the loss of the transmembrane form [7].

Our laboratory first reported DA neurodegeneration that occurs with age in *zi* rats [5]. In particular, the nigrostriatal DA pathway shows the most severe progressive neurodegeneration. In the substantia nigra pars compacta (SNc), a significant decrease in the number of DA neurons is detected from 2 months of age in *zi* rats, whereas no difference is detected at 1 month of age between *zi* rats and wild-type SD rats [8, 9]. With age, the number of DA neurons decreases significantly [8] (**Figure 1**). Loss of DA neurons in the SNc results in a decrease in the number of DA fibers and terminals in the dorsolateral caudate putamen (CPu), which receives DA input from the SNc. Consequently, the level of dopamine in the CPu of *zi* rats at 12 months of age is decreased to one-seventh of that in age-matched SD rats [8].

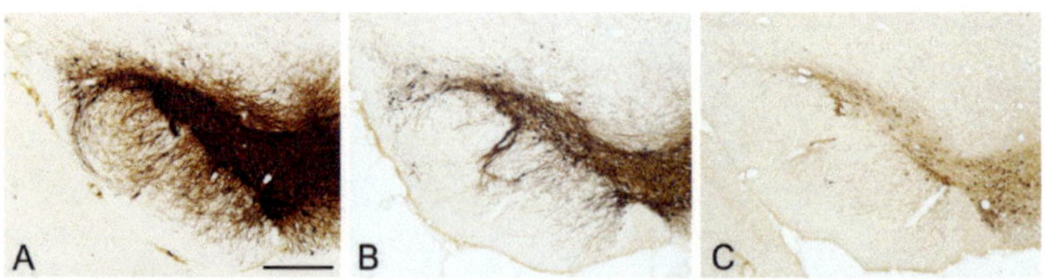

Figure 1. Progressive dopaminergic neurodegeneration with age in *zi* rats. Tyrosine hydroxylase-immunoreactive cells in the substantia nigra at 1 month (A), 6 months (B), and 12 months (C) of age. Scale bar: 500 μm.

Previous studies have indicated that *zi* rats show abnormal activities of some antioxidant enzymes in the brain and tend to accumulate reactive oxygen species (ROS) [10–13]. Examination of the ultrastructure of DA neurons in the SNc of *zi* rats reveals abnormal mitochondria with disrupted and enlarged cristae [9]. Additionally, *Atrn* null mice show reduced complex IV activity (cytochrome c oxidase activity) [14]. Complex IV is an enzyme in the respiratory electron transport chain in mitochondria. It was suggested that *Atrn* regulated ROS production in mitochondria. Therefore, we hypothesized that the neurodegeneration in *zi* rats is due to oxidative stress, and thus, we investigated whether antioxidants can protect against neurodegeneration in the mutant. Furthermore, to investigate whether *Atrn* is directly involved in regulation of the ROS-producing system in neurons, we established primary neuronal cultures from *zi* rats to represent *Atrn*-deficit neurons, and an *Atrn*-overexpressing cell line. Using these cells, we examined the viability and ROS accumulation under several oxidative stress conditions.

2. Materials and methods

2.1. Reagents

Materials for cultures were B27 supplement, B27 supplement minus antioxidants (AO (–)), neurobasal medium, Opti-MEM, and penicillin/streptomycin from Gibco (Life Technologies; Carlsbad, CA); MitoTracker Red CM-H_2Xros, MitoTracker green FM, and Lipofectamine Plus Reagent from Invitrogen (Life Technologies); cell proliferation reagent WST-1 from Roche Diagnostics (Basel, Switzerland); cytosine-arabinofuranoside, l-glutamine, and poly-l-lysine from Sigma-Aldrich (St. Louis, MO); pAcGFP1-N1 vector from Clontech Laboratories Inc. (Mountain View, CA). Reagents for the immunocytochemistry were purchased from the following sources: biotinylated horse anti-mouse IgG, normal goat serum, and vectastain ABC kit from Vector (Burlingame, CA); anti-tyrosine hydroxylase (TH) antibody from Incstar (Stillwater, MN); Alexa Fluor 488 goat anti-mouse IgG from Molecular Probes (Life Technologies).

2.2. *In vivo* study

Male *zitter* rats were housed in-groups of two or three in a cage with food and water ad libitum. The room was maintained at a constant temperature and humidity with a 12 h light/dark cycle in the Laboratory Animal Research Center at Dokkyo University School of Medicine. All procedures in this study were certified by the Animal Welfare Committee at Dokkyo University School of Medicine and were conducted in accordance with NIH guidelines. Between 1 and 10 months of age, we fed *zi* rats a diet supplied with vitamin E (500 mg d-, l-alpha-tocopherol/kg diet) or administered oral melatonin at dose of 0.5 mg/ml in drinking water, as previously reported [13, 15]. Tissue preparation and immunohistochemical procedure were described previously [5].

2.3. *Ex vivo* study

Ventral mesencephalic neurons were prepared from fetal *zi* and SD rats (Charles River Laboratories, Tsukuba, Japan) at gestation day 14. Cells were seeded in 24-well plates at a density of 2 × 10^5 cells/cm^2. Wells (for the cell viability assay and ROS assay) or cover glasses (for immunofluorescence, 15-mm diameter) were pre-treated with poly-l-lysine (0.1 mg/ml). After 2 h of initial plating, the medium was changed to neurobasal medium (containing penicillin/streptomycin and l-glutamine) supplemented with B27. Cultures were maintained at 37°C in a humidified 5% CO_2 incubator (Revco Ultima RCO5000T, Thermo Fisher Scientific; Asheville, NC). To obtain neuron-enriched cultures, cytosine-arabinofuranoside (7.5 μM) was added beginning at 2 days *in vitro* (DIV) to 6 DIV. At 6 DIV, neurons were divided into two groups and cultured in neurobasal medium supplemented with B27 (Cont) or B27 without antioxidants (AO (−)), consisting of B27 supplement without vitamin E, vitamin E acetate, superoxide dismutase (SOD), catalase, or glutathione (GSH). Cultures were used for experiments at 11 DIV. Over 95% of the cells in the cultures were neurons as determined by immunostaining for the neuron-specific marker microtubule-associated protein-2 (data not shown).

The cell viability assay was performed by using the cell proliferation reagent WST-1 according to the manufacturer's protocol. Cell viability was expressed as a percent of the values of SD-Cont.

ROS accumulation was monitored with a plate reader using MitoTracker Red CM-H_2Xros (MTR). Neurons were co-stained with 0.5 μM MTR and 0.2 μM MitoTracker green (MTG: mitochondria marker) in Opti-MEM for 30 min at 37°C and then assessed (MTR, excitation 535 nm, barrier filter 595 nm; MTG, excitation 485 nm, barrier filter 535 nm). The MTR/MTG ratio of each group was normalized to that of SD-Cont, which was used as an index of ROS content.

Immunofluorescence procedure was described previously [16].

2.4. *In vitro* study

Atrn cDNA, which encodes full-length membrane-type rat *Atrn*, was cleaved from pCAGGS-neo-*Atrn* (kind gift from Dr. Kenzo Sato, Tottori University) and inserted into the pAcGFP1-N1 vector as a ~4.3-kb *Eco* R1-*Bam* HI fragment. After cloning, insertion of the fusion sequence into the plasmid was confirmed. HEK293 cells (1.5 × 10^4 cells/10-mm glass bottom dish) were transfected with 0.1 μg *Atrn*-GFP or GFP (as a control) plasmid using Lipofectamine Plus Reagent. At 18 h after transfection, cells were incubated with 0.5 μM MTR for 30 min at 37°C. Fluorescence images of living cells were scanned with a confocal laser-scanning microscope (LSM 510 META; Carl Zeiss, Jena, Germany) using a 60× 1.4-NA oil-immersion objective. Under the microscope, cells were exposed to 1 mM H_2O_2 in Opti-MEM and observed for 60 min.

http://dx.doi.org/10.5772/63330

3. Results

3.1. The effect of antioxidants on DA neurodegeneration in *zi* rats

We treated *zi* rats with the antioxidants vitamin E and melatonin. Between 1 and 10 months of age, we fed *zi* rats a diet supplied with vitamin E, which is a lipid-soluble peroxyl radical scavenger. Chronic vitamin E feeding suppressed DA neuron death in the SNc (**Figure 2B**). The number of DA neurons in *zi* rats treated with vitamin E was 1.5 times higher than that in control *zi* rats [15]. However, vitamin E protected few DA fibers and terminals in the CPu of *zi* rats (data not shown).

Melatonin, which is a synthetic product of the pineal gland, is a direct free radical scavenger and an indirect antioxidant. Melatonin readily crosses the blood-brain barrier and plays a role in protecting against ROS in the brain. Chronic melatonin administration suppressed DA neuron death in the SNc of *zi* rats (**Figure 2C**). The number of DA neurons in *zi* rats treated with melatonin was two times higher than that in control *zi* rats [13]. In the CPu, DA fibers and terminals were protected by melatonin, and *zi* rats administered chronic melatonin showed twice as much dopamine as control *zi* rats [8, 13]. Melatonin protected DA neuronal somas, fibers, and terminals in both the SNc and the CPu of *zi* rats.

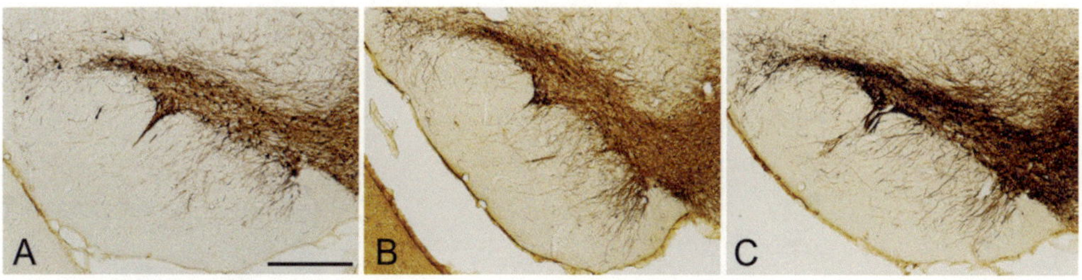

Figure 2. Antioxidants suppressed dopaminergic neurodegeneration in *zi* rats. Tyrosine hydroxylase-immunoreactive cells in the substantia nigra at 10 months of age in *zi* rats (A) or *zi* rats treated with vitamin E (B) or melatonin (C) for 9 months. Scale bar: 500 μm.

Antioxidants were effective for preventing DA neurodegeneration in *zi* rats, indicating that the DA neurodegeneration in the mutant rats is caused by oxidative stress.

3.2. Accumulation of ROS in *zi* mesencephalic neurons *ex vivo*

To investigate whether ROS accumulation in mesencephalic neurons is caused by a genetic factor of the *Atrn* mutation, we established primary mesencephalic neuronal cultures from *zi* rats and compared them with cultures from wild-type SD rats. Neurons were cultured under an individual condition with (Cont) or without antioxidants (AO (−)), consisting of B27 supplement without vitamin E, vitamin E acetate, SOD, catalase, or GSH. We analyzed the cell viability and ROS content according to two factors: genotype (*zi* or wild type) and supplement (AO (−) or Cont).

Cell viability was shown in **Figure 3A**. Two-way analysis of variance (ANOVA) revealed significant effects of the supplement ($P = 1.98 \times 10^{-8}$) and an interaction of genotype × supplement ($P = 8.73 \times 10^{-6}$), but no effect of genotype ($P = 0.493$). Mesencephalic neurons from *zi* rats showed significantly lower cell viability in AO (−) supplement compared to Cont supplement ($P < 1 \times 10^{-8}$). However, the cell viability of neurons from wild-type SD rats was significantly lower in AO (−) supplement ($P = 0.0085$), the decreasing rate was considerably less than that of *zi* rats.

Next, ROS accumulation in mitochondria was monitored using MTR, which produces intense fluorescence depending on ROS accumulation in mitochondria (**Figure 3B**). Two-way ANOVA revealed significant effects of genotype ($P = 6.21 \times 10^{-4}$), supplement ($P = 0.0016$), and an interaction of genotype × supplement ($P = 0.0026$). Mesencephalic neurons from *zi* rats showed significantly higher ROS content in AO (−) ($P = 0.0011$ compared with Cont supplement in *zi* rats), whereas that of the wild type showed low ROS content and no difference between AO (−) and Cont supplements ($P = 0.994$). With Cont supplement, the ROS content was not different according to genotype ($P = 0.875$ *zi* neurons vs. SD neurons).

Because the neurons from *zi* rats showed excessive ROS accumulation, we examined the morphology of DA neurons using immunofluorescence with anti-TH antibody (**Figure 3C**). With Cont supplement, TH-immunoreactive (TH-ir) neurons from *zi* rats had long processes similar to those from wild-type rats (**Figure 3C**, upper column). However, in AO (−), TH-ir neurons had no long processes and formed cell clusters (**Figure 3C**, lower column). These culture experiments revealed that mesencephalic neurons from *zi* rats accumulate excess ROS followed by DA neurodegeneration and death in the absence of exogenous antioxidants.

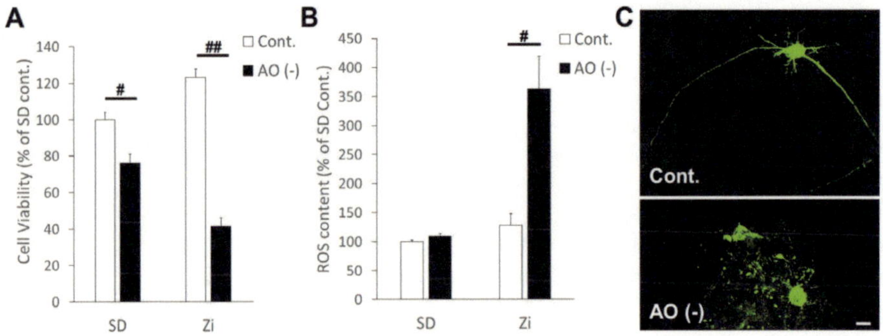

Figure 3. Effects of genotype and supplement factors in primary neuronal cultures from the ventral mesencephalon. Neurons from *zi* rats and wild-type rats (SD rats) were supplemented with B27 (Cont: open bars) or B27 without antioxidants (AO (−): closed bars) for 5 days. (A) Cell viability was measured with a plate reader using WST-1 assay. Data are the percent absorbance at 450 nm versus SD-Cont ($n = 4$). (B) ROS production by mitochondria was detected with a plate reader using MitoTracker Red CM-H_2Xros (MTR). Data are normalized to MitoTracker Green and represent the percent absorbance at 535 nm/485 nm versus SD-Cont ($n = 3$–4). All data are expressed as means ± SEM. Statistical analysis was performed with two-way ANOVA with Turkey post-hoc adjustment for multiple comparisons with a significant level set at #$P< 0.01$ and ##$P< 0.0001$. (C) Immunofluorescence demonstrating the morphological alteration of TH-immunoreactive neurons from *zi* rats in medium with B27 (Cont: upper column) or B27 without antioxidants (AO (−): lower column). Scale bar: 10 μm.

3.3. Suppression of ROS accumulation in *Atrn*-overexpressing cells *in vitro*

To investigate the function of *Atrn* during oxidative stress, ROS accumulation in mitochondria was observed in HEK293 cells that overexpressed *Atrn*-GFP.

ROS accumulation in *Atrn*-GFP-transfected cells was detected 30 min after MTR incubation (**Figure 4**). *Atrn*-GFP-transfected cells (**Figure 4A**) showed lower MTR intensity than the surrounding untransfected cells (**Figure 4C** and **D**).

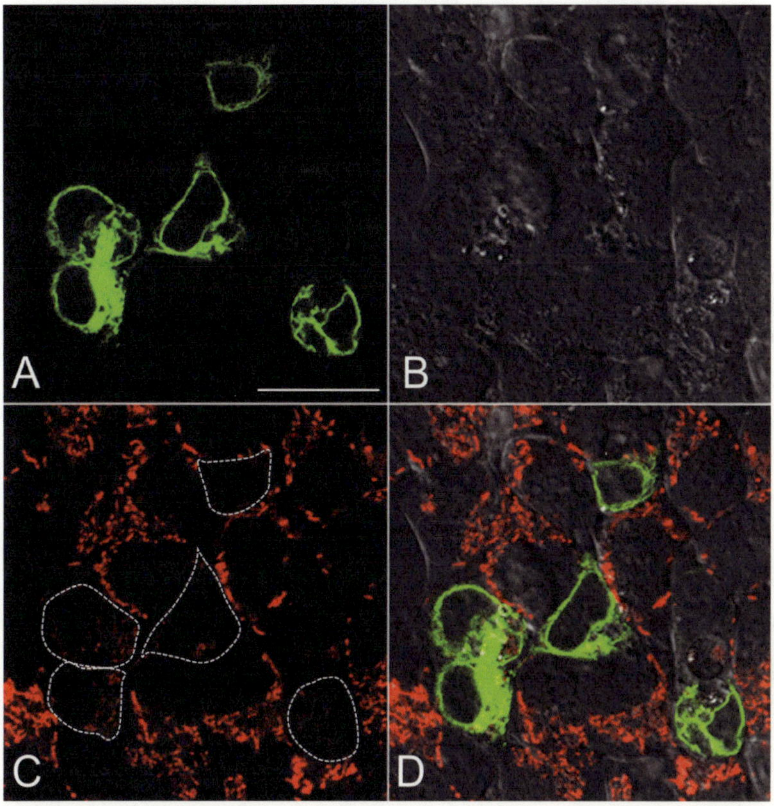

Figure 4. ROS accumulation in *Atrn*-GFP-transfected HEK293 cells. *Atrn*-GFP (A), the corresponding phase-contrast image (B), and MitoTracker Red CM-H_2Xros (C) were merged as shown in (D). White dotted lines (C) show the outline of *Atrn*-GFP-positive cells (A). Scale bar: 50 μm.

Under the microscope, the time of addition of H_2O_2 as a form of oxidative stress was set at 0 min, and live images were scanned at 0 and 60 min (**Figure 5**). *Atrn*-GFP-transfected cells showed little MTR fluorescent intensity at 0 min (**Figure 5C 2–3**) and faint intensity at 60 min (**Figure 5D 2–3**), whereas control transfected cells showed high MTR intensity at 0 min (**Figure 5A 2–3**) and markedly higher intensity at 60 min (**Figure 5B 2–3**). Compared with adjacent cells, *Atrn*-overexpressing cells maintained low MTR intensity under oxidative stress (**Figure 5D 2–3**).

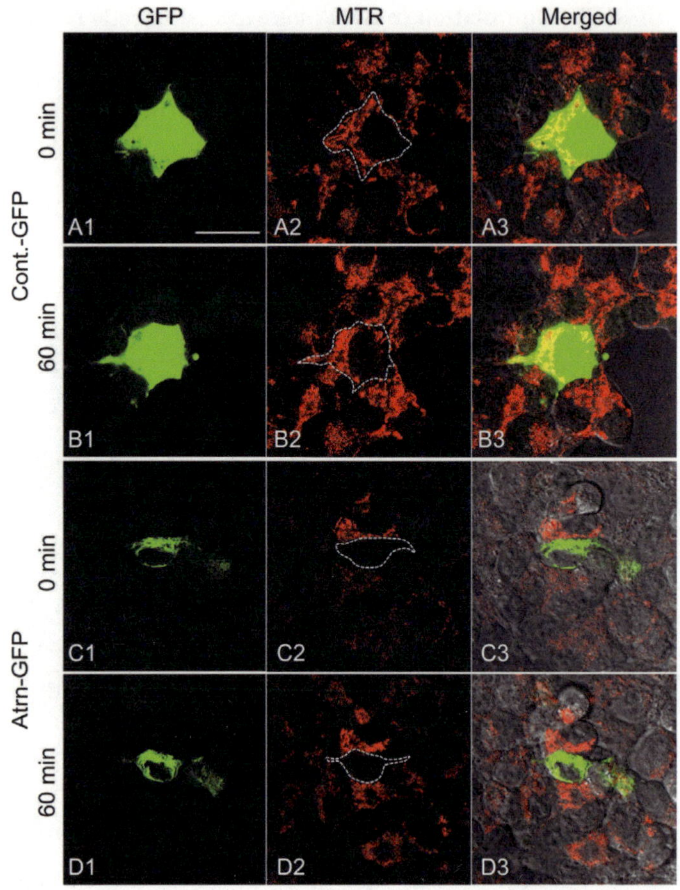

Figure 5. *Attractin* suppressed the accumulation of mitochondrial ROS under oxidative stress. HEK293 cells transfected with Cont-GFP (A, B) or *Atrn*-GFP (C, D) were incubated in medium containing 1 mM H_2O_2 for 60 min. Time-lapse images at 0 min (A, C) and 60 min (B, D) are shown. GFP (1), MitoTracker Red CM-H_2Xros: MTR (2), and the corresponding phase-contrast image were merged into (3). White dotted line (2) shows the outline of GFP-positive cells (1). Scale bar: 50 μm.

4. Discussion

This study revealed that the loss of *Atrn* led to ROS accumulation in mitochondria and resulted in DA neurodegeneration in *zi* rats.

Zi rats accumulate ROS and are vulnerable to oxidative stress, as observed with fibroblast cultures from the *zi/zi* kidney [11]. Moreover, DA neurons are particularly vulnerable to oxidative stress [1, 2]. Based on these observations, our previous studies revealed that the antioxidants vitamin E and melatonin suppress DA neurodegeneration in *zi* rats [5, 13, 15]. Therefore, we hypothesized that the DA neurodegeneration in *zi* rats was caused by oxidative stress. However, whether oxidative stress is directly caused by the genetic factor, *Atrn* gene mutation, was not clear. In the present study, we used *ex vivo* neuronal cultures and showed that this mutation directly led to ROS accumulation in mesencephalic neurons and caused DA neurodegeneration. B27 without the antioxidants vitamin E, vitamin E acetate, SOD, catalase, and GSH was used in this study. *In vivo,* SOD and catalase are produced by neurons, whereas vitamin E and vitamin E acetate are not synthesized in animal cells; GSH is mainly produced by astrocytes [17]. Thus, our result showing that wild-type neurons accumulate little ROS in medium without these five antioxidants indicates that the generated ROS is removed by scavenging agents including SOD and/or catalase in neurons. However, *zi* neurons accumulated significantly excessive ROS in the same medium, indicating that *zi* neurons have little or no endogenous scavenging agents and produce ROS levels that exceed their scavenging ability. This idea is consistent with previous assays using homogenates of *zi* brain tissues, which show abnormal H_2O_2 metabolism [10] and mitochondrial function [14]. In addition, morphological analysis using primary neuronal cultures from *zi* cerebral cortex shows protection from neurodegeneration by the antioxidants, vitamin E and catalase [11]. Additionally, *in vitro* study using DA neuroblastoma cell line shows that overexpressing *Atrn* protects against cell death induced by the neurotoxin 1-methyl-4-phenylpyridinium, which enhances ROS production [12]. Thus, *Atrn* may play a role in the activation of antioxidant enzymes in mitochondria. The observation that overexpression of *Atrn* suppressed ROS accumulation supports this hypothesis. We suggest that a deficiency in *Atrn* directly results in an abnormal antioxidant system and excess ROS accumulation in DA neurons. The findings in the present study will contribute to our understanding of the mechanism of not only DA neurodegeneration but also neurodegeneration of other neurons caused by oxidative stress. Further studies are needed to elucidate these possibilities.

Acknowledgements

This work was supported by research grant from Dokkyo Medical University (Investigator-Initiated Research Grant No.2014-01).

Author details

Ayuka Ehara[1*], Shin-ichi Sakakibara[2] and Shuichi Ueda[1]

*Address all correspondence to: aehara@dokkyomed.ac.jp

1 Departments of Histology and Neurobiology, Dokkyo Medical University School of Medicine, Mibu, Tochigi, Japan

2 Laboratory for Molecular Neurobiology, Graduate School of Human Sciences, Waseda University, Tokorozawa, Saitama, Japan

References

[1] Graham DG: Oxidative pathways for catecholamines in the genesis of neuromelanin and cytotoxic quinones. Mol Pharmacol 1978;14:633–643.

[2] Maker HS, Weiss C, Silides DJ, Cohen G: Coupling of dopamine oxidation (monoamine oxidase activity) to glutathione oxidation via the generation of hydrogen peroxide in rat brain homogenates. J Neurochem 1981;36:589–593.

[3] Cassarino DS, Fall CP, Swerdlow RH, Smith TS, Halvorsen EM, Miller SW, Parks JP, Parker WD, Jr, Bennett JP, Jr: Elevated reactive oxygen species and antioxidant enzyme activities in animal and cellular models of Parkinson's disease. Biochim Biophys Acta 1997;1362:77–86.

[4] Khan MM, Ahmad A, Ishrat T, Khan MB, Hoda MN, Khuwaja G, Raza SS, Khan A, Javed H, Vaibhav K, Islam F: Resveratrol attenuates 6-hydroxydopamine-induced oxidative damage and dopamine depletion in rat model of Parkinson's disease. Brain Res 2010;1328:139–151.

[5] Ueda S, Aikawa M, Ishizuya-Oka A, Yamaoka S, Koibuchi N, Yoshimoto K: Age-related dopamine deficiency in the mesostriatal dopamine system of zitter mutant rats: regional fiber vulnerability in the striatum and the olfactory tubercle. Neuroscience 2000;95:389–398.

[6] Rehm S, Mehraein P, Anzil AP, Deerberg F: A new rat mutant with defective overhairs and spongy degeneration of the central nervous system: clinical and pathologic studies. Lab Anim Sci 1982;32:70–73.

[7] Kuramoto T, Kitada K, Inui T, Sasaki Y, Ito K, Hase T, Kawagachi S, Ogawa Y, Nakao K, Barsh GS, Nagao M, Ushijima T, Serikawa T: *Attractin*/mahogany/zitter plays a critical role in myelination of the central nervous system. Proc Natl Acad Sci U S A 2001;98:559–564.

[8] Ueda S, Sakakibara S, Watanabe E, Yoshimoto K, Koibuchi N: Vulnerability of monoaminergic neurons in the brainstem of the zitter rat in oxidative stress. Prog Brain Res 2002;136:293–302.

[9] Nakadate K, Noda T, Sakakibara S, Kumamoto K, Matsuura T, Joyce JN, Ueda S: Progressive dopaminergic neurodegeneration of substantia nigra in the zitter mutant rat. Acta Neuropathol 2006;112:64–73.

[10] Gomi H, Ueno I, Yamanouchi K: Antioxidant enzymes in the brain of zitter rats: abnormal metabolism of oxygen species and its relevance to pathogenic changes in the brain of zitter rats with genetic spongiform encephalopathy. Brain Res 1994;653:66–72.

[11] Muto Y, Sato K: Pivotal role of *Attractin* in cell survival under oxidative stress in the zitter rat brain with genetic spongiform encephalopathy. Brain Res Mol Brain Res 2003;111:111–122.

[12] Paz J, Yao H, Lim HS, Lu XY, Zhang W: The neuroprotective role of *Attractin* in neurodegeneration. Neurobiol Aging 2007;28:1446–1456.

[13] Hashimoto K, Ueda S, Ehara A, Sakakibara S, Yoshimoto K, Hirata K: Neuroprotective effects of melatonin on the nigrostriatal dopamine system in the zitter rat. Neurosci Lett 2012;506:79–83.

[14] Sun K, Johnson BS, Gunn TM: Mitochondrial dysfunction precedes neurodegeneration in mahogunin (Mgrn1) mutant mice. Neurobiol Aging 2007;28:1840–1852.

[15] Ueda S, Sakakibara S, Nakadate K, Noda T, Shinoda M, Joyce JN: Degeneration of dopaminergic neurons in the substantia nigra of zitter mutant rat and protection by chronic intake of vitamin E. Neurosci Lett 2005;380:252–256.

[16] Sakakibara S, Nakadate K, Ookawara S, Ueda S: Non-cell autonomous impairment of oligodendrocyte differentiation precedes CNS degeneration in the Zitter rat: implications of macrophage/microglial activation in the pathogenesis. BMC Neurosci 2008;9:35.

[17] Allaman I, Belanger M, Magistretti PJ: Astrocyte-neuron metabolic relationships: for better and for worse. Trends Neurosci 2011;34:76–87.

Chapter 9

Oxidative Stress and Parkinson's Disease: Effects on Environmental Toxicology

Genaro Gabriel Ortiz, Fermín P. Pacheco-Moisés,
Mario A. Mireles-Ramírez, L. Javier Flores-Alvarado,
Héctor González-Usigli, Angélica L. Sánchez-López,
Lorenzo Sánchez-Romero,
Irma E. Velázquez-Brizuela,
Erika Daniela González-Renovato and
Erandis Dheni Torres-Sánchez

Additional information is available at the end of the chapter

http://dx.doi.org/10.5772/63794

Abstract

Epidemiological studies have found an increased risk of Parkinson's disease (PD) with environmental factors such as exposure to substances derived from industrial processes, use of agrochemicals, or living in a rural environment. The hypothesis that certain environmental toxins could be the source of the EP is supported by the discovery that chemicals such as herbicides paraquat, diquat, and the fungicide maneb are selectively toxic in nigrostriatal dopaminergic neurons. Also, one of the insecticides produced by plants, such as rotenone, and by-product of the synthesis of synthetic heroin MPTP (1-methyl-4-phenyl-1,2,3,6-tetrahydropyridine) can be reproduced in animal models where neurochemicals, histopathological, and clinical characteristic of PD can be found. Interestingly, there are similarities in the chemical structure of paraquat and MPTP. Recent evidence exhibited that inflammation and oxidative stress play an essential role in the development of PD. So, in our laboratory we found that in an animal model melatonin decreases the products of lipid oxidation, nitric oxide metabolites, and the activity of cyclooxygenase 2, which are induced by an intraperitoneal injection of MPTP. This suggests that the neuroprotective effects of melatonin are partially attributed to its antioxidant scavenging and anti-inflammatory action.

Keywords: dopaminergic neurons, melatonin, MPTP, paraquat, Parkinson, Parkinsonism

1. Introduction

Parkinson's disease (PD) is a neurodegenerative disorder characterized by tremor and disruptions to voluntary movement. The main neuropathology in PD involves the death of dopaminergic cells in the pars compacta of the substantia nigra with intracytoplasmic inclusions (Lewy bodies) in the remaining intact nigral neurons [1]. Neural loss in the substantia nigra increases with age in PD, consistent with a worsening prognosis and increased symptom severity in older patients. The substantia nigra is an anatomical region of the brain implicated in dopamine synthesis and voluntary motor control and is a part of the basal ganglia. Neural circuits in the basal ganglia, particularly the nigrostriatal pathway, appear to be crucial to the successful execution of both innate and learned motor behaviors [2].

PD primarily affects people of ages 50 and older, and the prevalence and risk of developing sporadic PD increases substantially with age and has an incidence rate of 18 per 100,000 per year [3]. As the disease progresses, significant motor disability is seen in PD patients even when treated with symptomatic medications. Symptoms like dysphagia, sialorrhoea, microphagia, and dystonia are also well-known. Nonmotor symptoms include cognitive impairment [4], neuropsychiatric symptoms (depression, psychosis, anxiety, and fatigue), sleep dysfunction (rapid eye movement sleep behavior disorder, sleep attacks, daytime sleepiness, advanced sleep phase syndrome, and early morning awakenings) [5], autonomic disturbances (constipation, nausea, orthostatic hypotension, and urogenital problems), and sensory disturbances (restless legs syndrome, visual changes, and decreased olfaction) [6]. Interestingly, increased mortality risk has been linked with both motor and nonmotor features in newly diagnosed PD patients, especially with features like postural instability, hallucinations, and cognitive impairment [7].

No definitive diagnostic test such as magnetic resonance imaging or computed topography scans or genetic tests can confirm PD. Its diagnosis is typically based on the presence of a combination of key motor features, such as associated and exclusionary symptoms, and response to levodopa [8].

The molecular mechanisms underlying the loss of these neurons still remain elusive. Different modes of cell death, apoptotic, necrotic, and autophagic, have been described to contribute to the neuronal loss occurring in PD [9]. Oxidative stress plays an important role in dopaminergic neurotoxicity. Mitochondrial complex I deficiencies of the respiratory chain account for the neuronal degeneration in PD. Neurotoxins and other environmental factors, such as pesticides, insecticides, dopamine metabolites, heavy metals, microbial toxins, and genetic mutations, in PD-associated proteins contribute to mitochondrial dysfunction [10, 11]. A byproduct of an illicit narcotic drug, 1-methyl-4-phenyl-1,2,3,6-tetrahydropyridine (MPTP) as well as its metabolite MPP+, has been shown to cause the same signs and symptoms as PD. In fact, inhibitors of mitochondrial complex 1 (MPTP, rotenone, and paraquat) are able to reproduce parkinsonism with selective dopaminergic neuronal loss in mice and primate models [12]. Furthermore, a chronic infusion of either rotenone [13] or MPTP [14] in rodents induces the formation of α-synuclein positive aggregates. These data support the suggestion that sporadic PD may be caused by a combination of genetic predisposition and environmental toxins, which

http://dx.doi.org/10.5772/63794

act via inhibition of the mitochondrial complex I to produce selective dopaminergic cell loss. Human epidemiological studies have implicated a higher incidence of PD in residents of rural environments with exposure to herbicides and pesticides [15].

2. Oxidative stress

The body is constantly exposed to the influence and attack of free radicals, which have been associated with various disorders of the nervous system such as Parkinson disease, the motor neuron disease, and other disorders of the central nervous system (CNS). A free radical is considered any molecule containing one or more unpaired electrons. It is produced by biochemical redox reactions occurring as a result of normal cellular metabolism (biochemical reactions with oxygen or produced as a result of oxidative stress), as well as by phagocytes in inflammatory reactions controlled in response to exposure to different environmental factors, including ionizing radiation, ultraviolet rays, smoking, air pollution, gamma radiation, hyperoxia, excessive exercise, ischemia, and toxic compounds such as cancer drugs, some anesthetics, and painkillers [16].

The main free radicals are superoxide anion (O_2•–), hydroxyl (OH•), nitric oxide (NO•), and peroxyl (ROO•) [17]. Some of them are considered highly reactive molecules that can cause cell damage and even death. Usually, the most damaged cellular components are unsaturated fatty acids in cell membranes and proteins such as enzymes conveying ions across membranes.

It is estimated that mitochondria are the main source of oxygen radicals (**Figure 1**) [18] in which anion superoxide (O_2•) is generated during electron transport. Superoxide dismutase (SOD) converts O_2•– to hydrogen peroxide (H_2O_2) by the Fenton reaction; the latter in the presence of Fe_2+ produces hydroxyl radical (OH•) by reacting Fe_2+ and Cu+. Then, the Fenton reaction is expressed as

$$O_2\bullet - + Fe^{3+} \_\_\_\_\_\_\_\_\_\_ Fe^{2+} + O_2$$

$$Fe^{2+} + H_2O_2 \_\_\_\_\_\_\_\_\_\_ Fe^{3+} + OH- + OH\bullet$$

$$O_2\bullet + H_2O_2 \_\_\_\_\_\_\_\_\_\_ OH- + OH\bullet + O_2$$

According to Burdon and Mattson 1995 and 1998, the O_2•– may also interact with nitric oxide (NO•) to form peroxynitrite (ONOO–). Of all free radicals, OH– is the most damaging free radical, since its presence–though is only a fraction of a second–is able to destroy proteolytic enzymes causing rupture of polysaccharide and lipid membrane peroxidation (LMP) altering its permeability and associated features [19] (**Figure 2**). Peroxynitrite (ONOO–) can cause direct damage to proteins and DNA, and is also a potent inducer of LMP that can destroy neurons, which are especially sensitive to this process. Oxidative stress can occur in different acute degenerative conditions such as cerebral ischemia, traumatic brain injury, and chronic degenerative processes such as Parkinson's disease [20]; it is observed, to a lesser extent, in neural circuits during normal physiological activity.

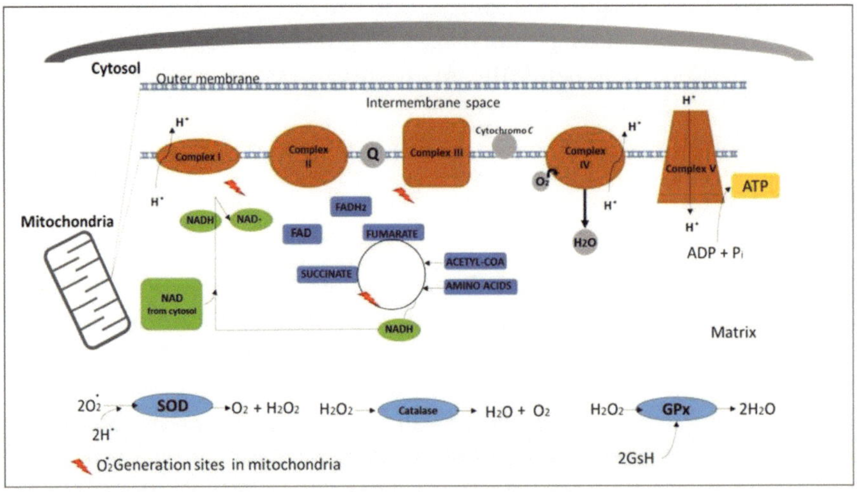

Figure 1. Mitochondria are considered the main source of free radicals, which come from the electron transport chain. Within mitochondria, $2O_2$+ is produced by the one-electron reduction of O_2. Therefore, it is the kinetic and thermodynamic factors underlying the interaction of potential one-electron donors with O_2 that control mitochondrial ROS production.

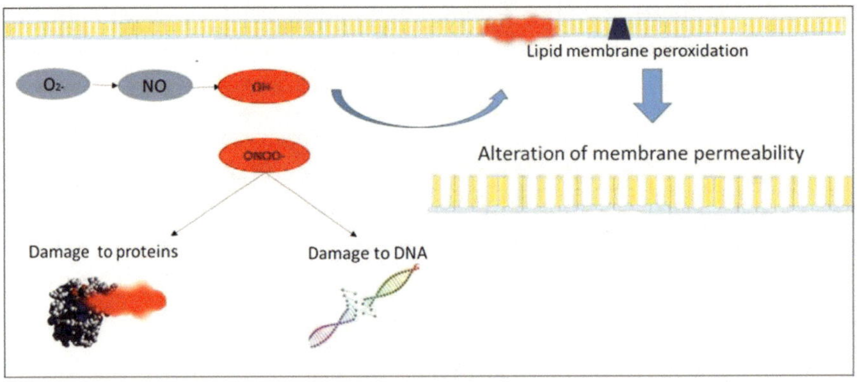

Figure 2. Damage generated by free radicals (ONOO-, OH-) directly affects proteins, membrane phospholipids, and DNA molecules. The resulting free radicals, such as superoxide anion (O_2-) and hydroxyl radical (OH•), as well as the nonradical hydrogen peroxide, can damage macromolecules, including DNA, proteins, and oxidized lipids have all been related in such damages. The superoxide radical, although it is unreactive in comparison with many other radicals, biological systems can convert it into other more reactive species, such as peroxyl (ROO•), alkoxyl (RO•), and hydroxyl (HO•) radicals.

On the other side, oxidative stress can cause the onset of a disturbance in cellular calcium homeostasis. This action is usually related to an effect on the receptor mobilizing Ca^{2+}, but the decrease of Ca^{2+} ATPase activity is also evident. Reactive oxygen species (ROS) also interfere with other transduction signal systems through the action of nitric oxide (NO) [21] (**Figure 3**). Reactive oxygen metabolites affect ligand binding to membrane receptors such as β-adrenergic, cholinergic, muscarinic, histamine, and serotonin. Some reactive oxygen species can affect enzymatic pathways such as the phospholipase A [22].

http://dx.doi.org/10.5772/63794

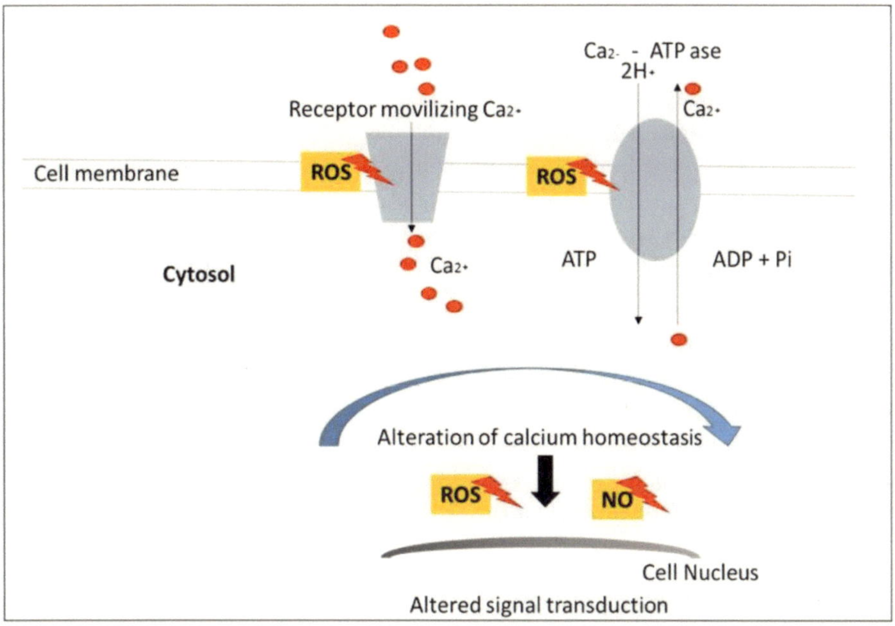

Figure 3. ROS can disrupt calcium homeostasis through its effect on receptors on the cell gate ionic membrane, calcium ATPase, and interfere with signal transduction. Interactions between Ca^{2+} and reactive oxygen species signaling coordinate signaling, which can be either beneficial or detrimental. In neurodegenerative disorders, cellular Ca^{2+}-regulating systems are compromised. Oxidative stress, perturbed energy metabolism, and alterations of disease-related proteins result in Ca^{2+}-dependent synaptic dysfunction.

Free radicals formed in the organism can initiate a series of chain reactions which continue, after several reactions, until removed with other free radicals or by the antioxidant system, which protects tissues from their deleterious effects. According to the mode of action, three main types of antioxidants are known: (a) those preventing the formation of new free radicals, (b) those making them less harmful before they can react, and (c) those preventing the formation of free radicals from other molecules.

The enzymes involved in the antioxidant system are superoxide dismutase glutathione peroxidase (GPx), catalase, glutathione reductase, glutathione S transferase, and other proteins that bind metals (ferritin, transferrin, and ceruloplasmin) limiting the availability of iron necessary to form the •OH radical.

Excessive ROS reactive nitrogen species (RNS) generation may contribute to cell injury and death. In particular, accumulation of nitrosative stress due to excessive generation of nitric oxide (NO) appears to be a potential factor contributing to neuronal cell damage and apoptosis. In this process, overstimulation of N-methyl-D-aspartate-type of glutamate receptors permit calcium influx Ca^{2+} to cell, increasing NO and promoting ROS formation through a process named S-nitrosylation which consists in a reaction between NO and cysteine thiol to form S-nitrosothiols (SNOS). In addition, NO can react with superoxide to generate peroxynitrite (ONOO–), which is highly toxic to cell, as well [23].

3. Clinical manifestations of Parkinson's disease

PD is a common neurodegenerative disorder characterized by progressive loss of *substantia nigra* dopaminergic neurons, and the concomitant loss of dopaminergic nerve terminals in the *caudo-putamen* nuclei, which is the main neuron projection area of the *substantia nigra*. PD affects about 1% of the population over 65 years, which increases to up to 4% after the age of 80 [24]. Its main symptoms were described in 1817 by James Parkinson in an essay called the "shaking palsy." From a clinical point of view, PD is characterized by tremor at rest, slow movements (bradykinesia), rigidity, postural instability, stiffness of the muscles, serious inability to initiate movement (akinesia), and mask-like face expression. Other symptoms may be a flexed posture, freezing (motor blocks), loss of arm swing on one side, loss of smell, or a persisting glabellar tap reflex. However, the above mentioned symptoms may not all be present in one patient [25]. Bradykinesia, slowness of movement, is the most characteristic symptom. PD patients may therefore show slowness in daily activities and slow reaction times and may have difficulties in fine motor control [26].

A number of nonmotor features can precede the motor symptoms of PD. These symptoms probably arise from extra-nigral structures. For instance, olfactory deficits [27] and cardiac sympathetic denervation [28, 29] are present in a very high proportion of patients presenting with the earliest motor signs, suggesting that such features probably precede the motor signs and may be more useful in characterizing early disease status. Other nonmotor symptoms include autonomic, mood, cognitive, and sensory dysfunctions, as well as sleep disturbances [30, 31]. Depression is the most frequent psychiatric complication in PD. Although depression often precedes motor symptoms in PD [32], it may still reflect impairments of the nigrostriatal dopaminergic circuit [33]. Anxiety is also comorbid with PD [34]. These nonmotor symptoms significantly contribute to the reduced quality of life in PD patients, but are frequently undiagnosed and left untreated [35, 36].

4. Physiopathology of Parkinson disease

One of the most surprising aspects of PD is the selective vulnerability of neuronal population to damage. PD can occur when an external or an internal toxin selectively destroys dopaminergic neurons. When the neurons which connect two specific brain regions, the compact part of the substantia nigra (SNPC) and the striatum, essential to maintain the motor function die, the dopaminergic pathway progressively degenerates, and the level of dopamine in the striatum decreases causing changes in brain circuitry and motor features of PD deficiencies appear.

The main pathological findings of PD are the loss of dopaminergic neurons and formation of fibril aggregates composed of α-synuclein, called Lewy bodies, in the remaining dopaminergic neurons located in substantia nigra pars compacta [37]. DA neurons of SNPC also have a tendency to degenerate with aging at a rate of approximately 5% per decade. In contrast, the rate of neurodegeneration in PD patients is about 10-fold faster and occurs mainly in the ventro-lateral part of SNPC [38].

The degeneration of neuronal cells may be the consequence of many pathogenic factors (toxic, infectious, genetic, metabolic, vascular, etc.) and the final consequence is apoptosis and cell death in which caspases (particularly caspase 3) and Bcl-2 protein families are central components with up and down regulatory mechanism that promotes apoptosis. Two main caspase-mediated pathways of cell death have been described in mammals: (a) the extrinsic or death receptor-mediated pathway, which has a critical role in the maintenance of tissue homeostasis, and (b) the intrinsic, mitochondria-dependent pathway that is mainly activated in response to extracellular cues and internal insults such as DNA damage, growth factor deprivation, cytoskeletal disruption, accumulation of unfolded proteins, hypoxia, and many others [12, 19–21, 39–42].

In vivo, the dysfunction of the proteasomal system in order to cleave misfolded α-syn due to lack of energy associated to mitochondrial damage, and problems with the autophagy-lysosomal degradation pathway, which disrupts damaged mitochondrial clearance, leads to the formation of protein inclusions and accumulation of damaged mitochondria, a major source of ROS, which activate the apoptotic cascade as has been mentioned. ROS accumulation may result in detrimental effects such as lipid peroxidation, protein oxidation, and further DNA damage. The maintenance of a pool of healthy mitochondria that can meet the bioenergetic demands of a neuron is therefore of critical importance; this is achieved by maintaining a careful balance between mitochondrial biogenesis, mitochondrial trafficking, mitochondrial dynamics, and mitophagy. Removal of damaged mitochondria through mitophagy can lead to the release of compartmentalized mitochondrial molecules. Once in the cytosol, some of these molecules, such as cyt-C, Smac/DIABLO, and HtrA2/OMI, are capable of activating apoptotic routines that lead to cell death. It is then reported that the failure of mitophagy results in the release of mtDNA into the cell cytosol contributing to mechanisms of cell death [43–47].

The central events in the mitochondrial-dependent cell death pathway are the activation of the mitochondrial permeability transition pore (mPTP) and the disruption of mitochondrial membrane potential, which cause the release of apoptogenic molecules and finally lead to cell death [48]. The protein α-syn is a small acidic protein containing 140 amino acids. This protein is able to undergo self-aggregation in a nucleation-dependent process to form nonfibrillar oligomers, protofibrils, and fibrillar aggregates with amyloid-like properties that are potentially cytotoxic to the neurons and it has been shown to be directly degraded *in vitro* by the 20S proteasome. Studies of the degradation of aggregated α-syn led us to suspect that oxidation of Met may play a role in α-syn degradation by the proteasome [46].

It is important to take into account that neuronal loss in PD is also associated to chronic neuroinflammation through microglial activation by some different mechanism including overexpression of inducible NOS (iNOS), COX-2, the cytokines tumor necrosis factor-alpha (TNF-α), and IL-1β and NO or accumulation of heat shock protein 60 (Hsp60) participating in DA cell death in PD via a mechanism unrelated to cytokine release and could serve as a signal of CNS injury through activation of microglial cells. Neuromelanin is released from dying dopaminergic neurons in the SNpc and activates microglia, provoking increase in the sensitivity of DA neurons to oxidative stress-mediated cell death. Parkinson's disease-associated proteins such as α-syn, parkin, LRRK2, and DJ-1 have also been reported to activate microglia, as well [11, 49].

One of the most surprising aspects of neurodegenerative diseases is the selective vulnerability of neuronal population to damage. Parkinson's disease can occur when an external or an internal toxin selectively destroys dopaminergic neurons. When the neurons which connect to two brain regions, the compact part of the substantia nigra (SNPC) and the striatum, essential to maintain the motor function die, the dopaminergic pathway progressively degenerates and the level of dopamine in the striatum decreases causing changes in brain circuitry, and motor features of PD deficiencies appear. The high vulnerability of the SNPC neurons to oxidative agents, compared to neurons in other cerebral regions, may be explained by a combination of different factors such as reduced antioxidant activity, increased iron concentration, increased susceptible to DA oxidation, and reduced activity of the mitochondrial complex I (NADH oxidoreductase) (**Figure 4**).

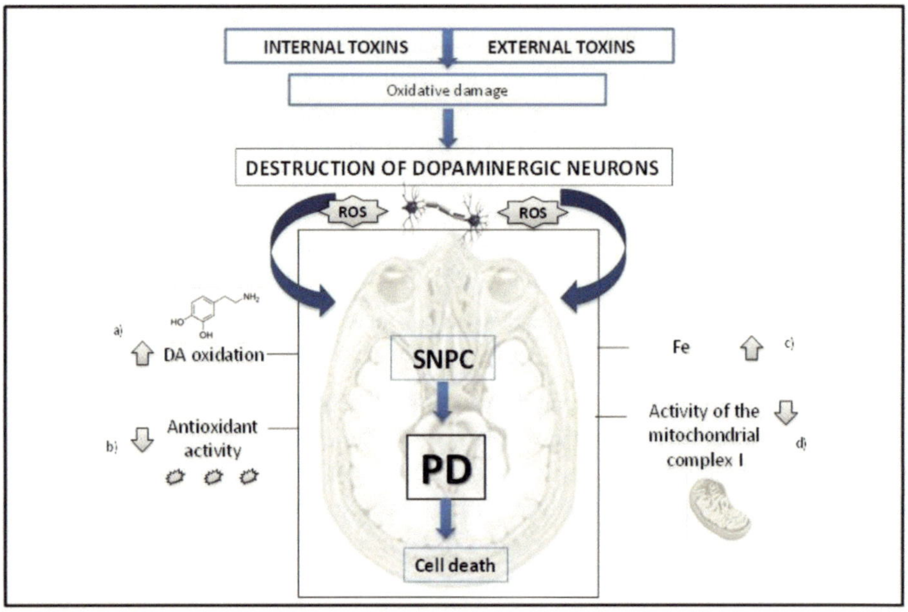

Figure 4. SNPC neurons and oxidative agents. External factors, such as neurotoxins, pesticides, insecticides, and endogenous factors such as dopamine (DA), and genetic mutations in PD-associated proteins contribute to oxidative damage and disruptions in the maintenance of the redox potential leading to destruction of dopaminergic neurons and cell death. Different pathways contribute to the substantia nigra pars compacta (SNPC) neurons vulnerability to oxidative damage including (a) high susceptibility of DA auto-oxidation, (b) reduced antioxidant activity such as glutathione, and (c) increased iron concentration d) deficits in mitochondrial complex I of the respiratory chain.

Biochemical abnormalities in the brain with PD show deficits in mitochondrial complex I, decreased extracellular thiols, increased oxidative iron in the substantia nigra, and oxidative damage, including DNA oxidation, nitration, and increased carbonyl groups of proteins. Lewy bodies inclusions contain phosphorylated neurofilaments and a protein called α-synuclein

[50]. Currently, there is evidence of properties of α-synuclein and its possible association with oxidative stress state present in PD. One such evidence is the notion that one type of amyloid aggregates of α-synuclein, similar to those observed *in vivo*, by coincubation with copper (II), Fe/hydrogen peroxide, or are induced cytochrome c/ hydrogen peroxide. Many motor characteristics defining the PD result primarily from the loss of substantia nigra neurons [28]. Deficiencies in mitochondrial function, increased oxidative stress, apoptosis, excitotoxicity, and inflammation, all of them are part of the processes that eventually result in neurodegeneration [51].

4.1. Genetic and Parkinson's disease

A relatively new theory explores the role of genetic factors in the development of Parkinson's disease. A total of 15–25% of Parkinson's patients have a close relative who had experienced parkinsonian symptoms (such as tremor).

There are many genes linked to familial forms of PD, which have produced advances in PD basic research, increasing our understanding of possible mechanism of dopaminergic cells damage in patients with this condition. These genes include those associated with α-syn, parkin, DJ-1, PINK-1, LRRK-2, ATP13A2, mitochondrial phosphatase, and phosphatase and tensin homolog (PTEN)-induced kinase gene, and they have been demonstrated to be involved in apoptosis regulation. Parkin is associated with the outer mitochondrial membrane (OMM) and prevents cell death by inhibiting mitochondrial swelling, cyt-C release, and caspase activation. Another finding in pathogenesis has been centered in the ATP13A2 gene, which regulates intracellular Mn^{2+} homeostasis, playing an important role in preventing damage induced by Mn^{2+} cytotoxicity. Overexposure of cells to Mn^{2+} may determine cell death by induction of DNA damage, oxidative stress, disruption of Ca^{2+}, iron homeostasis, and mitochondrial dysfunction. In an experimental model, monomeric α-Syn-expressing dopaminergic cells significantly attenuated Mn-induced neurotoxicity for initial exposures. However, overexposure to Mn produces precipitation of α-syn, which at the same time impairs antioxidative defense mechanism in this experimental model [39, 44, 52].

One important finding of PD is the presence of cytoplasmic inclusions containing α-synuclein and ubiquitin, known as Lewy bodies, in the SNPC and other brain regions. Some cases of familial PD are clearly attributed to mutations in the genes for α-synuclein and parkin.

4.2. Dopamine as a source of ROS in the CNS

Since the discovery that 1-methyl-4-phenyl-1,2,3,6-tetrahydrodropyridine infusion causes parkinsonism by selective inhibition of mitochondrial complex-1, raised the possibility that mitochondrial dysfunction is at the heart of PD [53].

In patients with PD, there is an excess amount of cytosolic DA outside of the synaptic vesicles due to damaged neurons with impaired reuptake, and a possible increased damage when an overload is related to levodopa treatment. Dopamine is easily metabolized via monoamine oxidase (MAO). Also DA suffers auto-oxidation to cytotoxic ROS producing mitochondrial impairment either by activation of the intrinsic apoptotic pathway or by inhibiting the respiratory chain. Also, the auto-oxidation of DA produces electron-deficient DA quinones or DA semiquinones, which, at the same time, modify some PD-related proteins, such as α-syn, parkin, DJ-1, superoxide dismutase-2 (SOD2), and UCH-L1. Additionally, DA quinones can be oxidized to aminochrome, whose redox-cycling leads to the generation of the superoxide radical and the depletion of cellular nicotinamide adenine dinucleotide phosphate-oxidase (NADPH), which ultimately forms the neuromelanin, contributing to this degenerative mechanism [11, 47] (**Figure 5**).

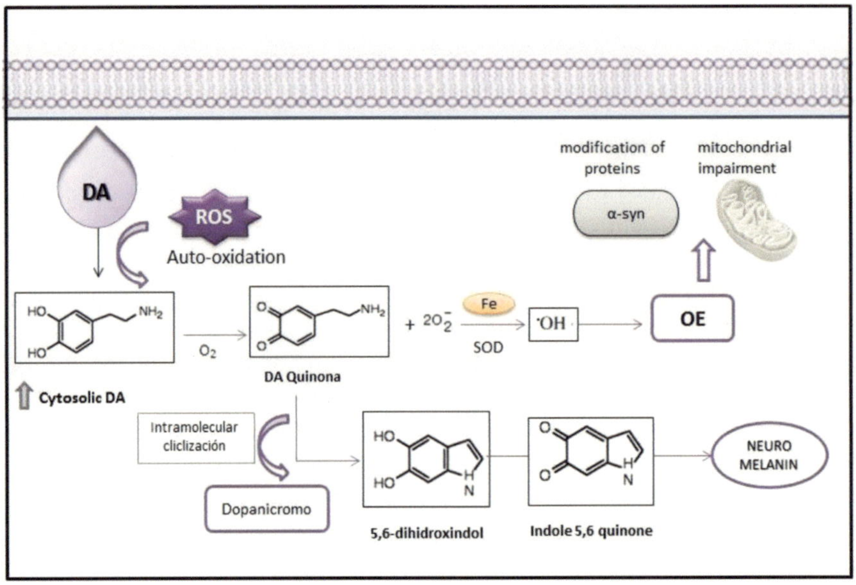

Figure 5. Dopamine as a source of ROS in the CNS. In patients with PD there is an excess amount of cytosolic dopamine (DA), this molecule is unstable and undergoes auto-oxidation to form dopamine quinones and free radicals that leads to modification of PD-related proteins such as α-syn and mitochondrial impairment. The products of dopamine oxidation, dopamine quinones, can also contribute to neurodegeneration. Dopamine quinones can cyclize to form dopaminocromo who is the precursor of neuromelanin, a brain pigment that may contribute to neurodegeneration.

The microtubule (MT) system may play an important role in PD pathogenesis, as well. It is crucial for many aspects of neuronal function, including motility, differentiation, and protein and organelle trafficking. In experimental models, both acute and chronic sub-lethal settings, 6OHDA-induced oxidative stress elicited significant alterations in microtubule (MT) dynamics; very important for axonal transportation; these includes reductions in MT growth rate, increased frequency of MT pauses/retractions, and increased levels of tubulin acetylation [54].

DA metabolism act as proneurotoxins in the development of PD. Certain components of snuff smoke can react with these proneurotoxins preventing its activation. This may explain the possible beneficial effect of smoking on the incidence of PD. The ROS generated by the auto-oxidation of dopamine have been implicated in the neuron loss; related to age and other neurodegenerative disorders such as PD. To date, there have been proposed two mechanisms by which the DA stimulates the production of ROS. These depend on the presence or absence of enzymatic mediators [55]. The DA in the substantia nigra and striatum is spread by the enzyme monoamine oxidase (MAO), located in the outer membrane of mitochondria [56], from this reaction results the superoxide and hydroxyl radicals plus hydrogen-peroxide production. Another derivative compound is 1,2,3,4 tetrahydropapaverolin DA (THP) obtained from enzymatic catabolism. TTP itself is capable of inducing necrosis in neuroblastoma cells and is related to the pathogenesis of PD [57].

DA is a molecule with a catechol group which cannot be easily enzymatically oxidized to form an array of electrochemical species (quinone type). First, the initial step in the oxidation of DA involves a reaction with molecular oxygen to form DA quinone and two molecules of superoxide anion. Second, the superoxide anions formation during autoxidation of DA leads to the production of hydrogen peroxide by the dismutation of superoxide. Third, in this way, iron mediated in substantia nigra showed high amounts of oxidative stress. Last, the total iron increased but does not necessarily mean an oxidative stress state as excess iron always store into the proteins, such as ferritin, which leaves the iron inert and harmless [58].

However, that state of iron stability can change by continuing entry and release of iron from ferritin to more active form entering the Fenton reaction generating the hydroxyl radical. The iron accumulates in astrocytes in the substantia nigra (experimental data), increasing the rate of Fe(III)/Fe(II) and reduced glutathione. Aging may be a factor which predisposes the brain to the PD, due to, according to our interpretation, the kidnapping by the mitochondria of Fe(II) in astroglia in the substantia nigra. Furthermore, there is evidence that the intracellular loss of redox balance results in aberrant dopamine oxidation in 6-hydroxydopamine, which in turn can undergo auto-oxidation to quinones and simultaneously generate superoxide. This cascade reaction, either by itself, or amplified by the generation of ROS, may explain the neuronal loss as an end result. The DA-o-quinone then undergoes intramolecular cyclization to form 5,6-dihydroxyquinoline, which is subsequently oxidized by the DA-o-quinone to form dopaminocromo; this compound undergoes a rearrangement to form 5,6-dihydroxyindole, which in turn is oxidized into a quinone indole. The following polymerization process finally leads to the generation of a dark pigment called neuromelanin. The dark appearance of the black substance is due to the presence of this pigment containing oxidation products of the cysteinyl-DA.

Dopaminergic neurons are particularly exposed to oxidative stress due to the metabolism of dopamine that causes a series of molecules that are potentially toxic if they are not adequately removed. Dopamine acts as a free radical generating compound, and can oxidize itself at physiological pH, generating dopamine-forming toxic quinones, superoxide radicals, and hydrogen peroxide [40]. It can also be enzymatically deaminated by monoamino oxidase (MAO) to 3,4-dihydroxyphenylacetic, a nontoxic metabolite acid (DOPAC), hydrogen peroxide [41], and by other oxidative processes. Thus, the metabolism of dopamine generates high concentrations of ROS, which can activate and induce apoptotic cell death cascades [19, 20]. ROS accumulation is toxic *per se*, and generates oxidative stress as a result of depletion of cellular antioxidants (e.g., vitamin E and reduced glutathione), increase the membrane lipid peroxidation, DNA damage, and oxidation alteration of protein folding [20]. Besides the general oxidative damage, there is evidence that the interaction between α-synuclein and dopamine metabolites determines the preferential neurodegeneration of dopaminergic neurons. Along with a number of possible changes, abnormal protein aggregates could also act as irritants, causing a chronic inflammatory reaction which can induce synaptic changes and neuronal death. Findings which suggest the existence of a chronic inflammation process include the presence of microglial activation and astrocytosis in the brain of these patients, particularly in the vicinity of protein aggregates. In PD, along with several toxic and genetic mechanisms producing neuronal damage, the compounds released from damaged neurons can induce microglial release of neurotoxic factors aggravating neurodegeneration [36]. Among those released is neuromelanin compound which is a strong iron chelator. The neuromelanin-ferrum complex activates microglia *in vitro*, causing the release of neurotoxic compounds such as tumor necrosis factor-alpha (TNF-α), interleukin-6 (IL-6), and nitric oxide (NO). Increased total iron concentration had been described in the substantia nigra of PD severe cases, although the underlying mechanism is not known [59]. Iron also contributes to increasing the generation of oxygen radicals (ROS), oxidative stress, and increased protein aggregation, including α-synuclein aggregation. The rapid aggregation of α-synuclein protein in turn can induce the formation of ROS. Lastly, dopamine stabilizes the protofibril form of α-synuclein, which would be toxic. Thus, in the oxidative atmosphere of a dopaminergic neuron, α-synuclein is involved in generating a vicious circle, which leads to neuronal death [59] (**Figure 6**).

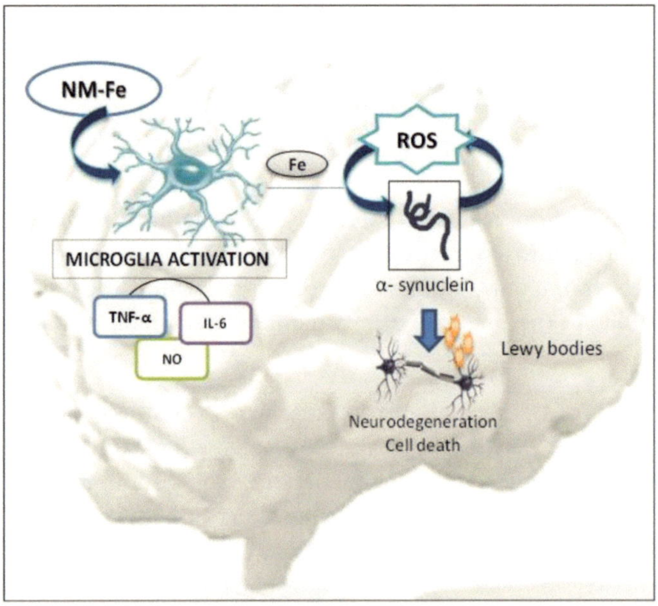

Figure 6. Interaction between α-synuclein and dopamine metabolites. Dopamine metabolites such as neuromelanin-Ferrum complex produce microglial activation that leads to chronic inflammation process, causing the release of interleukins, and free radicals. The reactive oxygen radicals interact with total iron concentration in the substantia nigra and increase the propensity of the α-synuclein to aggregate. This protein is present in Lewy bodies and the formation of aggregates is associated with increased oxidative stress, neurodegeneration, and cell death.

Finally, till date there have been at least five different mechanisms of death in neurons with dopaminergic dysfunction associated to oxidation of the dopamine (DA): (1) proteasome dysfunction, (2) mitochondrial dysfunction, (3) oxidative stress, (4) α-syn oligomers precipitation, and (5) lysosomal autophagy dysfunction.

Another possible mechanism implicated in neuronal destruction and death is associated with diminished neuroprotection due to the dysfunction of neuromelanin and diaphorase enzyme [45, 56].

4.3. MPTP and Parkinson's disease

In 1982 (California, USA), a group of recreational drugs were developed which severely causes parkinsonian syndrome days after injection; 1-methyl-4-phenyl-4-propionoxipiperidina (MPPP), a synthetic analog of meperidine, was used for that purpose. This analog-product, according to the analysis of samples provided by the seller, was contaminated by 1-methyl-4-phenyl-1,2,3,6 tetrahydropyridine, which was discovered to cause parkinsonism at a concentration of 2.5–2.9% by weight. Initial clinical symptoms shown by these patients were treated with carbidopa/L-dopa. In the following years, the clinical treatment was insufficient to halt the progression of the disease and died 12 and 16 years, respectively, after injection. Pathological analysis of their brains showed moderate to severe decrease of neurons in the substantia nigra without Lewy bodies. Besides, gliosis and clumping of microglia around nerve cells were found [60].

In 1991, an individual, 39 years old, tried to produce the MPPP following the instructions of a chemistry textbook and obtained, without knowing, the by-product MPTP. Approximately, 45 g of the drug in the course of a week were injected. At the end of this period, he had language problems, remained lethargic, and developed rigid posture. These symptoms worsened over the next week, so he had to be admitted to a hospital. In the next two weeks, he was treated with selegiline and carbidopa/L-dopa, which greatly improved their symptoms. Over the next 3.5 years, the patient responded transiently to treatment with carbidopa less/L-dopa and bromocriptine; however, his condition progressed to severe parkinsonism immobility and a significant hypophonia and died. Neuropathological analysis of this patient showed similar findings to those found in the brains of those patients studied from California. Besides, large amounts of extraneuronal melanin were found indicating a progressive death of nerve cells in response to a brief temporary aggression the nigrostriatal system. The above data show that the acute phase of parkinsonian syndrome is completed within a few days after administration of MPTP; however, neurodegeneration caused by MPTP silently continue for several years or even decades [61, 62].

From a neurochemical point of view there is a great similarity between the MPTP-induced parkinsonism and PD. The neurotoxic action of MPTP involving dopaminergic transmission produces a variety of neurochemical changes: (1) decrease in the concentration of dopamine and its metabolites (3,4-dihydroxyphenylacetic acid and homovanillic acid), (2) decrease activity of the enzyme tyrosine hydroxylase, and (3) alteration in the density of dopamine receptors.

Since the discovery of the effect of MPTP in human, extensive research in animal models, cell cultures, etc. was initiated to characterize in more detail the effects of the toxin.

MPTP produces selective death of dopaminergic neurons and parkinsonian syndrome in several species, including Rhesus monkeys, squirrel monkeys, and beagle dogs. The effects of MPTP, presented in a variety of nonhuman primates, consist in a very significant reduction in spontaneous activity, rigidity, tremor, and bradykinesia. Very few human subjects develop resting tremor characteristic of PD. MPTP initially produces temporary parkinsonian symptoms but become permanent with repeated administration of the toxin. The mechanisms involved in spontaneous recovery experienced by these animals are not known, but may be related to a transient alteration of other neurotransmitter systems other than nigrostriatal. On the other hand, rats and guinea pigs do not show permanent impairments of DA in the striatum nor they present movement disorders such as those observed in primates. In mice of the C57BL/6 strain MPTP induces toxic changes, but at higher concentrations.

There is no evidence that MPTP induces alterations in the cholinergic, GABAergic, and glutamatergic systems in primates. However, the levels of various neuropeptides, substance P, dynorphin, and enkephalin in striatum, substantia nigra, and globus pallidus are reduced in animals chronically treated with MPTP. These same abnormalities have been described in patients with PD. However, it is not known whether they are due to the degeneration of neurons containing these peptides or represent adaptive nigrostriatal denervation to changes.

The susceptibility of different animal species to MPTP may be related to differences in the metabolism of MPTP, cerebral distribution, and retention of the final metabolite [63].

4.4. Metabolism of MPTP

MPTP metabolism is a complex process, after systemic administration it readily crosses the blood brain barrier due to their lipophilicity. Once in the brain, it is transformed extraneuronally in astrocytes, a monoamine oxidase B rich cells, into the intermediate, 1-methyl-4-phenyl-2,3-dihydropyridinium (MPDP+). This is a very reactive ion undergoing autoxidation to the radical 1-methyl-4-phenyl pyridinium (MPP+) with the formation of superoxide anion (O_2•). Besides, the MPDP+ readily crosses the cell membrane and into the extracellular space to form MPP+ and O_2•. Extracellular MPP+ is leaking from astrocytes and used by the presynaptic DA system uptake, resulting in an energy-dependent concentration in dopaminergic neurons [64].

Intraneuronal concentration of MPP+ increases by binding to neuromelanin and then brought into the mitochondrial matrix through active transport system, which acts as a potent inhibitor of complex I of oxidative phosphorylation system. This effect is due MPP+ binding to complex I at a distal sulfur iron site core and near the binding site of ubiquinone Q10. This leads to the cessation of oxidative phosphorylation, ATP level is depleted and decreases the concentration of the major cellular antioxidant, reduced glutathione. This also leads to changes in cellular calcium, altered transmembrane potential, and ultimately neuronal death is manifested [65].

The inhibition of mitochondrial complex I can increase oxidative stress induced by MPP+, since the electrons inside the mitochondria may contribute to the toxic effects of MPTP. For example, it has been demonstrated that MPP+ induced lipid peroxidation in cultured cells and the DA is blocked by specific inhibitors of lipid peroxidation [66] (see **Figure 2**).

4.5. Toxicology of paraquat

The LD50 of paraquat in humans is about 3–5 mg/kg, which represents only 10–15 ml in a 20% solution. Although paraquat is regarded as moderately hazardous substance and the Environmental Protection Agency classifies it as a possible human carcinogen and weakly genotoxic, the toxic potential of this herbicide is very high [67].

The genotoxic potential of paraquat has been studied in our research group through induced micronuclei in erythrocytes and bone marrow of mice. Paraquat (15 or 20 mg/kg) was injected intraperitoneally at an interval of 24 hours and then every 6 hours until completion of the study (72 hours). We found that treatment with paraquat increases the number of polychromatic erythrocytes micronucleus cells in blood and bone marrow. Also in this work, it was found that the administration of melatonin, an efficient free radical scavenger, at doses of 2 or 10 mg/kg, 30 min before injection of paraquat partially reverses micronucleus formation [68].

The widespread use of paraquat carries great risk potential for misuse and also for accidental and intentional poisonings. Therefore, the label for minimum safety should be increased because recommendations for it use is not strictly followed. Particularly to protect the skin, equipment is required for face and hands. Poisoning usually occurs in the first instance through the skin when in direct contact with the backpack spray of the herbicide. The eyes and nose may also be exposed to the herbicide. Toxic effects include mild irritation, blistering, peeling, necrosis, dermatitis, and dermatitis of hands and sometimes of the scrotum. Severe exposure to the hands causes localized discoloration or temporary loss of nails. Splashes in the eyes can cause irritation and inflammation of eyelids and decreased visual acuity. Although the intact human skin is relatively impermeable to paraquat, some fatalities as a result of dermal exposure are documented. The presence of scratches, cuts, wounds, or severe dermatitis can substantially increase the risks [69].

The lungs are the first target of paraquat, and pulmonary effects represent the most lethal and least treatable manifestation. The inhalation toxicity is rare. The main mechanism of cell damage is the generation of free radicals that oxidize lung tissue. Although acute pulmonary edema and lung damage after several hours of severe acute exposures may occur, delayed pulmonary fibrosis is the usual cause of death that commonly occurs 7–14 days after ingestion. In some patients, ingestion of a large amount of concentrated paraquat form (20%) died more rapidly due to circulatory failure (within 48 hours). Lung cells appear to selectively accumulate paraquat which generates free radicals causing lipid peroxidation and cell damage. Hemorrhage, fluids, and leukocytes infiltrates into the alveolar spaces, followed by fibroblast proliferation. There is a progressive decrease in arterial oxygen tension and diffusion capacity of CO_2. Such deterioration in gas exchange causes progressive proliferation of fibrous connective tissue in the alveoli eventually causing death by asphyxiation and tissue anoxia [70].

In the gastrointestinal tract, toxicity first occurs at the mucosal layers after paraquat ingestion. This causes swelling, edema, and painful ulceration of the mouth, pharynx, esophagus, stomach, and intestine. At high doses of paraquat, hepatocellular damage occurs, which is manifested by increased serum liver enzymes. Also, the deterioration of renal function may play an important role in determining the outcome of paraquat poisoning. Normal tubular cells secrete paraquat in urine quickly, efficiently removing it from the blood. However, high blood concentrations of poison affect the secretory mechanism and may destroy the cells.

Ingestion or accidental or deliberate exposure to paraquat has been responsible for many deaths. In one study, done in 1989 in Sri Lanka, found that out of 669 cases of poisoning, agrochemicals were responsible for 59% of toxicity and paraquat was the most common agent with a fatality rate of 68%. Even in the United Kingdom, in the years 1990–1991 there were 44 deaths with paraquat.

In Sweden, Denmark, Finland, and Austria, the use of paraquat is prohibited. In 2003, Syngenta pursued the Standing Committee on the Food Chain and Animal Health of the European Commission to include the authorization policy of EU pesticides. Subsequently, in August 2005, Austria, Finland, and Denmark opposed the use of paraquat. This is because it has sufficient evidence linking chronic use of paraquat with Parkinson's disease (PD) as described below. Moreover, paraquat residues in food are usually not detectable, except when this herbicide is used before getting the harvest of crops such as cereals, pineapple, etc. These foods have been reported to have levels of up to 0.2 mg/kg, whereas the acceptable daily intake is 0.004 mg/kg.

In the case of smoking marijuana contaminated with paraquat, the toxic effects are rare or nonexistent. Most paraquat that contaminates marijuana is pyrolyzed during the combustion of cigarette becoming bipyridyl, which is known to be very less toxic [71].

4.6. Toxicology of diquat

In humans, diquat is not systemically selectively absorbed nor concentrated in the lung tissue, as paraquat do, therefore, lung injury caused by diquat is less. However, diquat has severe toxic effects on the central nervous system that are not typical of paraquat poisoning. In many cases of human diquat poisoning, the medical signs and symptoms of neurological toxicity are the most important. These include nervousness, irritability, restlessness, combativeness, disorientation, nonsensical statements, diminished reflexes, and inability to recognize friends or family members. Neurologic effects may progress to coma, accompanied by tonic-clonic convulsions resulting in death. Also, parkinsonism was reported after skin exposure to diquat.

Another interesting aspect is the recognition of the role of inflammation and oxidative stress in the pathogenesis of PD. For example, in postmortem studies of some patients who were exposed to MPTP activation of microglia around neurons was found. So in our laboratory, we investigated the effect of MPTP over the activity of cyclooxygenase 2 (COX-2) using mice from the C57/BL6 strain. Our data indicate that a single dose of MPTP in mice had the following effects: a significant increase in the peroxidase activity of COX-2 in midbrain, compared with controls and increased nitrite levels and lipoperoxides in serum. These effects were presented after 24 hours of treatment. We also found that melatonin partially reverses the effects of MPTP on the activity of COX-2 and levels of nitrites and lipoperoxides in serum. The oxidative stress induced by MPTP in the mouse midbrain is also reflected in the serum, suggesting a systemic MPTP damage, which is reversed by melatonin, due to its antioxidant action. The action of melatonin can be attributed to the decrease of oxidizing species like dopamine-quinone. It has been further suggested that the cytotoxicity of neuronal COX-2 can come from the formation of reactive oxygen species generated during the catalysis of peroxidase activity of the enzyme [72].

4.7. Herbicides and Parkinson's disease

Structural similarity of the MPP+ and paraquat suggested that this herbicide could be toxic to dopaminergic neurons. In 1985, it was found that paraquat produced a parkinsonian behavior in leopard frogs (*Rana pipiens*). Whereas in mice of strain C57BL/6 systemic administration of paraquat resulted in a loss of dopaminergic neurons, degeneration of striatal dopaminergic fibers, and a reduction in ambulatory activity. Subsequently, in humans, the incidence of PD positively correlates with exposure to pesticides, including paraquat, in patients from some regions of Canada, Taiwan, and elsewhere.

Paraquat neurotoxicity is associated with their ability to induce the formation of free radicals, to induce the fibrillation α-synuclein, and to induce cell death by apoptosis [72].

4.8. Other pesticides and Parkinson's disease

Another class of chemicals associated with PD in humans is certainly having dithiocarbamates, such as maneb. *In vitro* studies show that neurotoxicity induced by maneb is related to the enzymatic inhibition of mitochondrial complex III and the oxidation of catecholamines. Systemic administration of paraquat and maneb induce a synergistic decrease in the content of DA in the striatum, SNPC degeneration, and motor abnormalities. Moreover, neonatal exposure of both pesticides increases the susceptibility of nigrostriatal dopaminergic system in maturity [73, 74].

Several plants (Derris elliptica, Lonchocarpus, and Tephrosia) contain the insecticide rotenone, which is a specific inhibitor of mitochondrial complex I. Its exposure to humans has been associated with PD. In rats, continuous systemic administration of rotenone reproduces the key aspects of PD including the selective degeneration of the nigrostriatal dopaminergic system, like the formation of cytoplasmic inclusions, Lewy bodies, and movement disorders. The effect of rotenone is mediated by the enzyme activity of microglial NADPH oxidase, which is the main source of $O_2\bullet$ radical [75, 76].

Also, organochlorine insecticides such as dieldrin are associated with motor disorders observed in ducks, pigeons, and rats. Furthermore, dieldrin residues detected in brains of PD patients, in cultured cells *in vitro*, shows selective dopaminergic neurotoxicity, which is mediated by the formation of oxygen-free radicals, lipid peroxidation, and fibril formation, α-synuclein. Also, some organophosphorus insecticides are associated with PD in humans.

It remains to be determined whether exposure to pesticides explains some cases of PD. A valuable tool to help determine this has been studies in which high doses of the pesticide are used for short periods and chronic application of these toxic in animal models [77].

4.9. Medical treatment of Parkinson's disease

Medical treatment of PD is usually based on anticholinergics, amantadine, levodopa, and other dopaminergic drugs. These agents maintain a good quality of life for most patients; however, when the disease progresses, it usually becomes ineffective and can cause adverse effects. So far, the most potent treatment of PD is L-dopa. However, L-dopa motor complications of chronic administration have emerged as a major limitation in response to treatment. That is why, in the future, neuroprotective therapies would slow the progression of the disease and delay the L-dopa need. There is insufficient evidence that L-dopa therapy prevents the progressive death of nigrostriatal neurons, but instead there is speculation that it may contribute to the progressive disease course. In the past years, they have contributed new knowledge about the mechanisms of neurodegeneration present in the PD [78].

4.10. Mitochondria and Parkinson's disease

Mitochondria participate in numerous cellular functions including ion homeostasis, heme and steroid synthesis, calcium signaling, and apoptosis [79, 80]. The well-known role of this organelle is to generate energy for cellular metabolism by the oxidative phosphorylation system. Electrons derived from cellular metabolism reach the mitochondria through two key coenzymes. Then they undergo a passage throughout the electron transport chain that consists of five protein complexes located in the inner mitochondrial membrane. Electrons pass through complexes I, III, and IV thanks to a proton gradient generated by the transport of these complexes to the outer side of the inner mitochondrial. In this process, the electron leakage from the respiratory chain induces the conversion of oxygen (0.4–4%) in superoxide radicals. As a consequence mitochondria are the primary source of ROS [81].

In the mitochondrial respiratory chain, the complexes I and III are the major sites of superoxide production. Partially reduced forms of oxygen are highly active; they chemically interact with biological molecules, resulting in oxidation of protein, DNA and RNA, and peroxidation of lipids. The damaging effects of ROS are counteracted by endogenous antioxidant enzymes such as catalase, superoxide dismutase, glutathione peroxidase, and glutathione reductase, and by molecules such as glutathione, metallothionein, and vitamins A, C, and E. Then cell death may be as well associated with decreasing capability to clear ROS by mitochondria [82–84].

Complex I of the respiratory enzyme is decreased in substantia nigra in patients with PD, possibly causing electron leakage from the electron transport system and increasing in the generation of peroxide anion (O_2–). This produces increasing activity in the manganese-superoxide dismutase (Mn-SOD), which is demonstrated in autopsied parkinsonian brains. Therefore, it indicates an increase in the generation of O_2– in the mitochondria, resulting in an increase in the generation of hydrogen peroxide. Levels of cytokines, such as TNF- or, interleukin-1/3, and interleukin-6, are elevated in the striatum, indicating activation of astrocytes and/or microglial cells. The activation in the microglial cells increases the nitric oxide (NO–) formation through the diaphorase system, and diffused to nerve terminals and dopaminergic cells in the central nervous system. NO– reacts with O_2– to produce peroxynitrate. On the other hand, iron is accumulated in astrocytes and microglia and NO– provokes ferric ion conjugation with ferritin, which is slowly released from cells to the intercellular space. Other proposed mechanism of oxidation is union of iron to oxygen and L-DOPA to iron (or copper) in the complex 27 of the mitochondrial chain, possibly initiating a lipid peroxidation in the cell membrane [85].

The genes linked to familial forms of PD include those associated with α-syn, parkin, DJ-1, PINK-1, LRRK-2, ATP13A2, mitochondrial phosphatase, and phosphatase and tensin homolog (PTEN)-induced kinase gene, between others, and they have been demonstrated to be involved in apoptosis regulation. Parkin is associated with the outer mitochondrial membrane and prevents cell death by inhibiting mitochondrial swelling, cyt-C release, and caspase activation. Another finding in pathogenesis has been centered in the ATP13A2 gene, which regulates intracellular Mn^{2+} homeostasis, playing an important role in preventing damage induced by Mn^{2+} cytotoxicity. Overexposure of cells to Mn^{2+} may determine cell death by induction of DNA damage, oxidative stress, disruption of Ca^{2+} and iron homeostasis, and mitochondrial dysfunction. In an experimental model, monomeric α-Syn-expressing dopaminergic cells significantly attenuated Mn-induced neurotoxicity for initial exposures. However, overexposure to Mn produces precipitation of α-syn, which at the same time impairs antioxidative defense mechanism in this experimental model [86–88].

Other findings suggested that mitochondrial dysfunction is at the heart of PD. For instance, MPTP infusion causes parkinsonism by selective inhibition of mitochondrial complex-1 [89]. In patients with PD there is an excess amount of cytosolic dopamine outside of the synaptic vesicles due to damaged neurons with impaired reuptake, with a possible increased damage when an overload is related to levodopa treatment. Dopamine then is easily metabolized via monoamine oxidase or by auto-oxidation to cytotoxic ROS provoking mitochondrial impairment by activating the intrinsic apoptotic pathway or by inhibiting the respiratory chain. Also, the auto-oxidation of DA produces electron-deficient DA quinones or DA semiquinones, which at the same time can modify some PD-related proteins, such as α-syn, parkin, DJ-1, superoxide dismutase-2, and UCH-L1. Additionally, DA quinones can be oxidized to aminochrome, whose redox-cycling leads to the generation of the superoxide radical and the depletion of cellular nicotinamide adenine dinucleotide phosphate-oxidase (NADPH), which ultimately forms the neuromelanin, contributing to this degenerative mechanism [11].

5. Conclusion

There are many proposed mechanisms that may produce damage to dopaminergic neurons, but all of them finally converge in a common pathway involving ROS/RNS and mitochondrial dysfunction that promotes apoptosis. Exposure to environmental factors or mutations in PD-associated genes of patients with either sporadic or familial PD may cause mitochondrial dysfunction that ultimately results in PD. In the near future, neuroprotection may coincide with reductions in intracellular reactive oxygen species, lipid peroxidation, and DNA damage in the effort to save neurons from death avoiding neurodegeneration to advance until the point of neither manifesting PD symptoms nor producing advanced symptoms in a patient with evident motor PD.

Author details

Genaro Gabriel Ortiz[1*], Fermín P. Pacheco-Moisés[2], Mario A. Mireles-Ramírez[3], L. Javier Flores-Alvarado[4], Héctor González-Usigli[3], Angélica L. Sánchez-López[1], Lorenzo Sánchez-Romero[1], Irma E. Velázquez-Brizuela[1], Erika Daniela González-Renovato[1] and Erandis Dheni Torres-Sánchez[1]

*Address all correspondence to: genarogabriel@yahoo.com

1 Laboratory of Mitochondria-Oxidative Stress and Pathology, Neurosciences Division, West Biomedical Research Center of the Mexican Social Security Institute, Guadalajara, Jalisco, México

2 Department of Chemistry, Exact Sciences and Engineering Center, University of Guadalajara, Guadalajara, Jalisco, México

3 Department of Neurology, High Specialty Medical Unit, Western National Medical Center of the Mexican Social Security Institute, Guadalajara, Jalisco, México

4 Department of Biochemistry, Health Science Center, University of Guadalajara, Guadalajara, Jalisco, México

References

[1] Braak H, Braak E. Pathoanatomy of Parkinson's disease. J Neurol. 2000; 247 (Suppl 2):II3–II10.

[2] Groenewegen H. J. The basal ganglia and motor control. Neural Plast. 2003; 10:107–120. doi:10.1155/NP.2003.107.

[3] Twelves D, Perkins KS, Counsell C. Systematic review of incidence studies of Parkinson's disease. Mov Disord. 2003 Jan; 18(1):19–31.

[4] Aarsland D, Andersen K, Larsen JP, Lolk A, Nielsen H, Kragh-Sorensen P. Risk of dementia in Parkinson's disease: a community-based, prospective study. Neurology. 2001; 56:730–736.

[5] Fenelon G. Psychosis in Parkinson's disease: phenomenology, frequency, risk factors, and current understanding of pathophysiologic mechanisms. CNS Spectr. 2008; 13:18–25.

[6] Park S, Stacy M. Non-motor symptoms in Parkinson's disease. J Neurol. 2009; 256 (Suppl 3):S293–S298.

[7] Fénelon G, Mahieux F, Huon R, Ziégler M. Hallucinations in Parkinson's disease: prevalence, phenomenology and risk factors. Brain. 2000 Apr; 123 (Pt 4):733–745.

[8] Rao G, Fisch L, Srinivasan S, D'Amico F, Okada T, Eaton C, et al. Does this patient have Parkinson disease? JAMA 2003; 289(3):347–353.

[9] von Bohlen und Halbach O, Schober A, Krieglstein K. Genes, proteins, and neurotoxins involved in Parkinson's disease. Prog Neurobiol. (2004); 73:151–177.

[10] Anne-Marie Arel-Dubeau F, Fanny Longpré L, Bournival J, Tremblay C, Demers-Lamarche J, et al. Cucurbitacin E has neuroprotective properties and autophagic modulating activities on dopaminergic neurons. Oxid Med Cell Longev.. 2014; 425496:1–15.

[11] Blesa J, Trigo-Damas I, Quiroga-Varela A, Jackson-Lewis VR. Oxidative stress and Parkinson's disease. Front Neuroanat. 2015; 8(9):91.

[12] Seniuk NA, Tatton WG, Greenwood CE. Dose-dependent destruction of the coeruleus-cortical and nigral-striatal projections by MPTP. Brain Res. 1990; 527: 7–20.

[13] Betarbet R, Sherer TB, MacKenzie G, Garcia-Osuna M, Panov AV, Greenamyre JT. Chronic systemic pesticide exposure reproduces features of Parkinson's disease. Nat Neurosci. 2000; 3:1301–1306.

[14] Fornai F, Schluter OM, Lenzi P, Gesi M, Ruffoli R, Ferrucci M, Lazzeri G, Busceti CL, Pontarelli F, Battaglia G, Pellegrini A, Nicoletti F, Ruggieri S, Paparelli A, Sudhof TC. Parkinson-like syndrome induced by continuous MPTP infusion: convergent roles of the ubiquitin-proteasome system and alpha-synuclein. Proc Natl Acad Sci USA. 2005; 102: 3413–3418.

[15] Ortiz GG, Pacheco-Moises FP, Gomez-Rodriguez VM, Gonzalez-Renovato ED, Torres-Sanchez ED, et al. Fish oil, melatonin and vitamin E attenuates midbrain cyclooxygenase-2 activity and oxidative stress after the administration of 1-methyl-4-phenyl-1,2,3,6-tetrahydropyridine. Metab Brain Dis 2013.

[16] Chen X, Guo C, Kong J. Oxidative stress in neurodegenerative diseases*. Neural Regen Res. 2012; 376–385.

[17] Valko M, Leibfritz D, Moncol J, Cronin MT, Mazur M, Telser J. Free radicals and antioxidants in normal physiological functions and human disease. Int J Biochem Cell Biol [Internet]. 2007; 39(1):44–84.

[18] Murphy MP. How mitochondria produce reactive oxygen species. Biochem J. 2009; 417(1):1–13.

[19] Lobo V, Patil A, Phatak A, Chandra N. Free radicals, antioxidants and functional foods: impact on human health. Pharmacogn Rev [Internet]. 2010; 4(8):118. Available from: http://www.phcogrev.com/text.asp?2010/4/8/118/70902

[20] Uttara B, Singh A V, Zamboni P, Mahajan RT. Oxidative stress and neurodegenerative diseases: a review of upstream and downstream antioxidant therapeutic options. Curr Neuropharmacol. 2009; 7:65–74.

[21] Zündorf G, Reiser G. Calcium dysregulation and homeostasis of neural calcium in the molecular mechanisms of neurodegenerative diseases provide multiple targets for neuroprotection. Antioxid Redox Signal. 2011; 14(7):1275–1288.

[22] Van der Vliet A, Bast A. Effect of oxidative stress on receptors and signal transmission. Chem Biol Interact [Internet]. 1992 Dec; 85(2–3):95–116. Available from: http://www.ncbi.nlm.nih.gov/pubmed/1493612

[23] Radi EPF. Apoptosis and oxidative stress in neurodegenerative diseases. J Alzheimer's Dis. 2014; 42:S125–152.

[24] Gazewood JD, Richards DR, Clebak K. Parkinson's disease: an update. Am Family Phys. 2013; 87(4):267–273.

[25] Davie CA. A review of Parkinson's disease. Br Med Bull. 2008; 86(1): 109–127.

[26] Jankovic J. Parkinson's disease: clinical features and diagnosis. J Neurol Neurosurg Psychiat. 2008; 79(4):368–376.

[27] Stiasny-Kolster K, Doerr Y, Moller JC, et al. Combination of 'idiopathic' REM sleep behaviour disorder and olfactory dysfunction as possible indicator for α-synucleinopathy demonstrated by dopamine transporter FP-CIT-SPECT. Brain 2005; 128:126–137.

[28] Takatsu H, Nishida H, Matsuo H, et al. Cardiac sympathetic denervation from the early stage of Parkinson's disease: clinical and experimental studies with radiolabeled MIBG. J Nucl Med. 2000; 41:71–77.

[29] Druschky A, Hilz MJ, Platsch G, et al. Differentiation of Parkinson's disease and multiple system atrophy in early disease stages by means of I-123-MIBG–SPECT. J Neurol Sci. 2000; 175:3–12.

[30] Langston JW. The Parkinson's complex: parkinsonism is just the tip of the iceberg. Ann Neurol. 2006; 59:591–596.

[31] Chaudhuri KR, Schapira AH. Non-motor symptoms of Parkinson's disease: dopaminergic pathophysiology and treatment. Lancet Neurol. 2009; 8:464–474.

[32] Aarsland D, Pahlhagen S, Ballard CG, Ehrt U, Svenningsson P. Depression in Parkinson disease–epidemiology, mechanisms and management. Nat Rev Neurol. 2011; 8:35–47.

[33] Frisina P, Haroutunian V, Libow L. The neuropathological basis for depression in Parkinson's disease. Parkinsonism Relat Disord. 2009; 15:144–148.

[34] Martinez-Martin P, Damian J. Parkinson disease: depression and anxiety in Parkinson disease. Nat Rev Neurol. 2010; 6:243–245.

[35] Soh S, Morris M, McGinley J. Determinants of health-related quality of life in Parkinson's disease: a systematic review. Parkinsonism Relat Disord. 2011; 17:1–9.

[36] Hemmerle A, Herman J, Seroog K. Stress, depression and Parkinson's disease. Exp Neurol. 2012; 233:79–86.

[37] Schulz JB, Falkenburger BH. Neuronal pathology in Parkinson's disease. Cell Tissue Res. 2004; 318:135–147.

[38] Fearnley JM, Lees AJ. Ageing and Parkinson's disease: substantia nigra regional selectivity. Brain. 1991; 114(Pt 5):2283–2301.

[39] Radi E, Formichi P, Battisti C, Federico A. Apoptosis and oxidative stress in neurodegenerative diseases. J Alzheimers Dis [Internet]. 2014 ;42(Suppl 3):S125–S152. Available from: http://www.ncbi.nlm.nih.gov/pubmed/25056458.

[40] Choi MS, Nakamura T, Cho S-J, Han X, Holland EA, Qu J, et al. Transnitrosylation from DJ-1 to PTEN attenuates neuronal cell death in Parkinson's disease models. J Neurosci [Internet]. 2014; 34(45):15123–15131. Available from: http://www.jneurosci.org/cgi/doi/10.1523/JNEUROSCI.4751-13.2014

[41] Pereira C, Miguel Martins L, Saraiva L. LRRK2, but not pathogenic mutants, protects against H2O2 stress depending on mitochondrial function and endocytosis in a yeast model. Biochim Biophys Acta Gen Subj [Internet]. 2014 Jun; 1840(6):2025–2031.

[42] Sanders LH, McCoy J, Hu X, Mastroberardino PG, Dickinson BC, Chang CJ, et al. Mitochondrial DNA damage: molecular marker of vulnerable nigral neurons in Parkinson's disease. Neurobiol Dis [Internet]. 2014; 70:214–223. Available from: http://dx.doi.org/10.1016/j.nbd.2014.06.014

[43] Arel-Dubeau A-M, Longpré F, Bournival J, Tremblay C, Demers-Lamarche J, Haskova P, et al. Cucurbitacin E has neuroprotective properties and autophagic modulating activities on dopaminergic neurons. Oxid Med Cell Longev [Internet]. 2014; 2014:1–15.

[44] Celardo I, Martins LM, Gandhi S. Unravelling mitochondrial pathways to Parkinson's disease. Br J Pharmacol. 2014; 171(8):1943–1957.

[45] Segura-Aguilar J, Kostrzewa RM. Neurotoxin mechanisms and processes relevant to Parkinson's disease: an update. Neurotox Res [Internet]. 2015; 27(3):328–354.

[46] Alvarez-Castelao B, Gorostidi A, Ruíz-Martínez J, De Munain AL, Castaño JG. Epitope mapping of antibodies to alpha-synuclein in LRRK2 mutation carriers, idiopathic parkinson disease patients, and healthy controls. Front Aging Neurosci. 2014; 6(July): 1–9.

[47] Alberio T, Bondi H, Colombo F, Alloggio I, Pieroni L, Urbani A, et al. Mitochondrial proteomics investigation of a cellular model of impaired dopamine homeostasis, an early step in Parkinson's disease pathogenesis. Mol Biosyst [Internet]. 2014; 10:1332–1344.

[48] Li D-W, Yao M, Dong Y-H, Tang M-N, Chen W, Li G-R, et al. Guanosine exerts neuroprotective effects by reversing mitochondrial dysfunction in a cellular model of Parkinson's disease. Int J Mol Med [Internet]. 2014 Aug 19.

[49] Lee JA, Kim JH, Woo SY, Son HJ, Han SH, Jang BK, et al. A novel compound VSC2 has anti-inflammatory and antioxidant properties in microglia and in Parkinson's disease animal model. Br J Pharmacol [Internet]. 2015 Feb; 172(4):1087–1100.

[50] Keane PC, Kurzawa M, Blain PG, Morris CM. Mitochondrial dysfunction in Parkinson's disease. Parkinsons Dis [Internet]. 2011; 2011:1–18.

[51] Shukla V, Mishra SK, Pant HC. Oxidative stress in neurodegeneration. Adv Pharmacol Sci [Internet]. 2011; 2011:1–13.

[52] Harischandra DS, Jin H, Anantharam V, Kanthasamy A, Kanthasamy AG. Synuclein protects against manganese neurotoxic insult during the early stages of exposure in a dopaminergic cell model of Parkinson's disease. Toxicol Sci [Internet]. 2015 Feb 1; 143(2):454–468.

[53] Kim H-J, Kim HJ, Jeong J-E, Baek JY, Jeong J, Kim S, et al. N-terminal truncated UCH-L1 prevents Parkinson's disease associated damage. PLoS One [Internet]. 2014; 9(6):e99654.

[54] Patel VP, Chu CT. Decreased SIRT2 activity leads to altered microtubule dynamics in oxidatively-stressed neuronal cells: implications for Parkinson's disease. Exp Neurol [Internet]. 2014 Jul; 257(9):170–181.

[55] Hastings TG. The role of dopamine oxidation in mitochondrial dysfunction: implications for Parkinson's disease. J Bioenerg Biomembr. 2009; 41(6):469–472.

[56] Cohen G, Farooqui R, Kesler N. Parkinson disease: a new link between monoamine oxidase and mitochondrial electron flow. Proc Natl Acad Sci U S A [Internet]. 1997; 94(10):4890–4894.

[57] Marchitti SA, Deitrich RA, Vasiliou V. Neurotoxicity and metabolism of the catecholamine-derived 3,4-dihydroxyphenylacetaldehyde and 3,4-dihydroxyphenylglycolaldehyde: the role of aldehyde dehydrogenase. Pharmacol Rev [Internet]. 2007 Mar 22; 59(2):125–150.

[58] Kell DB. Towards a unifying, systems biology understanding of large-scale cellular death and destruction caused by poorly liganded iron: Parkinson's, Huntington's, Alzheimer's, prions, bactericides, chemical toxicology and others as examples. Arch Toxicol [Internet]. 2010; 84(11):825–889.

[59] Hirsch EC, Hunot S. Neuroinflammation in Parkinson's disease: a target for neuroprotection? Lancet Neurol [Internet]. 2009 Apr; 8(4):382–397.

[60] Davis GC, Williams AC, Markey SP, Ebert MH, Caine ED, Reichert CM, et al. Chronic Parkinsonism secondary to intravenous injection of meperidine analogues. Psychiatry Res. 1979; 1:249–254.

[61] Langston JW, Ballard P, Tetrud J, Irwin I. Chronic parkinsonism in humans due to a product of meperidine-analog synthesis. Science. 1983; 219:979–980.

[62] Langston JW, Forno LS, Tetrud J, Reeves AG, Kaplan JA, Karluk D. Evidence of active nerve cell degeneration in the substantia nigra of humans years after 1-methyl-4-phenyl-1,2,3,6-tetrahydropyridine exposure. Ann Neurol 1999; 46:598–605.

[63] Przedborski S, Jackson-Lewis V. Mechanisms of MPTP toxicity. Mov Disord. 1998; 13 (Suppl. 1):35–38.

[64] Przedborski S, Teismann T, Tieu K, Choi DK, Wu DC, Naini A, et al. Cyclooxygenase-2 is instrumental in Parkinson's disease neurodegeneration. Proc Natl Acad Sci U S A. 2003; 100:5473–5478.

[65] Pearce RK, Owen A, Daniel S, Jenner P, Marsden CD. Alterations in the distribution of glutathione in the substantia nigra in Parkinson's disease. J Neural Transm. 1997; 104:661–677.

[66] Kass GEN, Wright JW, Nicotera P, Orrenius S. The mechanism of 1-methyl-4-phenyl-1,2,3,6-tetrahydropyridine toxicity: role of intracellular calcium. Arch Biochem Biophys. 1988; 260:789–797.

[67] Pond SM. Manifestations and management of paraquat poisoning. Med J Aust. 1990; 152:256–259.

[68] Ortiz GG, Reiter RJ, Zúñiga G, Melchiorri D, Sewerynek E, Pablos MI, et al. Genotoxicity of paraquat: micronuclei induced in bone marrow and peripheral blood are inhibited by melatonin. Mutat Res Jan. 2000; 24;464:239–245.

[69] Vale JA, Meredith TJ, Buckley BM. Paraquat poisoning: clinical features and immediate general management. Hum Toxicol. 1987; 6:41–47.

[70] Smith P, Heath D. The pathology of the lung in paraquat poisoning. J Clin Pathol Suppl. 1975; 9:81–93.

[71] Bismuth C, Garnier R, Baud FJ, Muszynski J, Keyes C. Paraquat poisoning. An overview of the current status. Drug Safety. 1990; 5:243–251.

[72] Sechi GP, Agnetti V, Piredda M. Acute and persistent Parkinsonism after use of diquat. Neurology. 1992; 42:261–263.

[73] Ferraz HB, Bertolucci PH, Pereira JS, Lima JG, Andrade LA. Chronic exposure to the fungicide maneb may produce symptoms and signs of CNS manganese intoxication. Neurology. 1988; 38:550–553.

[74] Thiruchelvam M, Richfield EK, Goodman BM, Baggs RB, Cory-Slechta DA. Developmental exposure to the pesticides paraquat and maneb and the Parkinson's disease phenotype. Neurotoxicology. 2002; 23:621–633.

[75] Gao HM, Hong JS, Zhang W, Liu B. Distinct role for microglia in rotenone-induced degeneration of dopaminergic neurons. J Neurosci. 2002; 22:782–790.

[76] Alam M, Schmidt WJ. Rotenone destroys dopaminergic neurons and induces parkinsonian symptoms in rats. Behav Brain Res. 2002; 136:317–324.

[77] Fleming L, Mann JB, Bean J, Briggle T, Sanchez-Ramos JR. Parkinson's disease and brain levels of organochlorine pesticides. Ann Neurol. 1994; 36:100–103.

[78] Katunina EA, Titova N V, Malykhina EA, Gasanov MG, Makarova AA, Voronina TA, et al. [Oxidative stress and Parkinson's disease: mechanisms and perspectives of treatment]. Zhurnal Nevrol i psikhiatrii Im SS Korsakova/Minist Zdr i meditsinskoĭ promyshlennosti Ross Fed Vserossiĭskoe Obs Nevrol [i] Vserossiĭskoe Obs psikhiatrov [Internet]. 2015; 115(7):141–145.

[79] Hajnóczky G, Csordás G, Das S, Garcia-Perez C, Saotome M, Sinha Roy S, et al. Mitochondrial calcium signalling and cell death: approaches for assessing the role of mitochondrial Ca^{2+} uptake in apoptosis. Cell Calcium. 2006; 40(5–6):553–560.

[80] Rosier MF. T channels and steroid biosynthesis: in search of a link with mitochondria. Cell Calcium. 2006; 40(2):155–164.

[81] Murphy MP. How mitochondria produce reactive oxygen species. Biochem J. 2009; 417:1–13.

[82] Celardo I, Martins LM, Gandhi S. Unravelling mitochondrial pathways to Parkinson's disease. Br J Pharmacol. 2014; 171:1943–1957.

[83] Radi EPF. Apoptosis and oxidative stress in neurodegenerative diseases. J Alzheimer's Dis. 2014; 42:S125–S152.

[84] Antunes MS, Goes AT, Boeira SP, Prigol M, Jesse CR. Protective effect of hesperidin in a model of Parkinson's disease induced by 6-hydroxydopamine in aged mice. Nutrition. 2014 Nov-Dec; 30(11–12):1415–1422.

[85] Kindo T. Parkinson's disease and free radicals mechanism of neurodegeneration and neuroprotection. Ann N Y Acad Sci. 1996; 15(786):206–216.

[86] Kostrzewa JS-A. Neurotoxin mechanisms and processes relevant to Parkinson's disease: an update. Neurotox Res. 2015; 27(3):328–354.

[87] Dilshan S, Harischandra HJ. a-Synuclein protects against manganese neurotoxic insult during the early stages of exposure in a dopaminergic cell model of Parkinson's disease. Toxicol Sci. 2015;143(2).

[88] Hee-Jung Kim HJ-E. N-terminal truncated UCH-L1 prevents Parkinson's disease associated damage. PLOS One. 2014; 9(6):1–17.

[89] Tiziana Alberio AH. Mitochondrial proteomics investigation of a cellular model of impaired dopamine homeostasis, an early step in Parkinson's disease pathogenesis. Mol BioSystems. 2014; 10:1332–1344.

Chapter 10

Nitroso-Redox Crosstalk in Diabetic Cardiomyopathy

Daniel R González, Adriana V Treuer and
Ulises Novoa

Additional information is available at the end of the chapter

http://dx.doi.org/10.5772/63668

Abstract

Diabetes mellitus is one of the most common chronic diseases worldwide. Diabetic cardiomyopathy (DM) is the deterioration of the myocardial function and morphology produced by the altered glucose metabolism imposed in diabetes. This process of cardiac deterioration involves the generation of oxidative species. In the diabetic heart, several sources contribute to the observed oxidative stress, such as xanthine oxidoreductase (XOR), nicotinamide adenine dinucleotide phosphate (NADPH), nitrogen oxidases (NOX), mitochondria, and uncoupled nitric oxide synthases (NOS). A direct consequence of the increased production of reactive oxygen species (ROS) is NOS uncoupling. This is the aftermath of the oxidation of tetrahydrobioterin (BH4), an essential cofactor for NOS activity. When NOS is uncoupled, its activity is redirected toward the production of superoxide, instead of nitric oxide (NO), further contributing to the oxidative process. This nitroso-redox disarrangement has a direct impact on the excitation-contraction-coupling machinery of the myocyte, in the mitochondrial stability impairing energy production and favoring apoptosis, myocardial fibrosis, ultimately reducing cardiac function. This review focuses on the impact of superoxide sources in the diabetic heart and the pharmacological approaches that are currently under investigation as possible therapeutic tools.

Keywords: Superoxide, nitric oxide, BH4, NOX, XOR

1. Introduction

Diabetes mellitus is one of the most common chronic diseases worldwide [1] and continues to increase in numbers and significance, with characteristics of an epidemic [2], as modern lifestyles lead to reduced physical activity and increased obesity.

Diabetic cardiomyopathy is the manifestation in the myocardium of the alterations produced by the altered homeostasis of glucose metabolism [3], independent of coronary artery disease and hypertension. This cardiomyopathy is characterized initially by diastolic dysfunction and cardiac hypertrophy, with preserved ejection fraction [4]. As diabetes progress, systolic dysfunction and reduced ejection fraction are developed [5]. This process of cardiac deterioration in diabetes includes oxidative stress [6] that results in apoptosis [7–9] and fibrosis that further deteriorate the myocardium. Despite the importance of diabetic cardiomyopathy as a clinical entity, the pathological cellular and molecular mechanisms driving the adverse changes in diabetic myocardial structure and function have not been fully resolved, but the development and progression of diabetic complications is frequently attributed to increased oxidative stress [6].

Reactive oxygen species (ROS) consist of a variety of highly reactive oxygen-based molecules that consist of both free radicals and chemicals capable of generating free radicals, such as superoxide, H_2O_2, and peroxynitrite ($ONOO^-$) [10]. Although in health the primary source of ROS is the mitochondria [11], they are also produced by a range of other sources such as xanthine oxidase, NADPH oxidases and uncoupled nitric oxide synthase (NOS). Oxidative stress takes place when the rate of production of ROS overrides the degradation by antioxidant enzymes. An increase in ROS levels leads to a constellation of harmful consequences by producing damage by oxidative modifications, diminishing of nitric oxide (NO) bioavailability, and by inducing alteration in the intracellular-signaling pathways [12]. In a variety of studies in animal models of diabetes and humans with diabetic cardiomyopathy, it has been shown that increased ROS levels [11, 13] have been associated with the pathophysiology of heart failure, including from cardiac remodeling and mechanical impairment [14]. This ROS-induced damage is probably a consequence of oxidative damage to cardiac proteins and also by inducing cell death in the myocardium [8, 13, 15].

In diabetes, the resultant hyperglycemia, hyperlipidemia, and insulin resistance enhance oxidative stress in the diabetic heart [16]. Altered glucose flux, mitochondrial dysfunction, and nitric oxide synthase uncoupling jeopardize the diabetic myocardium, increasing the risk of cardiac remodeling and the transition toward heart failure [3].

In the diabetic heart, the alterations in the excitation-contraction coupling machinery are profound [17]. The levels of the sarcoendoplasmic reticulum Ca^{2+} pump (SERCA) are reduced [18], and total phospholamban (PLB) is increased [19], while phosphorylated phospholamban is reduced. Phospholamban is a 5 kDa protein that tonically inhibits the activity of SERCA2. Upon activation, phospholamban is phosphorylated (by PKA or CamKII, for instance), oligomerizes, and releases SERCA of its inhibition [20]. In this condition, Ca^{2+} is transported back into the sarcoplasmic reticulum at a higher rate. The expression of the calcium release channel ryanodine receptor (RyR2) and the sodium-calcium exchanger (NCX) are reduced in general [18, 19, 21–24]. Functionally, this pattern of protein expression is associated with impaired relaxation, increased sarcoplasmic reticulum calcium leak, and reduced contractility.

http://dx.doi.org/10.5772/63668

Altered calcium handling has been characterized in the diabetic cardiac myocytes [17]. Reduced capacity of the sarcoplasmic reticulum Ca^{2+} pump SERCA2 results in a diminished storage capacity of Ca^{2+} that impairs cardiac contractility [18, 19, 25]. Importantly, it also alters cardiac relaxation, which is evidenced in the diastolic dysfunction.

Oxidative stress may affect Ca^{2+} handling in the heart, at the level of the ryanodine receptor (RyR2) [26–28], which is the Ca^{2+} release channel of the sarcoplasmic reticulum. This channel is particularly redox sensitive and has been described that oxidative modification alters it function, leading to diastolic leak of Ca^{2+}, with a negative impact of contractility and relaxation [28–30].

In diabetes, several sources may contribute to the observed oxidative stress, such as xanthine oxidoreductase (XOR) [31, 32], NADPH oxidases (NOX) [33–35], mitochondria [11], and uncoupled nitric oxide synthases (NOS) [36, 37]. Apparently, the main source of superoxide in the diabetic heart corresponds to XOR and NOX. These latter enzymes are present in the heart, mainly with the isoforms NOX2 and NOX4.

A direct consequence of the increased production of ROS is the uncoupling of nitric oxide synthase [38]. This is due to the oxidation of tetrahydrobioterin, an essential cofactor for NOS activity [39]. When NOS is uncoupled, its activity is redirected toward the production of superoxide, instead of NO [26], further contributing to the oxidative process.

2. NADPH oxidases NOX

Nicotinamide adenine dinucleotide phosphate oxidase enzymes (NADPH oxidases or NOX) received growing attention as a source of ROS and particularly for their involvement in redox signaling [40]. NOX exist in several isoforms (NOX1, 2, 4, and 5) [41]. These enzymes catalyze for electron transfer from NADPH to molecular oxygen, resulting in the generation of oxygen-free radicals. NADPH oxidase is increased in both failing and diabetic rodent hearts [42–44]. In diabetic rodents, the upregulation of NADPH oxidase correlates with morphological evidence of cardiac hypertrophy and upregulation of pro-fibrotic genes [42, 43, 45].

NOX2 is formed by the membrane-associated $p22^{phox}$ and one $gp91^{phox}$. The translocation of the cytosolic regulatory subunits $p40^{phox}$, $p47^{phox}$, $p67^{phox}$ and the small G protein Rac1 (the isoform expressed in the cardiomyocyte) or Rac2 is necessary for the occurrence of electron transfer from NADPH to oxygen. Under stimulation, for instance, with high levels of glucose or AngII, PKC is activated, leading to phosphorylation of $p47^{phox}$, an event that promotes the association of cytosolic subunits with p22phox and gp91phox [41] (**Figure 1**). In the cardiovascular system, these enzymatic components are expressed in endothelial cells, smooth muscle, cardiomyocytes, and fibroblasts [41, 46].

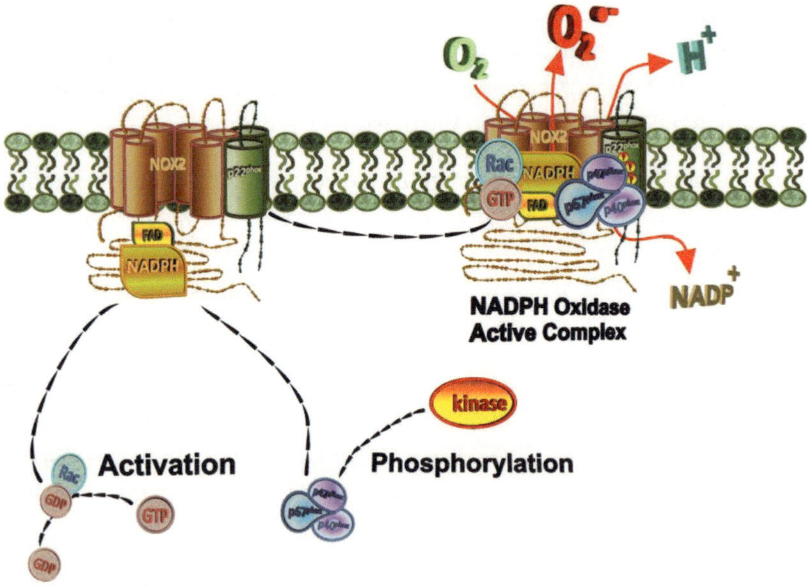

Figure 1. Mechanism of NADPH oxidase activation. Upon proper stimulus, Rac is activated and p47[phox] is phosphorylated. Then p47[phox] binds p40[phox] and p67[phox] and along with Rac, translocate to the cell membrane, where they activate NOX2 superoxide production.

2.1. NOX in diabetes

Several reports indicate that an increased activity of NOX, particularly NOX2 [34, 43, 47, 48] and NOX4 [35], may be implicated in the pathophysiology of diabetic cardiomyopathy. Hyperglycemia induces O_{2-} generation in the heart primarily by disruption of the electron transport chain in mitochondria, activation of NOX and uncoupling of NOS. In type-2 diabetes, a state of permanent oxidative stress alters mitochondrial function, impairing energy production and ultimately producing cardiomyocyte dysfunction. Elevated glucose levels have been shown to stimulate NOX activity, increasing NOX-derived superoxide production in cardiac cells [48].

2.2. Physiological functions of NOX2

Recently, Prosser *et al.* elegantly demonstrated a physiological role for NOX2 in the cardiac myocytes, demonstrating that NOX2 activity is required to stimulate RyR2 in conditions of physiological stretching (preload). NOX2 activation upon stretching sensitizes RyR2 increasing the rate of Ca^{2+} sparks [49]. This mechanism becomes dysregulated in dystrophic cardiomyopathy [50]. Furthermore, more recently, it has been published that NOX2 in conjunction with NOS1 are absolutely required for another cardiac physiological response to an increase in afterload (Anrep effect) [51]. NOX2 oxidase has been implicated in the cardiac dysfunction observed in ob/ob cardiac myocytes [34, 52].

http://dx.doi.org/10.5772/63668

2.3. NOX2 and diabetic cardiomyopathy

Several lines of evidence showed a role of NOX2 in the diabetic cardiomyopathy [53, 54]. First, NOX2 is activated and its subunits are upregulated in several models of diabetes and insulin resistance, streptozotocin-treated mice, ob/ob and db/db mice, and fructose-fed rats, with increased oxidative stress as a consequence.

Using streptozotocin-treated mice, Roe *et al.* [55] described that pharmacological inhibition of NADPH oxidase with apocynin reduced part of the cardiac damage and it improved heart functional evaluated as fractional shortening, and cardiomyocytes mechanics, associated with a reduction in nitrosative and oxidative stress. Nevertheless, since apocynin is not a specific inhibitor for NOX2, these results might be ascribed also to NOX4, which is also present in the cardiomyocyte.

Evidence for a more specific and crucial role for NOX2 came from studies using knock out for Rac1, one of the cytosolic components of the holoenzyme complex. In cardiac-specific Rac-1 knockout mice, induction of diabetes by streptozotocin treatment showed reduced apoptosis, fibrosis and improved cardiac function compared to wild-type animals [56, 57]. The mechanisms of reduced cardiac damage involves a reduction in NADPH oxidase activity, a reduction in mitochondrial ROS production that attenuates fetal gene program, reduces the inflammatory process, and reduces endoplasmic reticulum stress. In addition, cardiomyocyte-specific deletion of Rac-1 reduces cardiac damage in diabetic mice after ischemia-reperfusion by reducing calpain proteolictic activity [58].

2.4. NOX4

NOX4 is expressed constitutively in the heart and its activity has been ascribed as mitochondrial [59]. Its physiological role has not been clarified. On the contrary, there are descriptions of NOX4 in pathological conditions that are both beneficial [60] and deleterious [44]. Indeed, Sadoshima's group has shown that NOX4 is an important source of oxidative stress in a mouse model of pressure overload (by aortic constriction). In this study, NOX4 deletion was associated with preserved ejection fraction and reduced hypertrophy, apoptosis, and mitochondrial function compared to wild-type animals [44]. Nevertheless, these results are contrary to those observed by Shah's group. These investigators reported a protective role for NOX4, using the same strategy (pressure overload in a cardiomyocyte-specific knock-out mouse for NOX4), with the difference that they additionally used a mouse with cardiomyocyte-targeted increase in NOX4, which showed an increased angiogenesis in response to overload [60].

Regarding diabetic cardiomyopathy, Maalouf *et al.* reported that NOX4 plays a pivotal role in the cardiac damage in streptozotocin-treated rats. They found that NOX4 was up upregulated and when silenced using antisense oligonucleotides, this was reversed, along with the induction of fetal program genes and fibrosis, as well as cardiac function [35].

3. Xanthine oxidoreductase

Xanthine oxidoreductase (XOR) is a highly conserved member of the molybdoenzyme family. It consists of a 150 kDa homodimer that is involved in the purine degradation pathway, producing superoxide as a secondary metabolite. This precursor may further divert in the formation of two enzymatic activities, xanthine dehydrogenase (XDH) and xanthine oxidase (XO). XO is derived from XDH as a result of proteolisis or reversible oxidation of cysteines of XDH. Whereas XDH reduces NAD^+ to NADH, XO utilizes molecular oxygen as electron acceptor. They differ in that XO only reduces oxygen, whereas XDH can reduce either O_2 or NAD^+. Both forms catalyze the conversion of hypoxanthine to xanthine and xanthine to uric acid. In both steps, O_{2-} and H_2O_2 are produced [61]. Normally, in the cardiac myocyte, XOR is located in the sarcoplasmic reticulum, where it regulates some features of calcium handling and also myofilament calcium sensitivity. We have reported that XOR is upregulated in dilated cardiomyopathy, producing oxidative stress that interferes with NO signaling, resulting in dysregulated RyR2 activity, ultimately producing diastolic calcium leak and reducing contractility [28]. It is probably that in diabetes, XOR may impact negatively calcium handling, but this has not been clarified.

XOR has been implicated in the pathophysiology of streptozotocin-induced diabetic cardiomyopathy and its inhibition with allopurinol, oxypurinol, and antioxidants yielded some positive results that included improvement in cardiac function, reduction in oxidative stress, reduced cardiac apoptosis, fibrosis (collagen I), and hypertrophy [31, 33, 62]. In obese (ob/ob mice), XOR is upregulated and its activity increased, leading to alterations in the redox state of the heart, such as diminished GSH/GSSG ratio and decreased levels of NO metabolites [32].

Importantly, XOR has been shown to be increased in type-1 diabetic patients [63]. In addition, in a study in patients with type-2 diabetes and left ventricular hypertrophy, the treatment with allopurinol reduced left ventricular mass modestly but significantly in a period of 9 months of treatment, in a dosage that reduced plasma uric acid by ~50% [64].

4. Mitochondria

Due to their high-energy demand, cardiomyocytes are abundant in mitochondria. However, mitochondria are also an important source of ROS and NO [65, 66].

In physiological conditions, most of the reducing equivalents of the electron transport chain are directed toward the production of ATP and about 0.1% leak and produces superoxide [11].

Diabetes induces a series of metabolic derangements in myocardial mitochondria [12]. Under conditions of hyperglycemia, the mitochondrial inner membrane hyperpolarizes and inhibits the electron transport in complex III, generating superoxide [67].

Myocardial diabetic damage is reduced by overexpression of Mn SOD and catalase [57, 68] and by pharmacological inhibition of mitochondrial ROS by a mitochondrial-directed SOD

http://dx.doi.org/10.5772/63668

mimetic, mito-Tempo [69]. Noteworthy, besides being a source of ROS, mitochondria may suffer the consequences of increase oxidative stress as well [70]. High levels of ROS may sensitize the mitochondrial permeability transition pore (mPTP), releasing cytochrome C, and Smac/DIABLO ultimately inducing apoptosis [71]. The mitochondrial permeability transition pore is constituted by the adenine nucleotide translocase (ANT), the voltage-dependent anionic channel (VDAC), and cyclophilin D, which under stress conditions such as high Ca^{2+} or increased ROS make the mitochondrial membrane permeable to ions and molecules <1500 Da, dissipating the mitochondrial membrane potential [72]. In human atrial tissue from patients with diabetes, Anderson *et al.* [73] found increased H_2O_2 production, with increased sensitivity to Ca^{2+}-induced mPTP opening compared with nondiabetic patients and also in the heart of Zucker rats [74].

The components of the mPTP contain several redox-sensitive sites that can be oxidized or *S*-nitrosylated [71, 72]. *S*-Nitrosylation generally prevents mPTP opening, while oxidation sensitizes to opening (**Figure 2**). This is consistent with the fact that NO donors, at low concentrations, protect the mPTP from opening [72, 75, 76]. For instance, cyclophilin D has been shown to undergo *S*-nitrosylation in cysteine 203, preventing the oxidative-induced opening of the pore [77]. High NO donor concentrations, on the other, promote mPTP opening, associated with oxidation rather than hypernytrosylation. Nevertheless, the role of *S*-nitrosylation of mPTP in conditions of diabetic cardiomyopathy remains to be determined.

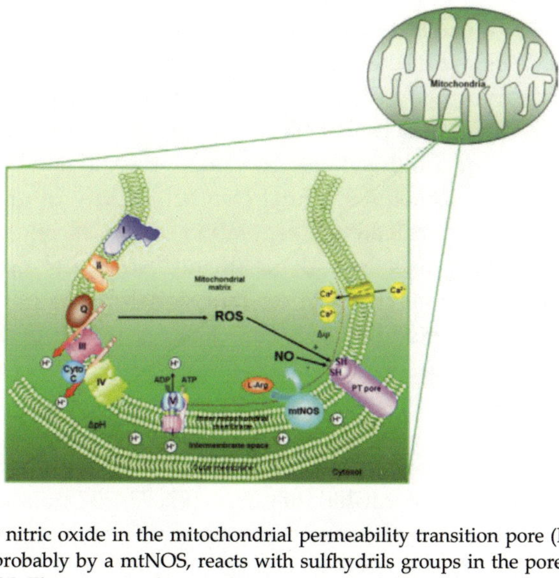

Figure 2. Potential role for nitric oxide in the mitochondrial permeability transition pore (PT). Nitric oxide produced within the mitochondria, probably by a mtNOS, reacts with sulfhydrils groups in the pore, *S*-nitrosylating them and preventing oxidation by ROS. This prevents the pore from opening and dissipating mitochondrial protons gradient.

In addition, mitochondria appear to play a central role in diabetic cardiomyopathy through alterations in the process of authopagie, and this process is clearly influenced by the mitochondrial oxidative status [15, 78–81].

5. Nitric oxide

Nitric oxide (NO) is a free radical that is produced by a family of NO synthases (NOSs), using NADPH, the amino acid L-arginine and oxygen as substrates. NOSs are homodimers and each subunit contains one flavin mononucleotide (FMN), one flavin adenine dinucleotide , one tetrahydrobiopterin (BH_4), and one Fe(3)-heme cofactor that facilitates the 5-electron oxidation of L-arginine to yield NO. In biological systems, NO exerts it effects by redox reactions (such as *S*-nitrosylation) or by inducing the production of cGMP as a second messenger [27, 82, 83].

Nitric oxide plays several important roles in the physiology of the myocardium, both in cardiomyocytes and in blood vessels [83–85]. NOS1 (former neuronal NOS) and eNOS (or NOS3) are expressed constitutively in the heart structures, particularly in the cardiomyocyte, NOS1 participates in the regulation of contractility [86, 87] by regulating RyR2 *S*-nitrosylation [29, 30] and phospholamban phosphorylation [88, 89]. NOS1 regulates the β-adrenergic [86, 90] and force-frequency response [29, 91] in the heart. Also NOS1 prevents cardiac dysfunction after a myocardial infarction and pressure overload [92–95]. For these reasons, the role for NO in diabetic cardiomyopathy has gained attention [96–98].

5.1. NOS1

Our group has recently identified specific stimulatory influences of NOS1 on both β-adrenergic inotropic responses and Ca^{2+} transients ($[Ca^{2+}]_i$) using NOS1$^{-/-}$ mice. These results are consistent with *in vitro* studies indicating that NO regulates SR Ca^{2+} release via the RyR by *S*-nitrosylation of a specific thiol moiety. RyR2 activation via nitrosylation is highly sensitive to ROS. We demonstrated non-cGMP related, redox-sensitive positive inotropic effects in isolated heart preparations [82] and demonstrated the role of NOS1 specifically in SR Ca^{2+} cycling [29, 99]. The interplay between NO and ROS is also of critical importance for Ca^{2+} handling. In the SR, NO augments RyR activity via *S*-nitrosylation in a manner regulated by ROS [100, 101]. ROS also activates the RyR2 but promotes maximal channel activity in an irreversible manner, reducing the ability of NO to exert feedback regulation of SR Ca^{2+} release. Such a situation is likely to lead to an increased Ca^{2+} leak through the SR and "futile" Ca^{2+} cycling, which increases ATP expenditure. It is also conceivable that oxidant signaling may directly regulate cross-bridge cycling kinetics, thereby modulating the efficiency of contraction.

5.2. NOS1 and cardioprotection

It has been consistently documented that NOS1 exerts a protective role in the myocardium in several model of stress, such as myocardial infarction [92, 93, 95], pressure overload [94, 102], ischemia-reperfusion [103], and dystrophic cardiomyopathy [104], just to mention the most relevant. Mechanistically, NOS1 nitrosylates several proteins, including ion channels [27, 29, 105] and mitochondrial components [106], and reduces oxidative stress [107].

A key hallmark of diabetic cardiomyopathy is hypertrophy. In this process, NO may play a role; furthermore, it has been shown that eNOS uncoupling (rather than the absence of NO) induces hypertrophy in the model of pressure overload [108]. Recoupling eNOS with BH_4

reverses this process, but not the use of tempol, a ROS scavenger [109, 110]. In ob/ob mice, myocardial hypertrophy has been documented [111], along with reduced NO bioavailability associated with reduced levels of NOS1 and increased NADPH [34] and XOR activity [32].

The activity of NOS1 is required for basal phospholamban phosphorylation in the mouse heart [88, 89], with NOS1 uncoupling resulting in an impaired ventricular relaxation and diastolic dysfunction, as observed in a model of hypertension [112]. Conversely, an increased production of BH_4 by cardiac-specific overexpression of GTP cyclohydrolase 1 (GCH1, the rate-limiting enzyme for BH4 biosynthesis), accelerates myocardial relaxation [113]. NOS1 uncoupling in mdx cardiomyocytes is probably the result of the NOX2-derived oxidative stress, which ultimately leads to tetrahydrobioterin oxidation. With this in mind, one possibility is that NOS1 is found in a monomeric form resulting in uncoupling. This uncoupling has been proposed as the aftermath of excessive tetrahydrobioterin (BH_4), oxidation to dihydrobioterin (BH_2).

5.3. NOS2

Inducible nitric oxide synthase (iNOS or NOS2) appears to play a central role in the pathophysiology of the diabetic cardiomyopathy [54]. In the heart, like in most tissues, iNOS is not constitutively expressed. Inflammatory conditions trigger the activation of the nuclear factor kappa beta (NF-κB). The activity of iNOS has been usually ascribed as part of the nitrosative stress. Since iNOS activity is much higher than the constitutive isoforms (NOS1 and 3), it reacts with superoxide, producing peroxynitrite [83]. This oxidant reacts with the aromatic ring of tyrosine residues, generating nitrotyrosine, one of the most widespread markers of nitrosative and oxidative stress [114]. iNOS-derived NO depresses cardiac contractility and function [115], and has been described to be upregulated in patients with diabetic cardiomyopathy [116].

iNOS expression has been manipulated pharmacologically in diabetes, using resveratrol, a natural polyphenol present in red wine and grapes. Reveratrol reduces the oxidative stress, improves myocardial relaxation [117] and reduces iNOS expression in type-2 diabetes models, by reducing the activation of NF-κB [118].

5.4. NOS uncoupling

In physiological conditions, NOS catalyze the reaction of oxidation of L-arginine to produce NO and L-citrulline, in the presence of NADPH, oxygen, and the cofactor 6R-5,6,7,8-tetrahydrobioterin (BH_4). In the absence of BH_4, electrons coming from NADPH flow to molecular oxygen, but uncoupled of L-arginine, producing superoxide instead of NO [26]. Apparently, BH_4 stabilizes the NOS configuration as a dimer that favors the proper flow of electrons to L-arginine. In its absence, NOS monomerizes and only maintains its oxidase activity [119]. BH_4 and BH_2 have been shown to bind to NOS with similar affinity (Kd ~80 nM). Tetrahydrobiopterin essential cofactor for aromatic amino acid hydroxylases and NOS. BH_4 can be synthesized by two pathways: *de novo* or recycled from its oxidized forms (**Figure 3**). For *de novo* synthesis, GTP cyclohydrolase I (GTPCH), 6-pyruvoyl tetrahydrobioterin synthase (PTPS), and sepiapterin reductase (SR) convert GTP to BH_4. In the first reaction catalyzed by GTPCH, guanosine

5'triphosphate (GTP) is reduced to 7,8-dihydroneopterin 3'triphosphate (DNTP), being the rate-limiting reaction. Next, the conversion of DNTP to 6-pyrovoyl tetrahydrobioterin (PTP) is catalyzed by PTPS. The final reactions are two successive propyl side-chain reductions catalyzed by SR [39, 120].

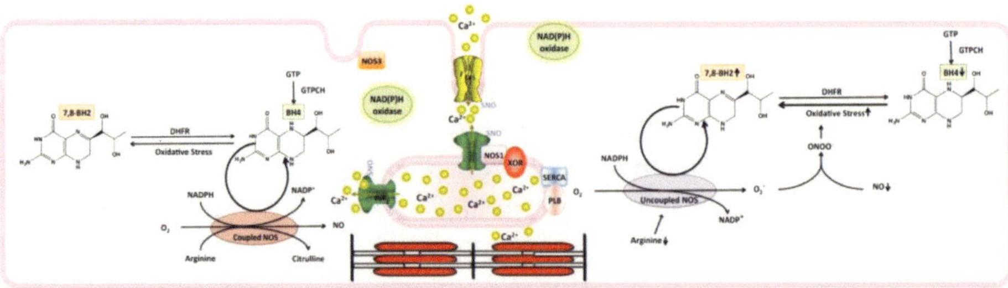

Figure 3. NOS uncoupling in the cardiomyocyte. Upon increased oxidative stress, BH_4, which normally couples L-arginine and NADPH oxidation and NO production, oxidized to BH_2, which is unable to couple this reaction, with the NADPH electrons passing directly to oxygen, producing superoxide.

When BH_4 is oxidized to BH_2, is reduced back to BH_4 by the enzyme dihydrofolate reductase (DHFR), in the salvage pathway. It is worth mentioning that during NOS catalysis BH_4 is not consumed, indicating that BH_2 formation is probably the result of other oxidative processes such as oxidative stress [39, 120].

5.5. NOS uncoupling in diabetes

It has been reported that NOS uncoupling takes places in diabetes, particularly in the vasculature [121]. For this reason, it has been associated with NOS3 [36, 37], the NOS isoform that is dominant in the endothelium. Given that oxidative stress is increased and that cardiac relaxation is impaired in diabetes, it is reasonable to think that NOS1 is uncoupled in the diabetic cardiomyocyte, since this isoform is related to phospholamban phosphoryaltion. Interestingly, it has been reported in the gastrointestinal system that diabetes produces NOS1 uncoupling, which is restored upon treatment with BH_4 [122] and sepiapterin, a BH_4 precursor [123].

The first report relating NOS uncoupling and diabetes was performed in cardiomyocytes exposed to high glucose concentration [124]. In these conditions, treatment with BH_4 restored the mechanic parameters in cardiomyocytes toward normal, an effect that could not be obtained using tetrahydroneopterin, which also shares ROS-scavenging properties as BH_4. Furthermore, the treatment of normal myocytes with the GTP cyclohydrolase I inhibitor 2,4-diamino-6-hydroxy-pryrimidine (DAHP) resembled the features of myocytes under hyperglycemic conditions.

The same group described that treatment of insulin-resistant mice with the BH_4 precursor folic acid was able to produce NOS recoupling. These effects were associated with improved cardiac function and reduction of sarcoplasmic reticulum calcium leak in isolated cardiomyocytes [125].

Furthermore, Jo *et al.* described that treatment of streptozotocin-induced diabetic mice with the BH_4 precursor sepiapterin was able to restore the intracardiac BH_4 levels and restored the BH_4/BH_2 ratio in diabetic mice. This treatment recoupled NOS in wild type, eNOS- and nNOS-deficient mice, but not in iNOS-deficient mice, suggesting that iNOS uncoupling was responsible for the oxidative stress observed in type-1 diabetic mice. Importantly, this treatment restored ventricular function except in iNOS mice [126]. Apparently, NOS uncoupling is related to the increased activity of NADPH oxidase in streptozotocin-induced diabetic mice [55]. Furthermore, a recent report describes that in db/db mice, a model of type-2 diabetes, the coadministration of sepiapterin and L-citrulline,a precursor of L-arginine restored cardiac function in diabetic hearts and improved their response after ischemia-reperfusion [127].

6. Conclusion

In the diabetic heart, an increased hyperglycemia induced the mitochondrial production of ROS, which favors apoptosis. Concomitantly, diabetes induces the activation of NOX that further impairs mitochondrial function. In addition, the diabetic state induces the expression of iNOS, which in conjunction with an increased ROS production leads to the generation of peroxynitrite, a highly oxidizing species. These elements create a feed-forward system that deteriorates cardiac function at several levels. Furthermore, increased ROS production may oxidize BH4, producing NOS uncoupling, further aggravating the oxidative damage.

Despite the heavy burden that diabetes imposes to the heart, current therapeutic strategies do not specifically address diabetes-induced heart failure; therefore, novel pharmacological treatments might be of high relevance. Theoretically, a reduction in mitochondrial or NOX derived-oxidative stress in diabetic cardiomyopathy should be able to improve some of the features of diabetic cardiomyopathy. Nevertheless, indiscriminate NOX inhibition or ROS quenching may have detrimental effects if the protective role of NOX4 (as opposed as other NOXs) is disturbed, as it has been suggested in several stress conditions for the myocardium. On the other hand, inhibitors of mitochondrial ROS production are still in their infancy and have not been tested in humans. Therefore, pharmacological restoration of intracardiac BH_4 levels may offer a new therapeutic opportunity for diabetic cardiomyopathy, as they have been used in other pathologies, although the results have been somehow disappointing [128]. In addition, isoform-specific NOX inhibitors are needed as pharmacological tools against diabetic cardiomyopathy.

Acknowledgements

This work was supported in part by the grant 1150662 from Fondo Nacional de Desarrollo Científico y Tecnológico (Fondecyt) Chile, and Programa de Investigación en Química y Bioogánica de Recursos Naturales, Universidad de Talca, Talca, Chile.

Author details

Daniel R González*, Adriana V Treuer and Ulises Novoa

*Address all correspondence to: dagonzalez@utalca.cl

Department of Biomedical Sciences, School of Health Sciences, University of Talca, Talca, Chile

References

[1] Shaw JE, Sicree RA, Zimmet PZ. Global estimates of the prevalence of diabetes for 2010 and 2030. Diabetes Res Clin Pract 2010;87:4–14.

[2] Zimmet P, Alberti KG, Shaw J. Global and societal implications of the diabetes epidemic. Nature 2001;414:782–7.

[3] Pappachan JM, Varughese GI, Sriraman R, Arunagirinathan G. Diabetic cardiomyopathy: pathophysiology, diagnostic evaluation and management. World J Diabetes 2013;4:177–89.

[4] Asghar O, Al-Sunni A, Khavandi K, Khavandi A, Withers S, Greenstein A, et al. Diabetic cardiomyopathy. Clin Sci (Lond) 2009;116:741–60.

[5] Falcao-Pires I, Leite-Moreira AF. Diabetic cardiomyopathy: understanding the molecular and cellular basis to progress in diagnosis and treatment. Heart Fail Rev 2012;17:325–44.

[6] Ansley DM, Wang B. Oxidative stress and myocardial injury in the diabetic heart. J Pathol 2013;229:232–41.

[7] Barouch LA, Gao D, Chen L, Miller KL, Xu W, Phan AC, et al. Cardiac myocyte apoptosis is associated with increased DNA damage and decreased survival in murine models of obesity. Circ Res 2006;98:119–24.

[8] Frustaci A, Kajstura J, Chimenti C, Jakoniuk I, Leri A, Maseri A, et al. Myocardial cell death in human diabetes. Circ Res 2000;87:1123–32.

[9] Rota M, LeCapitaine N, Hosoda T, Boni A, De AA, Padin-Iruegas ME, et al. Diabetes promotes cardiac stem cell aging and heart failure, which are prevented by deletion of the p66shc gene. Circ Res 2006;99:42–52.

[10] Giordano FJ. Oxygen, oxidative stress, hypoxia, and heart failure. J Clin Invest 2005;115:500–8.

[11] Bugger H, Abel ED. Mitochondria in the diabetic heart. Cardiovasc Res 2010;88:229–40.

http://dx.doi.org/10.5772/63668

[12] Lorenzo O, Ramirez E, Picatoste B, Egido J, Tunon J. Alteration of energy substrates and ROS production in diabetic cardiomyopathy. Mediators Inflamm 2013;2013:461967.

[13] Kaneto H, Katakami N, Kawamori D, Miyatsuka T, Sakamoto K, Matsuoka TA, et al. Involvement of oxidative stress in the pathogenesis of diabetes. Antioxid Redox Signal 2007;9:355–66.

[14] Murdoch CE, Grieve DJ, Cave AC, Looi YH, Shah AM. NADPH oxidase and heart failure. Curr Opin Pharmacol 2006;6:148–53.

[15] Ouyang C, You J, Xie Z. The interplay between autophagy and apoptosis in the diabetic heart. J Mol Cell Cardiol 2014;71:71–80.

[16] Mandavia CH, Aroor AR, Demarco VG, Sowers JR. Molecular and metabolic mechanisms of cardiac dysfunction in diabetes. Life Sci 2013;92:601–8.

[17] Belke DD, Dillmann WH. Altered cardiac calcium handling in diabetes. Curr Hypertens Rep 2004;6:424–9.

[18] Zhao SM, Wang YL, Guo CY, Chen JL, Wu YQ. Progressive decay of Ca2+ homeostasis in the development of diabetic cardiomyopathy. Cardiovasc Diabetol 2014;13:75.

[19] Choi KM, Zhong Y, Hoit BD, Grupp IL, Hahn H, Dilly KW, et al. Defective intracellular Ca(2+) signaling contributes to cardiomyopathy in Type 1 diabetic rats. Am J Physiol Heart Circ Physiol 2002;283:H1398–408.

[20] Mattiazzi A, Kranias EG. The role of CaMKII regulation of phospholamban activity in heart disease. Front Pharmacol 2014;5:5.

[21] Lacombe VA, Viatchenko-Karpinski S, Terentyev D, Sridhar A, Emani S, Bonagura JD, et al. Mechanisms of impaired calcium handling underlying subclinical diastolic dysfunction in diabetes. Am J Physiol Regul Integr Comp Physiol 2007;293:R1787–97.

[22] Shao CH, Wehrens XH, Wyatt TA, Parbhu S, Rozanski GJ, Patel KP, et al. Exercise training during diabetes attenuates cardiac ryanodine receptor dysregulation. J Appl Physiol (1985) 2009;106:1280–92.

[23] Stolen TO, Hoydal MA, Kemi OJ, Catalucci D, Ceci M, Aasum E, et al. Interval training normalizes cardiomyocyte function, diastolic Ca2+ control, and SR Ca2+ release synchronicity in a mouse model of diabetic cardiomyopathy. Circ Res 2009;105:527–36.

[24] Zhang L, Cannell MB, Phillips AR, Cooper GJ, Ward ML. Altered calcium homeostasis does not explain the contractile deficit of diabetic cardiomyopathy. Diabetes 2008;57:2158–66.

[25] Vasanji Z, Dhalla NS, Netticadan T. Increased inhibition of SERCA2 by phospholamban in the type I diabetic heart. Mol Cell Biochem 2004;261:245–9.

[26] Crabtree MJ, Smith CL, Lam G, Goligorsky MS, Gross SS. Ratio of 5,6,7,8-tetrahydrobiopterin to 7,8-dihydrobiopterin in endothelial cells determines glucose-elicited

changes in NO vs. superoxide production by eNOS. Am J Physiol Heart Circ Physiol 2008;294:H1530–40.

[27] Gonzalez DR, Treuer A, Sun QA, Stamler JS, Hare JM. S-Nitrosylation of cardiac ion channels. J Cardiovasc Pharmacol 2009;54:188–95.

[28] Gonzalez DR, Treuer AV, Castellanos J, Dulce RA, Hare JM. Impaired S-nitrosylation of the ryanodine receptor caused by xanthine oxidase activity contributes to calcium leak in heart failure. J Biol Chem 2010;285:28938–45.

[29] Gonzalez DR, Beigi F, Treuer AV, Hare JM. Deficient ryanodine receptor S-nitrosylation increases sarcoplasmic reticulum calcium leak and arrhythmogenesis in cardiomyocytes. Proc Natl Acad Sci U S A 2007;104:20612–7.

[30] Wang H, Viatchenko-Karpinski S, Sun J, Gyorke I, Benkusky NA, Kohr MJ, et al. Regulation of myocyte contraction via neuronal nitric oxide synthase: role of ryanodine receptor S-nitrosylation. J Physiol 2010;588:2905–17.

[31] Rajesh M, Mukhopadhyay P, Batkai S, Mukhopadhyay B, Patel V, Hasko G, et al. Xanthine oxidase inhibitor allopurinol attenuates the development of diabetic cardiomyopathy. J Cell Mol Med 2009;13:2330–41.

[32] Saraiva RM, Minhas KM, Zheng M, Pitz E, Treuer A, Gonzalez D, et al. Reduced neuronal nitric oxide synthase expression contributes to cardiac oxidative stress and nitroso-redox imbalance in ob/ob mice. Nitric Oxide 2007;16:331–8.

[33] Gao X, Xu Y, Xu B, Liu Y, Cai J, Liu HM, et al. Allopurinol attenuates left ventricular dysfunction in rats with early stages of streptozotocin-induced diabetes. Diabetes Metab Res Rev 2012;28:409–17.

[34] Li SY, Yang X, Ceylan-Isik AF, Du M, Sreejayan N, Ren J. Cardiac contractile dysfunction in Lep/Lep obesity is accompanied by NADPH oxidase activation, oxidative modification of sarco(endo)plasmic reticulum Ca2+-ATPase and myosin heavy chain isozyme switch. Diabetologia 2006;49:1434–46.

[35] Maalouf RM, Eid AA, Gorin YC, Block K, Escobar GP, Bailey S, et al. Nox4-derived reactive oxygen species mediate cardiomyocyte injury in early type 1 diabetes. Am J Physiol Cell Physiol 2012;302:C597–604.

[36] Heitzer T, Krohn K, Albers S, Meinertz T. Tetrahydrobiopterin improves endothelium-dependent vasodilation by increasing nitric oxide activity in patients with type II diabetes mellitus. Diabetologia 2000;43:1435–8.

[37] Katakam PV, Snipes JA, Steed MM, Busija DW. Insulin-induced generation of reactive oxygen species and uncoupling of nitric oxide synthase underlie the cerebrovascular insulin resistance in obese rats. J Cereb Blood Flow Metab 2012;32:792–804.

[38] Landmesser U, Dikalov S, Price SR, McCann L, Fukai T, Holland SM, et al. Oxidation of tetrahydrobiopterin leads to uncoupling of endothelial cell nitric oxide synthase in hypertension. J Clin Invest 2003;111:1201–9.

[39] Tejero J, Stuehr D. Tetrahydrobiopterin in nitric oxide synthase. IUBMB Life 2013;65:358–65.

[40] Bedard K, Krause KH. The NOX family of ROS-generating NADPH oxidases: physiology and pathophysiology. Physiol Rev 2007;87:245–313.

[41] Cave AC, Brewer AC, Narayanapanicker A, Ray R, Grieve DJ, Walker S, et al. NADPH oxidases in cardiovascular health and disease. Antioxid Redox Signal 2006;8:691–728.

[42] Grieve DJ, Byrne JA, Siva A, Layland J, Johar S, Cave AC, et al. Involvement of the nicotinamide adenosine dinucleotide phosphate oxidase isoform Nox2 in cardiac contractile dysfunction occurring in response to pressure overload. J Am Coll Cardiol 2006;47:817–26.

[43] Huynh K, Kiriazis H, Du XJ, Love JE, Gray SP, Jandeleit-Dahm KA, et al. Targeting the upregulation of reactive oxygen species subsequent to hyperglycemia prevents type 1 diabetic cardiomyopathy in mice. Free Radic Biol Med 2013;60:307–17.

[44] Kuroda J, Ago T, Matsushima S, Zhai P, Schneider MD, Sadoshima J. NADPH oxidase 4 (Nox4) is a major source of oxidative stress in the failing heart. Proc Natl Acad Sci U S A 2010;107:15565–70.

[45] Huynh K, Bernardo BC, McMullen JR, Ritchie RH. Diabetic cardiomyopathy: mechanisms and new treatment strategies targeting antioxidant signaling pathways. Pharmacol Ther 2014;142:375–415.

[46] Cai H, Griendling KK, Harrison DG. The vascular NAD(P)H oxidases as therapeutic targets in cardiovascular diseases. Trends Pharmacol Sci 2003;24:471–8.

[47] Lei S, Liu Y, Liu H, Yu H, Wang H, Xia Z. Effects of N-acetylcysteine on nicotinamide dinucleotide phosphate oxidase activation and antioxidant status in heart, lung, liver and kidney in streptozotocin-induced diabetic rats. Yonsei Med J 2012;53:294–303.

[48] Zhang M, Kho AL, Anilkumar N, Chibber R, Pagano PJ, Shah AM, et al. Glycated proteins stimulate reactive oxygen species production in cardiac myocytes: involvement of Nox2 (gp91phox)-containing NADPH oxidase. Circulation 2006;113:1235–43.

[49] Prosser BL, Ward CW, Lederer WJ. X-ROS signaling: rapid mechano-chemo transduction in heart. Science 2011;333:1440–5.

[50] Gonzalez DR, Treuer AV, Lamirault G, Mayo V, Cao Y, Dulce RA, et al. NADPH oxidase-2 inhibition restores contractility and intracellular calcium handling and reduces arrhythmogenicity in dystrophic cardiomyopathy. Am J Physiol Heart Circ Physiol 2014;307:H710–H721.

[51] Jian Z, Han H, Zhang T, Puglisi J, Izu LT, Shaw JA, et al. Mechanochemotransduction during cardiomyocyte contraction is mediated by localized nitric oxide signaling. Sci Signal 2014;7:ra27.

[52] Dong F, Zhang X, Ren J. Leptin regulates cardiomyocyte contractile function through endothelin-1 receptor-NADPH oxidase pathway. Hypertension 2006;47:222–9.

[53] Kowluru A, Kowluru RA. Phagocyte-like NADPH oxidase [Nox2] in cellular dysfunction in models of glucolipotoxicity and diabetes. Biochem Pharmacol 2014;88:275–83.

[54] Soskic SS, Dobutovic BD, Sudar EM, Obradovic MM, Nikolic DM, Djordjevic JD, et al. Regulation of inducible nitric oxide synthase (iNOS) and its potential role in insulin resistance, diabetes and heart failure. Open Cardiovasc Med J 2011;5:153–63.

[55] Roe ND, Thomas DP, Ren J. Inhibition of NADPH oxidase alleviates experimental diabetes-induced myocardial contractile dysfunction. Diabetes Obes Metab 2011;13:465–73.

[56] Li J, Zhu H, Shen E, Wan L, Arnold JM, Peng T. Deficiency of rac1 blocks NADPH oxidase activation, inhibits endoplasmic reticulum stress, and reduces myocardial remodeling in a mouse model of type 1 diabetes. Diabetes 2010;59:2033–42.

[57] Shen E, Li Y, Li Y, Shan L, Zhu H, Feng Q, et al. Rac1 is required for cardiomyocyte apoptosis during hyperglycemia. Diabetes 2009;58:2386–95.

[58] Shan L, Li J, Wei M, Ma J, Wan L, Zhu W, et al. Disruption of Rac1 signaling reduces ischemia-reperfusion injury in the diabetic heart by inhibiting calpain. Free Radic Biol Med 2010;49:1804–14.

[59] Ago T, Kuroda J, Pain J, Fu C, Li H, Sadoshima J. Upregulation of Nox4 by hypertrophic stimuli promotes apoptosis and mitochondrial dysfunction in cardiac myocytes. Circ Res 2010;106:1253–64.

[60] Zhang M, Brewer AC, Schroder K, Santos CX, Grieve DJ, Wang M, et al. NADPH oxidase-4 mediates protection against chronic load-induced stress in mouse hearts by enhancing angiogenesis. Proc Natl Acad Sci U S A 2010;107:18121–6.

[61] Berry CE, Hare JM. Xanthine oxidoreductase and cardiovascular disease: molecular mechanisms and pathophysiological implications. J Physiol 2004;555:589–606.

[62] Kumar S, Prasad S, Sitasawad SL. Multiple antioxidants improve cardiac complications and inhibit cardiac cell death in streptozotocin-induced diabetic rats. PLoS One 2013;8:e67009.

[63] Desco MC, Asensi M, Marquez R, Martinez-Valls J, Vento M, Pallardo FV, et al. Xanthine oxidase is involved in free radical production in type 1 diabetes: protection by allopurinol. Diabetes 2002;51:1118–24.

[64] Szwejkowski BR, Gandy SJ, Rekhraj S, Houston JG, Lang CC, Morris AD, et al. Allopurinol reduces left ventricular mass in patients with type 2 diabetes and left ventricular hypertrophy. J Am Coll Cardiol 2013;62:2284–93.

[65] Dedkova EN, Blatter LA. Characteristics and function of cardiac mitochondrial nitric oxide synthase. J Physiol 2009;587:851–72.

[66] Gonzalez DR, Treuer AV, Dulce RA. Neuronal nitric oxide synthase in heart mitochondria: a matter of life or death. J Physiol 2009;587:2719–20.

[67] Teshima Y, Takahashi N, Nishio S, Saito S, Kondo H, Fukui A, et al. Production of reactive oxygen species in the diabetic heart. Roles of mitochondria and NADPH oxidase. Circ J 2014;78:300–6.

[68] Ye G, Metreveli NS, Donthi RV, Xia S, Xu M, Carlson EC, et al. Catalase protects cardiomyocyte function in models of type 1 and type 2 diabetes. Diabetes 2004;53:1336–43.

[69] Ni R, Cao T, Xiong S, Ma J, Fan GC, Lacefield JC, et al. Therapeutic inhibition of mitochondrial reactive oxygen species with mito-TEMPO reduces diabetic cardiomyopathy. Free Radic Biol Med 2015;90:12–23.

[70] Tocchetti CG, Caceres V, Stanley BA, Xie C, Shi S, Watson WH, et al. GSH or palmitate preserves mitochondrial energetic/redox balance, preventing mechanical dysfunction in metabolically challenged myocytes/hearts from type 2 diabetic mice. Diabetes 2012;61:3094–105.

[71] Mailloux RJ, Jin X, Willmore WG. Redox regulation of mitochondrial function with emphasis on cysteine oxidation reactions. Redox Biol 2014;2:123–39.

[72] Bernardi P, Di LF. The mitochondrial permeability transition pore: molecular nature and role as a target in cardioprotection. J Mol Cell Cardiol 2015;78:100–6.

[73] Anderson EJ, Rodriguez E, Anderson CA, Thayne K, Chitwood WR, Kypson AP. Increased propensity for cell death in diabetic human heart is mediated by mitochondrial-dependent pathways. Am J Physiol Heart Circ Physiol 2011;300:H118–24.

[74] Riojas-Hernandez A, Bernal-Ramirez J, Rodriguez-Mier D, Morales-Marroquin FE, Dominguez-Barragan EM, Borja-Villa C, et al. Enhanced oxidative stress sensitizes the mitochondrial permeability transition pore to opening in heart from Zucker Fa/fa rats with type 2 diabetes. Life Sci 2015;141:32–43.

[75] Leite AC, Oliveira HC, Utino FL, Garcia R, Alberici LC, Fernandes MP, et al. Mitochondria generated nitric oxide protects against permeability transition via formation of membrane protein S-nitrosothiols. Biochim Biophys Acta 2010;1797:1210–6.

[76] Ohtani H, Katoh H, Tanaka T, Saotome M, Urushida T, Satoh H, et al. Effects of nitric oxide on mitochondrial permeability transition pore and thiol-mediated responses in cardiac myocytes. Nitric Oxide 2012;26:95–101.

[77] Nguyen TT, Stevens MV, Kohr M, Steenbergen C, Sack MN, Murphy E. Cysteine 203 of cyclophilin D is critical for cyclophilin D activation of the mitochondrial permeability transition pore. J Biol Chem 2011;286:40184–92.

[78] Sciarretta S, Zhai P, Shao D, Zablocki D, Nagarajan N, Terada LS, et al. Activation of NADPH oxidase 4 in the endoplasmic reticulum promotes cardiomyocyte autophagy and survival during energy stress through the protein kinase RNA-activated-like endoplasmic reticulum kinase/eukaryotic initiation factor 2alpha/activating transcription factor 4 pathway. Circ Res 2013;113:1253–64.

[79] Varga ZV, Giricz Z, Liaudet L, Hasko G, Ferdinandy P, Pacher P. Interplay of oxidative, nitrosative/nitrative stress, inflammation, cell death and autophagy in diabetic cardiomyopathy. Biochim Biophys Acta 2015;1852:232–42.

[80] Sciarretta S, Volpe M, Sadoshima J. NOX4 regulates autophagy during energy deprivation. Autophagy 2014;10:699–701.

[81] Wang B, Yang Q, Sun YY, Xing YF, Wang YB, Lu XT, et al. Resveratrol-enhanced autophagic flux ameliorates myocardial oxidative stress injury in diabetic mice. J Cell Mol Med 2014;18:1599–611.

[82] Gonzalez DR, Fernandez IC, Ordenes PP, Treuer AV, Eller G, Boric MP. Differential role of S-nitrosylation and the NO-cGMP-PKG pathway in cardiac contractility. Nitric Oxide 2008;18:157–67.

[83] Treuer AV, Gonzalez DR. Nitric oxide synthases, S-nitrosylation and cardiovascular health: from molecular mechanisms to therapeutic opportunities (review). Mol Med Rep 2015; 11:1555–65.

[84] Tang L, Wang H, Ziolo MT. Targeting NOS as a therapeutic approach for heart failure. Pharmacol Ther 2014;142:306–15.

[85] Ziolo MT, Kohr MJ, Wang H. Nitric oxide signaling and the regulation of myocardial function. J Mol Cell Cardiol 2008;45:625–32.

[86] Barouch LA, Harrison RW, Skaf MW, Rosas GO, Cappola TP, Kobeissi ZA, et al. Nitric oxide regulates the heart by spatial confinement of nitric oxide synthase isoforms. Nature 2002;416:337–9.

[87] Sears CE, Bryant SM, Ashley EA, Lygate CA, Rakovic S, Wallis HL, et al. Cardiac neuronal nitric oxide synthase isoform regulates myocardial contraction and calcium handling. Circ Res 2003;92:e52–9.

[88] Wang H, Kohr MJ, Traynham CJ, Wheeler DG, Janssen PM, Ziolo MT. Neuronal nitric oxide synthase signaling within cardiac myocytes targets phospholamban. Am J Physiol Cell Physiol 2008;294:C1566–75.

[89] Zhang YH, Zhang MH, Sears CE, Emanuel K, Redwood C, El-Armouche A, et al. Reduced phospholamban phosphorylation is associated with impaired relaxation in left ventricular myocytes from neuronal NO synthase-deficient mice. Circ Res 2008;102:242–9.

[90] Ashley EA, Sears CE, Bryant SM, Watkins HC, Casadei B. Cardiac nitric oxide synthase 1 regulates basal and beta-adrenergic contractility in murine ventricular myocytes. Circulation 2002;105:3011–6.

[91] Khan SA, Skaf MW, Harrison RW, Lee K, Minhas KM, Kumar A, et al. Nitric oxide regulation of myocardial contractility and calcium cycling: independent impact of neuronal and endothelial nitric oxide synthases. Circ Res 2003;92:1322–9.

[92] Burger DE, Lu X, Lei M, Xiang FL, Hammoud L, Jiang M, et al. Neuronal nitric oxide synthase protects against myocardial infarction-induced ventricular arrhythmia and mortality in mice. Circulation 2009;120:1345–54.

[93] Dawson D, Lygate CA, Zhang MH, Hulbert K, Neubauer S, Casadei B. nNOS gene deletion exacerbates pathological left ventricular remodeling and functional deterioration after myocardial infarction. Circulation 2005;112:3729–37.

[94] Loyer X, Gomez AM, Milliez P, Fernandez-Velasco M, Vangheluwe P, Vinet L, et al. Cardiomyocyte overexpression of neuronal nitric oxide synthase delays transition toward heart failure in response to pressure overload by preserving calcium cycling. Circulation 2008;117:3187–98.

[95] Saraiva RM, Minhas KM, Raju SV, Barouch LA, Pitz E, Schuleri KH, et al. Deficiency of neuronal nitric oxide synthase increases mortality and cardiac remodeling after myocardial infarction: role of nitroso-redox equilibrium. Circulation 2005;112:3415–22.

[96] Jayakumari NR, Reghuvaran AC, Rajendran RS, Pillai VV, Karunakaran J, Sreelatha HV, et al. Are nitric oxide-mediated protein modifications of functional significance in diabetic heart? ye'S, -NO', wh'Y-NO't?. Nitric Oxide 2014;43:35–44.

[97] Khanna S, Singh GB, Khullar M. Nitric oxide synthases and diabetic cardiomyopathy. Nitric Oxide 2014;43:29–34.

[98] Pechanova O, Varga ZV, Cebova M, Giricz Z, Pacher P, Ferdinandy P. Cardiac NO signalling in the metabolic syndrome. Br J Pharmacol 2015;172:1415–33.

[99] Beigi F, Gonzalez DR, Minhas KM, Sun QA, Foster MW, Khan SA, et al. Dynamic denitrosylation via S-nitrosoglutathione reductase regulates cardiovascular function. Proc Natl Acad Sci U S A 2012;109:4314–9.

[100] Kyrychenko S, Polakova E, Kang C, Pocsai K, Ullrich ND, Niggli E, et al. Hierarchical accumulation of RyR post-translational modifications drives disease progression in dystrophic cardiomyopathy. Cardiovasc Res 2013;97:666–75.

[101] Niggli E, Ullrich ND, Gutierrez D, Kyrychenko S, Polakova E, Shirokova N. Posttranslational modifications of cardiac ryanodine receptors: Ca(2+) signaling and EC-coupling. Biochim Biophys Acta 2013;1833:866–75.

[102] Watts VL, Sepulveda FM, Cingolani OH, Ho AS, Niu X, Kim R, et al. Anti-hypertrophic and anti-oxidant effect of beta3-adrenergic stimulation in myocytes requires differential neuronal NOS phosphorylation. J Mol Cell Cardiol 2013;62:8–17.

[103] Burkard N, Williams T, Czolbe M, Blomer N, Panther F, Link M, et al. Conditional overexpression of neuronal nitric oxide synthase is cardioprotective in ischemia/reperfusion. Circulation 2010;122:1588–603.

[104] Lai Y, Zhao J, Yue Y, Wasala NB, Duan D. Partial restoration of cardiac function with DeltaPDZ nNOS in aged mdx model of Duchenne cardiomyopathy. Hum Mol Genet 2014;23:3189–99.

[105] Treuer AV, Gonzalez DR. NOS1AP modulates intracellular Ca(2+) in cardiac myocytes and is up-regulated in dystrophic cardiomyopathy. Int J Physiol Pathophysiol Pharmacol 2014;6:37–46.

[106] Piantadosi CA. Regulation of mitochondrial processes by protein S-nitrosylation. Biochim Biophys Acta 2012;1820:712–21.

[107] Khan SA, Lee K, Minhas KM, Gonzalez DR, Raju SV, Tejani AD, et al. Neuronal nitric oxide synthase negatively regulates xanthine oxidoreductase inhibition of cardiac excitation-contraction coupling. Proc Natl Acad Sci U S A 2004;101:15944–8.

[108] Takimoto E, Champion HC, Li M, Ren S, Rodriguez ER, Tavazzi B, et al. Oxidant stress from nitric oxide synthase-3 uncoupling stimulates cardiac pathologic remodeling from chronic pressure load. J Clin Invest 2005;115:1221–31.

[109] Moens AL, Takimoto E, Tocchetti CG, Chakir K, Bedja D, Cormaci G, et al. Reversal of cardiac hypertrophy and fibrosis from pressure overload by tetrahydrobiopterin: efficacy of recoupling nitric oxide synthase as a therapeutic strategy. Circulation 2008;117:2626–36.

[110] Moens AL, Leyton-Mange JS, Niu X, Yang R, Cingolani O, Arkenbout EK, et al. Adverse ventricular remodeling and exacerbated NOS uncoupling from pressure-overload in mice lacking the beta3-adrenoreceptor. J Mol Cell Cardiol 2009;47:576–85.

[111] Barouch LA, Berkowitz DE, Harrison RW, O'Donnell CP, Hare JM. Disruption of leptin signaling contributes to cardiac hypertrophy independently of body weight in mice. Circulation 2003;108:754–9.

[112] Silberman GA, Fan TH, Liu H, Jiao Z, Xiao HD, Lovelock JD, et al. Uncoupled cardiac nitric oxide synthase mediates diastolic dysfunction. Circulation 2010;121:519–28.

[113] Carnicer R, Hale AB, Suffredini S, Liu X, Reilly S, Zhang MH, et al. Cardiomyocyte GTP cyclohydrolase 1 and tetrahydrobiopterin increase NOS1 activity and accelerate myocardial relaxation. Circ Res 2012;111:718–27.

[114] Zhang YL, Wei JR. 3-nitrotyrosine, a biomarker for cardiomyocyte apoptosis induced by diabetic cardiomyopathy in a rat model. Mol Med Rep 2013;8:989–94.

[115] Song D, Kuo KH, Yao R, Hutchings SR, Pang CC. Inducible nitric oxide synthase depresses cardiac contractile function in Zucker diabetic fatty rats. Eur J Pharmacol 2008;579:253–9.

[116] Frustaci A, Ciccosanti F, Chimenti C, Nardacci R, Corazzari M, Verardo R, et al. Histological and proteomic profile of diabetic versus non-diabetic dilated cardiomyopathy. Int J Cardiol 2016;203:282–9.

[117] Zhang H, Morgan B, Potter BJ, Ma L, Dellsperger KC, Ungvari Z, et al. Resveratrol improves left ventricular diastolic relaxation in type 2 diabetes by inhibiting oxidative/nitrative stress: in vivo demonstration with magnetic resonance imaging. Am J Physiol Heart Circ Physiol 2010;299:H985–H994.

[118] Bagul PK, Deepthi N, Sultana R, Banerjee SK. Resveratrol ameliorates cardiac oxidative stress in diabetes through deacetylation of NFkB-p65 and histone 3. J Nutr Biochem 2015;26:1298–307.

[119] Reif A, Frohlich LG, Kotsonis P, Frey A, Bommel HM, Wink DA, et al. Tetrahydrobiopterin inhibits monomerization and is consumed during catalysis in neuronal NO synthase. J Biol Chem 1999;274:24921–9.

[120] Thony B, Auerbach G, Blau N. Tetrahydrobiopterin biosynthesis, regeneration and functions. Biochem J 2000;347 Pt 1:1–16.

[121] Alp NJ, Mussa S, Khoo J, Cai S, Guzik T, Jefferson A, et al. Tetrahydrobiopterin-dependent preservation of nitric oxide-mediated endothelial function in diabetes by targeted transgenic GTP-cyclohydrolase I overexpression. J Clin Invest 2003;112:725–35.

[122] Gangula PR, Mukhopadhyay S, Ravella K, Cai S, Channon KM, Garfield RE, et al. Tetrahydrobiopterin (BH4), a cofactor for nNOS, restores gastric emptying and nNOS expression in female diabetic rats. Am J Physiol Gastrointest Liver Physiol 2010;298:G692–9.

[123] Gangula PR, Mukhopadhyay S, Pasricha PJ, Ravella K. Sepiapterin reverses the changes in gastric nNOS dimerization and function in diabetic gastroparesis. Neurogastroenterol Motil 2010;22:1325–2.

[124] Esberg LB, Ren J. Role of nitric oxide, tetrahydrobiopterin and peroxynitrite in glucose toxicity-associated contractile dysfunction in ventricular myocytes. Diabetologia 2003;46:1419–27.

[125] Roe ND, He EY, Wu Z, Ren J. Folic acid reverses nitric oxide synthase uncoupling and prevents cardiac dysfunction in insulin resistance: role of Ca2+/calmodulin-activated protein kinase II. Free Radic Biol Med 2013;65:234–43.

[126] Jo H, Otani H, Jo F, Shimazu T, Okazaki T, Yoshioka K, et al. Inhibition of nitric oxide synthase uncoupling by sepiapterin improves left ventricular function in streptozotocin-induced diabetic mice. Clin Exp Pharmacol Physiol 2011;38:485–93.

[127] Baumgardt SL, Paterson M, Leucker TM, Fang J, Zhang DX, Bosnjak ZJ, et al. Chronic co-administration of sepiapterin and l-citrulline ameliorates diabetic cardiomyopathy and myocardial ischemia/reperfusion injury in obese type 2 diabetic mice. Circ Heart Fail 2016;9:e002424.

[128] Moens AL, Kass DA. Therapeutic potential of tetrahydrobiopterin for treating vascular and cardiac disease. J Cardiovasc Pharmacol 2007;50:238–46.

Chapter 11

Ubiquinone, Ezetimibe/Simvastatin and Rosuvastatin Effects on Mitochondrial Function in Diabetic Polyneuropathy

Luis M. Román-Pintos, Geannyne Villegas-Rivera,
Ernesto G. Cardona-Muñoz,
Adolfo D. Rodríguez-Carrizalez,
Fermín P. Pacheco-Moisés and
Alejandra G. Miranda-Díaz

Additional information is available at the end of the chapter

http://dx.doi.org/10.5772/63656

Abstract

Diabetic polyneuropathy (DPN) pathophysiologic findings include loss of multifocal and focal nerve fibers secondary to axonal degeneration and segmental demyelization due to oxidative stress and mitochondrial dysfunction induced by chronic hyperglycaemia.

Aim: To evaluate the effect of ubiquinone, ezetimibe/simvastatin and rosuvastatin on mitochondrial function in patients with diabetic polyneuropathy.

Methods: A randomized, double-blinded, placebo-controlled clinical trial was performed in patients with type 2 Diabetes Mellitus (T2DM) who had DPN, glycated haemoglobin (HbA1c) <12% (108 mmol/mol), previous exclusion of other type of neuropathy. Ninety-eight persons with T2DM were enrolled allocated 1:1:1:1 to either placebo, ubiquinone 400 mg, ezetimibe/simvastatin 10/20 mg or rosuvastatin 20 mg for 16 weeks. Primary outcomes were F0F1-ATP hydrolysis, erythrocyte and sub-mitochondrial platelet membrane fluidity. Results were expressed as mean ± SD or SEM and percentages.

Results: F0F1-ATP hydrolysis levels in healthy controls were 236.80±118.42 nmol/PO4; all patients with T2DM exhibited an increase, but only rosuvastatin demonstrated an improvement with baseline 463.37±47.07 nmol/PO4 vs. after 340.61±37.80 nmol/PO4 treatment ($p<0.05$). Plasma and sub-mitochondrial membrane fluidity did not experience any significant changes.

Conclusions: Rosuvastatin was found to improve mitochondrial function by reducing F0F1-ATP hydrolysis. No changes in sub-mitochondrial platelets particles or erythrocytes ghosts were found.

Keywords: ubiquinone, statins, diabetic polyneuropathy, oxidative stress, mitochondrial dysfunction

1. Introduction

Nerve dysfunction system in patients with diabetes is known as diabetic neuropathy and is considered as the most prevalent microvascular complication—up to 60%—in diabetes mellitus (DM) subjects [1]. Diabetic polyneuropathy (DPN) comprise ≈70% of all cases [2]. Diabetic sensorimotor polyneuropathy is the most common for these complications, occurring in patients with type 1 and 2 diabetes mellitus, as well as in those with prediabetes and glucose intolerance [3]. Its diagnosis is established by means of validated scores based on clinical features and abnormal nerve conduction studies (NCS) [4]. Pathophysiologic findings include loss of multifocal and focal nerve fibers secondary to axonal degeneration and segmental demyelization, basically due to oxidative stress and mitochondrial dysfunction induced by chronic hyperglycemia, which leads to neural apoptosis [5, 6]. Mitochondrial dysfunction leads to free radical excessive production through imbalance between hydrogen ions and electron transport carriers, which takes place in the inner mitochondrial membrane and could be evaluated indirectly by membrane fluidity and F0F1-ATPase hydrolysis [7, 8].

Ubiquinone (coenzyme Q10) is a potent antioxidant acting as an electron carrier in the mitochondrial electron transport chain, thus reducing free radical production with high concentrations present in high metabolic activity tissues such as heart, kidney, liver, and skeletal muscle [9]. Ezetimibe diminishes cholesterol ester content in chylomicrons by reducing liver cholesterol intake that in consequence increases LDL uptake and plasma depuration; when combined with simvastatin, cholesterol reduction is potentially increased [10]. Pleiotropic effects of statins include an increase in nuclear factor kappa B activity and amelioration of superoxide (O^{2-}) ions after 12-week treatment [11]. Another HMG-CoA inhibitor, rosuvastatin, has an antioxidant effect by acting as free radical carrier diminishing mitochondrial and cellular Lipid peroxidation (LPO) production [12].

We conducted this study to evaluate the effect of ubiquinone, ezetimibe/simvastatin, and rosuvastatin on mitochondrial function in patients with DPN.

2. Subjects, materials, and methods

2.1. Study design

A randomized, double blinded, placebo controlled phase II clinical trial was performed in the Clinic and Experimental Therapeutics Institute, University of Guadalajara, Mexico. Subjects were assigned to four group treatments by blocks with a parallel sequence 1:1:1:1 by means of a randomized computer-based list, generated by a different researcher who was unaware of drugs given to patients. Patients were divided into the following groups: control group that received placebo and three experimental groups that were assigned to ubiquinone, ezetimibe/simvastatin, and rosuvastatin as a daily single dose for 16 weeks.

2.2. Study population

Participants were eligible based on Dyck et al. characteristics for DPN [4]. Inclusion criteria were subjects ≥18 years old, T2DM (T2DM) according to ADA (American Diabetes Association) criteria, HbA1c <12%, and informed consent signed. Patients were excluded if they had renal or hepatic failure, pregnant or nursing women, and other neuropathies rather than diabetic (alcohol-induced, radiculopathy, autoimmune, cancer-related). They were eliminated once admitted if lack of adherence to treatment evaluated when <80% of drug intake, and/or severe adverse drug reaction. Patients were selected by invitation in forums, outpatients recruited from primary care clinics, and database collected previously by our research Institute, Guadalajara residents from February 2010 to 2012. Patients were instructed to take their drugs only by night at the same time every day as follows: placebo 100 mg, ubiquinone 400 mg, ezetimibe/simvastatin 10/20 mg, and rosuvastatin 20 mg. All drugs were similar in physical characteristics and presented in dark vials, carefully filled by another group researcher who placed a respective tag with the patient code. Moreover, patients were provided with a diary where they could write down the date and time of drug administration, and drug adverse reactions felt. Such information was collected and registered after every 4 weeks. Primary outcomes were mitochondrial function parameters: F0F1-ATPase hydrolysis, erythrocyte ghosts, and submitochondrial platelet membrane fluidity. We also measured other metabolic and safety measures: fasting glucose, HbA1c, total cholesterol, high and low density lipoproteins (HDL, LDL), and triglycerides. Safety profile was assessed with drug adverse reactions, renal (urea, creatinine), and hepatic [alanine and aspartate aminotransferase (ALT, AST), gamma glutamil-transferase (GGT), and bilirubin and phosphokinase (CPK)] laboratory variables.

2.3. Healthy subjects

We included an additional group consisting of nine subjects randomly selected from a preventive medicine first contact clinic to establish a cutoff point for the below-mentioned parameters. Healthy age and sex-matched volunteers without DM were included in the control group.

2.4. Mitochondrial function markers

Hydrolytic activity of mitochondrial F0F1-ATPase was obtained by spectrophotometry, from release of inorganic phosphate in serum samples of platelets isolated according to the method described by Baracca et al. [13]. Thirty microliters of the sample and 20 μL of ATP (100 mM) were added to 1 mL of ATPase buffer [125 mM KCl, 40 mM of Mops (pH 8), 3 mM MgCl2], and then agitated, followed by incubation at 40°C for 10 minutes. ATPase activity was stopped with 200 μL of 30% trichloroacetic acid, and samples were centrifuged for 10 minutes at 3500 rpm. Then, 1 mL of 3.3% ammonium molybdate and 100 μL of 10% ferrous sulfate were added to 800 μL of the supernatant, and samples were incubated for 20 minutes at room temperature to finally read absorbance at 660 nm. Results are expressed in nmol/PO4.

Membrane fluidity of erythrocyte ghosts and submitochondrial membrane in platelets was performed once obtained by centrifuging whole blood from patients at 4°C for 15 minutes at 3500 rpm. Supernatant was removed from the residue and 200 μL of cold buffer was added (NaCl 140 mM, KCl 4.7 mM, MgCl 1.2 mM, KH_2PO_4 1.2 mM, dextrose 11 mM and HEPES 15 mM), and homogenized. Platelets (70 μL) were isolated and stored at −80°C. Evaluation of membrane fluidity was performed by incorporation of 1,3-dipyrenylpropane (DPyP) to biological membranes [14]. Two milliliters of Tris-HCL buffer with a pH of 7.8 (10 mM) was added to 35 μL of the mitochondrial membranes and mixed at 24°C. Using fluorescent spectrophotometer (Perkin Elmer L550B), the fluorescent intensity of the monomer (Im) and excimer (Ie) were measured at 395 and 494 nm, respectively. Immediately, 5 μL (0.1 μg) of DPyP was added and incubated at room temperature in darkness for 3 hours, in order to allow the incorporation of the DPyP to membranes. The second measurement was performed at the same wavelengths and the Ie/Im ratio of the fluorescence intensity was calculated.

2.5. Ethical considerations

Study was approved by the Research and Ethics Committee of the Health Science University Center, University of Guadalajara, Mexico. Identification codes were assigned to each participant to guarantee patient confidentiality, and an informed consent form was signed before entering the protocol, according to national and international laws (National Institutes of Health) with clinical trial identifier NCT02129231 and also as stipulated by the Helsinki Statements in 2000.

2.6. Statistical analysis

Sample size determination was described elsewhere [15] taking into account a 95% confidence interval, 80% potency, and two-tailed $p < 0.05$, which resulted in 21 for each group. Quantitative variables were expressed as mean ± standard deviation. Wilcoxon tests were realized before and after measurements, and Kruskal-Wallis with Mann-Whitney´s *U* test as post hoc analysis for between-group comparisons. Qualitative variables were expressed as frequencies and percentages. The McNemar test was used to evaluate differences in dichotomy variables before and after treatment, between-group comparisons were determined by Fisher´s exact test and χ^2 as needed. The significance level was established with *p*-value <0.05.

3. Results

In the scrutiny phase, 155 patients were assessed, of which 63 were not eligible and 98 were included as follows: placebo 24, ubiquinone 24, ezetimibe/simvastatin 25, and rosuvastatin 25 (**Figure 1**).

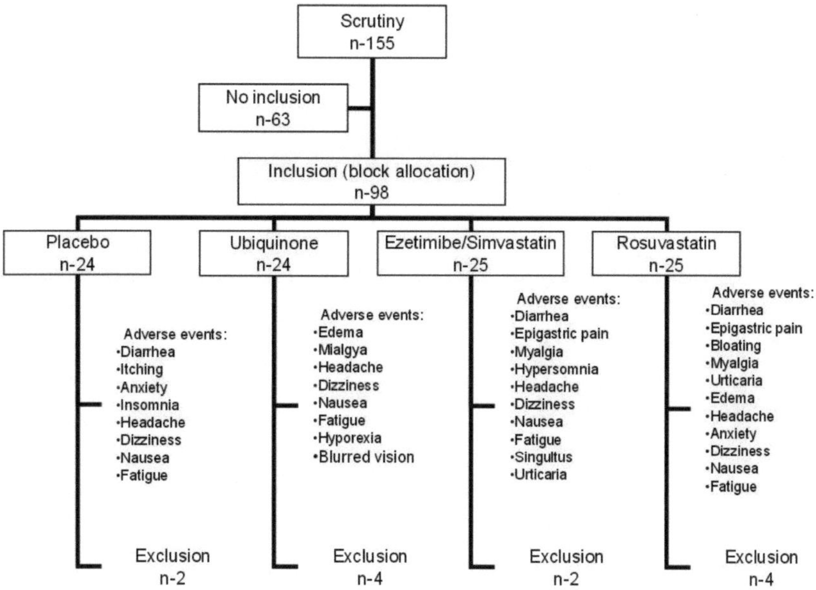

Figure 1. Flow diagram for patients follow-up.

Demographic features were homogeneous at baseline without significant differences between groups. Notably, there were a greater number of women above 50 years old and more than 10 years with T2DM. Overweight and obesity was found in all treatment groups (**Table 1**).

3.1. Mitochondrial function markers

F0-F1-ATPase in HS was 236.80 ± 118.42 nmol/PO4, those with placebo had 416.23 ± 38.39 nmol/PO4 ($p = 0.094$ vs. HS), for ubiquinone 535.86 ± 65.14 nmol/PO4 ($p < 0.05$ vs. HS), ezetimibe/simvastatin 447.09 ± 56.91 nmol/PO4 ($p = 0.065$ vs. HS), and rosuvastatin with 463.37 ± 47.07 nmol/PO4 ($p < 0.05$ vs. HS). There was no significant difference between treatment groups ($p = 0.583$, Kruskal-Wallis). At the end of treatment, placebo group had 443.41 ± 42.86 nmol/PO4 ($p = 0.783$, baseline vs. final), ubiquinone 391.30 ± 42.08 nmol/PO4 ($p = 0.823$, baseline vs. final), ezetimibe/simvastatin 328.50 ± 36.38 nmol/PO4 ($p = 0.426$, baseline vs. final), and rosuvastatin group had a significant reduction with 340.61 ± 37.80 nmol/PO4 ($p < 0.05$, baseline vs. final; **Figure 2A**).

Erythrocyte ghost membrane fluidity in HS was 0.80 ± 0.19 Ie/Im, while baseline levels on placebo group were 0.97 ± 0.10 Ie/Im ($p = 0.293$ vs. HS), ubiquinone 1.05 ± 0.18 Ie/Im ($p = 0.571$ vs. HS), ezetimibe/simvastatin had 1.23 ± 0.30 Ie/Im ($p = 0.936$ vs. HS), and rosuvastatin 0.98 ± 0.19 Ie/Im ($p = 0.936$ vs. HS); moreover, no significant differences were observed between treatment groups ($p = 0.632$, Kruskal-Wallis). After treatment period, there was no evident change in either group with placebo 1.13 ± 0.31 Ie/Im ($p = 0.836$, baseline vs. final), ubiquinone 1.21 ± 0.25 Ie/Im ($p = 0.245$, baseline vs. final), ezetimibe/simvastatin 1.14 ± 0.19 Ie/Im ($p = 0.983$ baseline vs. final), and rosuvastatin 0.99 ± 0.17 Ie/Im ($p = 0.778$, baseline vs. final), without difference between groups (p = 0.837, Kruskal-Wallis). There was no change in membrane fluidity after 16-week treatment, probably due to short-period intervention or this particular membrane property is not involved *y* pathogenic alterations noted in DM patients (**Figure 2B**).

	Placebo (n=24)	Ubiquinone (n=24)	Ezetimibe/ Simvastatin (n=25)	Rosuvastatin (n=25)
Gender (M/F), n (%)	7/17 (29/71)	9/15 (38/62)	10/15 (40/60)	12/13 (48/52)
Age (years)	54.7±9.6	58.8±9.2	55.0±12.0	54.0±10.5
Weight (kilograms)	73.7±11.4	73.8±8.6	75.4±13.9	76.9±18.7
Height (meters)	1.59±0.09	1.59±0.11	1.60±0.10	1.62±0.13
BMI (kg/m²)	29.3±4.3	29.3±7.3	29.4±4.1	29.0±4.7
Type 2 DM duration (years)	10.5±8.3	9.7±6.2	10.2±6.6	12.1±8.3
SBP (mmHg)	142±25	134±20	144±25	135±17
DBP (mmHg)	84±11	78±8	81±10	81±7
Smoking (Y/N), n (%)	9/15 (38/62)	10/14 (42/58)	8/17 (32/68)	12/13 (48/52)
Type 2 DM treatment, n (%)				
Insulin	1 (4.2)	1 (4.2)	2 (8.0)	
Metformin	5 (20.8)	5 (20.8)	5 (20.0)	4 (16.0)
Glyburide		1 (4.2)	1 (4.0)	3 (12.0)
Metformin/Glyburide	15 (62.5)	12 (50.0)	13 (52.0)	11 (44.0)
Metformin/Insulin	1 (4.2)	3 (12.5)	2 (8.0)	2 (8.0)
Metformin/Glyb/Insulin		1 (4.2)		3 (12.0)
Others	2 (8.3)	1 (4.2)	2(8.0)	2 (8.0)

Values in mean ± SD, unless otherwise specified.

Table 1. Demographic and clinical features.

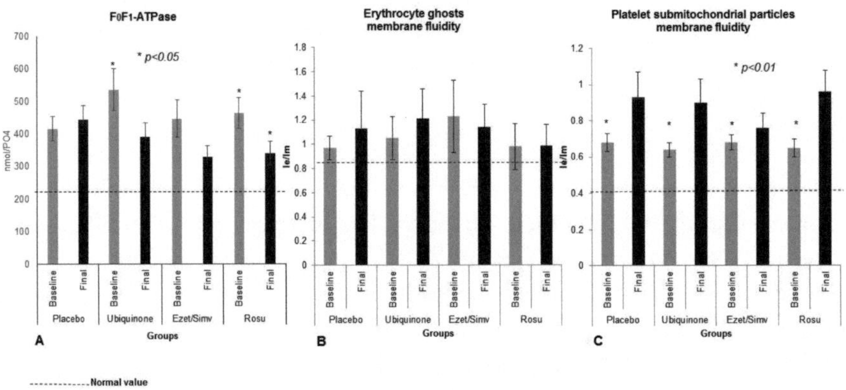

Figure 2. Mitochondrial dysfunction parameters in patients with DPN.

Submitochondrial platelet membrane fluidity in HS had 0.38 ± 0.03 Ie/Im, with increase in treatment groups; placebo control group had 0.68 ± 0.05 Ie/Im ($p < 0.01$ vs. HS), ubiquinone 0.64 ± 0.04 Ie/Im ($p < 0.01$ vs. HS), ezetimibe/simvastatin 0.68 ± 0.04 Ie/Im ($p < 0.01$ vs. HS), and rosuvastatin 0.65 ± 0.05 Ie/Im ($p < 0.01$ vs. HS); however, no statistical difference between treatment groups was found ($p = 0.675$, Kruskal-Wallis). After 16-week treatment there was no significant change in any group, those with placebo had 0.93 ± 0.14 Ie/Im ($p = 0.426$, baseline vs. final), ubiquinone 0.90 ± 0.13 Ie/Im ($p = 0.057$, baseline vs. final), ezetimibe/simvastatin 0.76 ± 0.08 Ie/Im ($p = 0.670$, baseline vs. final), and rosuvastatin 0.96 ± 0.12 Ie/Im ($p = 0.092$, baseline vs. final), without difference between groups ($p = 0.780$, Kruskal-Wallis). There is a significant difference in submitochondrial membrane fluidity when compared with healthy controls, probably because of underlying pathophysiologic changes in patients with diabetes, which cannot be resolved with short-time treatment (**Figure 2C**).

3.2. Metabolic and safety profile parameters

Serum transaminases were increased on experimental groups at baseline compared with placebo, without clinical relevance. A significant reduction in fasting glucose was noted for placebo and ubiquinone groups, probably due to lifestyle changes; however, no difference on HbA1c was observed. A reduction in the total bilirubin on ubiquinone and rosuvastatin treatments was also noted (–0.16 ± 0.27 and −0.17 ± 0.31 mg/dL, respectively), without significant difference compared with placebo. As expected, a significant reduction in TC, LDL, and TG was detected on statins (CT-82.8 ± 49.8 mg/dL and LDL-57.1 ± 48.4 mg/dL for ezetimibe/simvastatin ($p < 0.001$), and CT-73.3 ± 49.5 mg/dL, LDL-64.9 ± 44.0 mg/dL, and TG-41.1 ± 61.2 mg/dL) ($p < 0.001$, $p < 0.001$ and $p < 0.01$, respectively vs. placebo) for rosuvastatin (**Table 2**). Gastrointestinal, neurologic, dermatologic, and muscular adverse events related to drugs were reported, but only two patients were eliminated from the study for myopathy related to statins (one with ezetimibe/simvastatin and the other with rosuvastatin).

	Placebo (n=24)			**Ubiquinone (n=24)**			**Ezetimibe/ Simvastatin (n=25)**			**Rosuvastatin (n=25)**			***P* (Kruskal-Wallis)**
	Base line	**Final**	***p***	**Base line**	**Final**	***p***	**Base line**	**Final**	***p***	**Base line**	**Final**	***p***	
Glucose (mg/dL)	186.4± 14.48	150.2± 11.2	**0.004**	159.5± 11.05	138.1± 11	**0.020**	146.64± 9.92	152.6± 14	0.620	192.04± 12.73	179.2± 15.2	0.520	0.220
Urea (mg/dL)	29.5± 2.1	28.9± 2.2	0.520	29.23± 1.93	30.5± 2.5	0.170	30.03± 1.51	32.5± 1.9	0.280	31.22± 2.27	28.6± 2.2	0.300	0.440
Creatinine (mg/dL)	0.79± 0.04	0.84± 0.05	0.180	0.81± 0.05	0.80± 0.05	0.840	0.82± 0.04	0.85± 0.05	0.570	0.84± 0.04	0.80± 0.04	0.320	0.750
AST (U/L)	21.9± 1.89	21.8± 1.4	0.820	27.22± 2.5	**28± 2.4***	0.400	24.63± 0.99	**27.1± 2.5***	0.270	27.8± 1.91	**26.7± 1.2^**	0.700	**0.020**

	Placebo (n=24)			Ubiquinone (n=24)			Ezetimibe/ Simvastatin (n=25)			Rosuvastatin (n=25)			*P* (Kruskal-Wallis)
	Base line	Final	*p*	Base line	Final	*p*	Base line	Final	*p*	Base line	Final	*p*	
ALT (U/L)	20.2± 1.43	20.5± 1.9	0.990	29.5± 4.88	**30.3± 3.3***	0.730	28.57± 3.26	**28.4± 3.1***	0.570	31.22± 2.47	**30.3± 2.4^**	0.870	**0.010**
GGT (U/L)	34.73± 6.49	39.4± 8.6	0.270	55.22± 12.98	59.6± 17.9	0.600	39.83± 9.04	33.7± 3.7	0.780	44.33± 6.93	43.9± 7.7	0.260	0.800
Total Bilirubin (mg/dL)	0.70± 0.06	0.56± 0.05	0.052	0.77± 0.06	0.63± 0.08	**0.030**	0.61± 0.04	0.64± 0.06	0.800	0.83± 0.05	0.65± 0.07	**0.020**	0.790
Direct bilirubin (mg/dL)	0.11± 0.01	0.11± 0.01	0.780	0.12± 0.02	0.15± 0.03	0.290	0.10± 0.01	0.13± 0.01	0.080	0.15± 0.02	0.13± 0.02	0.420	0.830
Total cholesterol (mg/dL)	211.43 ±11.73	202.3 ±8	0.610	230.17 ±9.89	227.1± 8.3	0.330	210.56 ±9.94	**129.3± 9.7¥**	**0.001**	217.2± 8.04	**142.7± 8.8¥**	**0.001**	**0.001**
Low density cholesterol (mg/dL)	126.68 ±8.76	109.6± 7.8	**0.010**	134.19 ±8.08	132.5± 8.8	0.790	117.45 ±7.16	**61.7± 6.1¥**	**0.001**	133.56 ±7.96	**75± 8.1¥**	**0.001**	**0.001**
HDL cholesterol mg/dL)	36.95 ±2.61	39.7± 2.5	0.470	43.95± 3.69	43.4± 3.9	0.300	36.23± 2.06	32.7± 2.1	0.090	36.79± 1.91	36.5± 2.3	0.360	0.060
Trigly cerides (mg/dL)	240.13 ±27.41	242.4	0.590	260.25 ±36.59	263.1± 37.9	0.550	234.63 ±49.96	**161.9± 21.2***	0.055	220.6± 24.49	**168.4± 24.4***	**0.003**	**0.005**
CPK (U/L)	82.21± 13.78	82.8± 10.3	0.930	101.74± 18.42	00± 13.1	0.990	95.92± 14.4	86.4± 8.3	0.460	114.93 ±18.44	157.3± 35.1	0.190	0.100
A1c (%)	8.83± 0.36	9.2± 0.5	0.260	8.49± 0.36	7.9± 0.3	0.090	7.84± 0.32	8.1± 0.4	0.250	8.97± 0.40	**9.4± 0.4∞**	0.090	**0.030**

Median ± Standard error *$p<0.05$ ^$p<0.01$ ¥$p<0.001$ vs. Placebo ∞$p<0.01$ vs. Ubiquinone (Mann-Whitney's U test). A1c, glycated hemoglobin; ALT, alanine aminotransferase; AST, aspartate aminotransferase; CK, creatinine kinase; GGT, gamma glutamyl transferase; HDL, high-density cholesterol; LDL, low density cholesterol.

Table 2. Metabolic characteristics.

4. Discussion

Oxidative stress generates many of the pathophysiologic changes found in T2DM [16]; furthermore, free radical excessive production is involved in axonal degeneration and segmental demyelinization found in T2DM patients with DPN [17, 18]. Mitochondrial biogenesis is a complex process that involves more than 100 proteins coded by the nucleus and requires coordination with synthesis of 13 proteins coded by mitochondrial DNA. The integrity of this process is essential for normal oxidative phosphorylation, primary source of ATP production, O_2-, H_2O_2, and other ROS, which plays a fundamental role in the initiation and progression of diabetes. These products can overregulate the expression of proinflammatory cytokines and unchain death signals [19]. Mitochondria are very efficient by using glucose substrates to produce energy in the form of ATP. In this process, protons are pumped from the mitochondrial matrix to cross the inner mitochondrial membrane through the respiratory complexes forming the oxidative phosphorylation chain. Five complexes are implicated in ATP synthesis, culminating in complex V or ATP-synthase, and an inverse process occurs at the same time, named as ATP hydrolysis. An increase in F0F1-ATP hydrolysis has been found in rats with induced DM, probably induced by mitochondrial dysfunction [20], just as seen in treatment groups before intervention. Rosuvastatin demonstrated a reduction in F0F1-ATP hydrolysis after 16-week period, probably by reducing free radical production through improvement of NAD(P)H oxidase [21], constituting the first study to report this finding. We suppose an improvement in mitochondrial function by reduction in its catabolism, and probably reducing cell apoptosis.

The most important functions of erythrocyte membrane include (a) enzymatic activity, (b) ion transport of ions and anionic substances, (c) osmotic stability, (d) oxygen diffusion, and (e) membrane receptor activity, where a change in elasticity results in the deterioration of blood flow and worsens tissue perfusion [22]. Membrane fluidity of erythrocyte ghosts was slightly increased in patients with diabetes compared with HS. After intervention, all patients maintain almost the same values, probably due to T2DM chronicity, short-time treatment period, and/or not enough doses to improve this membrane property. In 2002, Koter et al. demonstrated a reduction in membrane fluidity with atorvastatin after 12 weeks of treatment in 31 hypercholesterolemic subjects [23]; however, T2DM consists in more complex physiopathologic components than lipid alterations as a single insult. More profound research must be conducted to establish the exact mechanisms that can be restored in order to improve erythrocyte membrane fluidity.

Submitochondrial particles are primarily composed of the internal mitochondrial membrane where oxidative phosphorylation and other enzymes are involved as metabolite carriers. Patients with T2DM had upper levels of platelet submitochondrial membrane fluidity when compared with HS, along with an increase after intervention. Until now, this was the first time to measure this particular platelet property. So, it is difficult to make a statement concerning its role on the pathogenesis of DPN. Previous studies on Alzheimer disease has shown low levels of platelet submitochondrial membrane fluidity due to increased levels of LPO [13]. So, we could speculate that an improvement in the mitochondrial function was achieved after treatment in all groups; however, no significant differences were found between them.

Metabolic outcomes were as expected, whereas no changes were observed on placebo and ubiquinone groups using statin-reduced TC, LDL, and TG. A recently published article (IMPROVE-IT) showed that ezetimibe combined with simvastatin enhances the lipid-lowering effect of this statin monotherapy, with the same security [24]. This study highlights the importance of LDL reduction in the improvement of cardiovascular events. Rosuvastatin showed a more intense reduction in LDL and TG, with an additional effect on F0F1-ATP hydrolysis, which raises the concern about the implication of oxidized LDL in the pathophysiology of T2DM microvascular complications.

A slight decrease in HbA1c was shown before and after intervention with ubiquinone, not enough to have a statistical inference but probably a larger number of patients and/or longer period of treatment would be needed to have a significant result. On the other hand, both placebo and ubiquinone had significant changes in fasting plasma glucose after treatment, probably due to tight control on lifestyle modifications. Finally, a slight increase in transaminases was observed with the three experimental groups compared with placebo, but levels were at normal range and there was no difference before and after 16-week intervention. So, it was considered as an incidental finding without clinically correlation.

In conclusion, patients with T2DM exhibit an increase in F0F1-ATP hydrolysis and membrane fluidity in erythrocytes and platelets, probably due to hypercatabolism secondary to hyperglycemia. A decreased mitochondrial membrane potential, dysfunction in intramitochondrial calcium regulation, and depletion of ATP production have been described previously; however, this is the first time, to our knowledge, that an increase in ATP hydrolysis is reported. These mechanisms, collectively, may lead to axon degeneration [19].

Alpha-lipoic acid (ALA) is the only effective treatment for neuropathological changes in DPN; for responders to initial 4-week high-dose (600 mg tid) administration of ALA, a subsequent treatment with ALA (600 mg qd) over 16 weeks effectively diminished neuropathic symptoms, whereas ALA withdrawal was associated with a higher use of rescue analgesic drugs in type 2 diabetic patients with symptomatic DPN [25]. However, ubiquinone and statins have proved a reduction in the oxidative stress status and neuropathic pain relief in previous publications [15, 26, 27].

We now demonstrate that all treatment groups had a diminishing effect on F0F1-ATP hydrolysis, but only rosuvastatin was found to improve mitochondrial function by significantly reducing F0F1-ATP hydrolysis. No changes in submitochondrial platelet particles or erythrocyte ghosts were found with this 16-week period treatment with ubiquinone, ezetimibe/simvastatin, or rosuvastatin; more research needs to be conducted to avoid bias, such as heterogeneity of antidiabetic drugs, lifestyle changes during the study, and reduced treatment period.

http://dx.doi.org/10.5772/63656

Author details

Luis M. Román-Pintos[1], Geannyne Villegas-Rivera[2], Ernesto G. Cardona-Muñoz[3], Adolfo D. Rodríguez-Carrizalez[3], Fermín P. Pacheco-Moisés[4] and Alejandra G. Miranda-Díaz[3*]

*Address all correspondence to: kindalex@outlook.com

1 Tonalá University Centre, University of Guadalajara, Guadalajara, Jalisco, México

2 Western Clinical Research Institute, Guadalajara, Jalisco, México

3 Clinical and Experimental Therapeutics Institute, Department of Physiology, Health Sciences University Centre, University of Guadalajara, Guadalajara, Jalisco, México

4 Department of Pharmacobiology, Engineering and Exact Sciences University Centre, University of Guadalajara, Guadalajara, Jalisco, México

References

[1] Dyck PJ, Kratz KM, Karnes JL, Litchy WJ, Klein R, Pach JM, et al. The prevalence by staged severity of various types of diabetic neuropathy, retinopathy, and nephropathy in a population-based cohort: the Rochester Diabetic Neuropathy Study. Neurology. 1993;43(4):817–824.

[2] Boulton AJM, Malik RA, Arezzo JC, Sosenko JM. Diabetic somatic neuropathies. Diabetes Care. 2004;27(6):1458–1486.

[3] Izenberg A, Perkins BA, Bril V. Diabetic neuropathies. Seminars in Neurology. 2015;35(4):424–430.

[4] Dyck PJ. Detection, characterization and staging of polyneuropathy: assessed in diabetics. Muscle Nerve. 1988;11:21–32.

[5] Dyck PJ, Giannini C. Pathologic alterations in the diabetic neuropathies of humans: a review. Journal of Neuropathology and Experimental Neurology. 1996;55(12):1181–1193.

[6] Vincent AM, Brownlee M, Russell JW. Oxidative stress and programmed cell death in diabetic neuropathy. Annals of the New York Academy of Science. 2002;959:368–383.

[7] Labrouche S, Freyburger G, Gin H, Boisseau MR, Cassagne C. Changes in phospholipid composition of blood cell membranes (erythrocyte, platelet, and polymorphonuclear) in different types of diabetes—clinical and biological correlations. Metabolism. 1996;145(1):57–62.

[8] Vinogradov AD. Steady-state and pre-steady-state kinetics of the mitochondrial F1F0 ATPase: is ATP synthase a reversible molecular machine? Journal of Experimental Biology. 2000;203:41–49.

[9] Bhagavan HN, Chopra RK. Coenzyme Q10: absorption, tissue uptake, metabolism and pharmacokinetics. Free Radicals Research. 2006;40(5):445–453.

[10] Neuvonen PJ, Niemi M, Backman JT. Drug interactions with lipid-lowering drugs: mechanisms and clinical relevance. Clinical Pharmacology Therapeutics. 2006;80(6): 565–581.

[11] Heart Protection Study Collaborative Group. MRC/BHF heart protection study of cholesterol lowering with simvastatin in 20 536 high-risk individuals: a randomised placebo controlled trial. Lancet. 2002;360:7–22.

[12] Ajith TA, Riji T, Anu V. In vitro anti-oxidant and DNA protective effects of the novel 3-hydroxy-3-methylglutaryl coenzyme A reductase inhibitor rosuvastatin. Clinical Experimental Pharmacology and Physiology. 2008;35:625–629.

[13] Baracca A, Barogi S, Carelli V, Lenaz G, Solaini G. Catalytic activities of mitochondrial ATP synthase in patients with mitochondrial DNA T8993G mutation in the ATPase 6 gene encoding subunit a. Journal of Biology and Chemistry. 2000;275(6):4177–4182.

[14] Ortiz GG, Pacheco-Moisés F, El Hafidi M, Jiménez-Delgado A, Macías-Islas MA, Rosales Corrala SA, et al. Detection of membrane fluidity in sub-mitochondrial particles of platelets and erythrocyte membranes from Mexican patients with Alzheimer disease by intramolecular excimer formation of 1,3 dipyrenylpropane. Disease Markers. 2008;24:151–156.

[15] Villegas-Rivera G, Román-Pintos LM, Cardona-Muñoz EG, Arias-Carvajal O, Rodríguez-Carrizalez AD, Troyo-Sanromán R, et al. Effects of ezetimibe/simvastatin and rosuvastatin on oxidative stress in diabetic neuropathy: a randomized, double-blind, placebo-controlled clinical trial. Oxidative Medicine and Cellular Longevity. 2015;2015; 756294, 10 pp. DOI: 10.1155/2015/756294.

[16] Singh RB, Niaz MA, Kumar A, Sindberg CD, Moesgaard S, Littarru GP. Effect on absorption and oxidative stress of different oral Coenzyme Q10 dosages and intake strategy in healthy men. Biofactors. 2005;25:219–224.

[17] Várkonyi T, Kempler P. Diabetic neuropathy: new strategies for treatment. Diabetes, Obesity and Metabolism. 2008;10:99–108.

[18] Kasznicki J, Kosmalski M, Sliwinska A, Mrowicka M, Stanczyk M, Majsterek I, Drzewoski J. Evaluation of oxidative stress markers in pathogenesis of diabetic neuropathy. Molecular Biology and Reproduction. 2012;39:8669–8678.

[19] Hernández-Beltrán N, Moreno CB, Gutiérrez-Álvarez AM. Contribution of mitochondria to pain in diabetic neuropathy. Endocrinología y Nutrición. 2013;60(1):25–32.

[20] Rücker B, Abreu-Vieira G, Bischoff LB, Harthmann AD, Sarkis JJ, Wink MR, Casali EA. The nucleotide hydrolysis is altered in blood serum of streptozotocin-induced diabetic rats. Archives of Physiology and Biochemistry. 2010;116(2):79–87.

[21] Mennickent S, Bravo M, Calvo C, Avello M. Efectos pleiotrópicos de las estatinas. Revista Médica de Chile. 2008;136:775–782.

[22] Kowalczyk E, Kowalski J, Błaszczyk J, Gwoździński Ł, Ciećwierz J, Sienkiewicz M. Estimation of cell membrane properties and erythrocyte red-ox balance in patients with metabolic syndrome. Molecular Biology and Reproduction. 2012;39(12):11113–11118.

[23] Koter M, Broncel M, Chojnowska-Jezierska J, Klikczynska K y Franiak I. The effect of atorvastatin on erythrocyte membranes and serum lipids in patients with type-2 hypercholesterolemia. European Journal of Clinical Pharmacology. 2002;58:501–506.

[24] IMPROVE-IT investigators. Ezetimibe Added to Statin Therapy after Acute Coronary Syndromes. New England Journal of Medicine. 2015;372(25):2387–2397.

[25] Garcia-Alcala H, Santos-Vichido CI, Islas-Macedo S, Genestier-Tamborero CN, Minutti-Palacios M, Hirales-Tamez O, et al. Treatment with α-lipoic acid over 16 weeks in type 2 diabetic patients with symptomatic polyneuropathy who responded to initial 4-week high-dose loading. Journal of Diabetes Research. 2015; 189857, 8 pp. DOI: http://dx.doi.org/10.1155/2015/189857

[26] Hernández-Ojeda J, Cardona-Muñoz EG, Román-Pintos LM, Troyo-Sanromán R, Ortiz-Lazareno PC, Cárdenas-Meza MA, Pascoe-González S, Miranda-Díaz AG. The effect of ubiquinone in diabetic polyneuropathy: a randomized double-blind placebo-controlled study. Journal of Diabetes and Its Complications. 2012;26(4):352–358.

[27] Hernández-Ojeda J, Román-Pintos LM, Rodríguez-Carrizalez AD, Troyo-Sanromán R, Cardona-Muñoz EG, Alatorre-Carranza MP, Miranda-Díaz. Effect of rosuvastatin on diabetic polyneuropathy: a randomized, double-blind, placebo-controlled Phase IIa study. Diabetes, Metabolic Syndrome and Obesity: Targets and Therapy. 2014;7:401–407.

Chapter 12

Involvement of Free Radicals in the Development and Progression of Alzheimer's Disease

Martha C. Rosales Hernández,

Maricarmen Hernández Rodríguez,

Jessica E. Mendieta Wejebe and José Correa Basurto

Additional information is available at the end of the chapter

http://dx.doi.org/10.5772/64708

Abstract

Alzheimer's disease (AD) is a major dementia related to an overproduction of free radicals (FRs), which leads to the generation of oxidative stress in brain tissue. Amyloid beta-peptide of 42 amino acid residues ($A\beta_{1-42}$) is the main source of FRs in patients with AD. βA_{1-42} results from hydrolysis of the amyloid precursor protein by β-secretase in a process known as the amyloidogenic pathway. During βA_{1-42} aggregation, the peptide interacts with various transition metals to produce hydrogen peroxide (H_2O_2) by the Fenton reaction, generating the hydroxyl radical ($^{\bullet}OH$), which damages lipids, proteins, and nucleic acids, thereby contributing to neurodegeneration. In addition, βA_{1-42} is recognized by microglial receptors; it activates these cells, causing overproduction of superoxide anion ($O_2^{\bullet -}$) by NADPH oxidase; $O_2^{\bullet -}$ is also converted into H_2O_2 and finally to $^{\bullet}OH$ in the Fenton reaction. Other factors that contribute to oxidative stress during microglial activation are the overproduction of nitric oxide and interleukins and the overexpression of some enzymes, including cyclooxygenase and inducible nitric oxide synthase, all of which contribute to FR production. Currently, various models *in vitro* and *in vivo* exist that permit quantification of $O_2^{\bullet -}$ and H_2O_2 and determination of the effects of these reactive oxygen species.

Keywords: Amyloid beta, NADPH oxidase, free radicals, oxidative stress

1. Introduction

Alzheimer's disease (AD) is a chronic pathology, the development and progression of which has been related to free radical (FR) production such as occurs in diabetes, cancer, and other diseases secondary to molecular damage. AD is characterized by neuronal damage associated with an overproduction of free radicals (FRs). Although several hypotheses have been advanced to explain the memory loss that occurs in AD, the most accepted theory is that neuronal damage is associated with the presence of aggregates of the amyloid beta peptide of 42 residues ($A\beta_{1-42}$) that is related to FR production.

It is known that Aβ aggregation contributes to FR production because Aβ molecules are able to bind metals such as copper (cupric ion, Cu^{2+}) that are present at high concentrations in the brains of patients with AD. Cu^{2+} leads to the formation of hydrogen peroxide (H_2O_2), which is a reactive oxygen specie (ROS). In turn, H_2O_2 reacts with other metals such as iron (Fe^{2+}) through the Fenton reaction, producing the hydroxyl radical ($^{\bullet}OH$), which damages membrane lipids, proteins, and other biomolecules. Here, it is important to remember that ROS include not only FRs such as $^{\bullet}OH$, superoxide anion ($O_2^{\bullet-}$), and others but also non-FRs such as H_2O_2, ozone (O_3), and hypochlorous acid (HOCl). One hypothesis suggests that the ROS produced during AD hydrolyze a significant amount of acetylcholine (ACh), reducing cholinergic neurotransmission and thereby contributing to memory loss [1]. This has justified the use of acetylcholinesterase (AChE) inhibitors to treat AD; however, these drugs have shown limited clinical results [2].

Brain tissue is especially susceptible to oxidative stress due to its high aerobic metabolic activity and high lipid content. Oxidative stress is defined as the loss of cell homeostasis provoked by an imbalance between the production of prooxidant molecules (ROS) and the activity of antioxidant defense systems. Under physiological conditions, ROS are present at low concentrations in tissues, where they act as signaling molecules during cell growth, cell proliferation, redox homeostasis, and cellular signal transduction (activating tyrosine kinases, MAPKs (mitogen-activated protein kinases), or Ras protein) [3]. However, higher concentrations of ROS lead to a pathophysiological condition produced by an oxidative stress state.

It has been reported that AD is associated with a high level of oxidative stress and lowered antioxidant defenses. Thus, AD may be due to the presence of FRs that alter metal metabolism and result in Aβ aggregation toxicity [4]. In recent years, considerable research has focused on the amyloid fibrils that are produced in AD, and it has been shown that the structures of these aggregates are more complex than the linear addition of monomers to fibrils; in fact, a variety of Aβ aggregates have been described. Furthermore, the amyloid fibrils cause the formation of several toxic intermediates, including soluble oligomers that bind to hippocampal neurons to produce dysfunctions in synaptic plasticity and consequently contribute to the development of AD [5]. Hence, great efforts have been made to find ways to prevent Aβ aggregation because the oligomers and fibrils are also able to activate the NADPH oxidase in microglial cells, which are "like macrophage cells" in the brain. NADPH oxidase can produce great quantities of $O_2^{\bullet-}$, which is converted to H_2O_2; this, in turn, can participate in the Fenton reaction, producing $^{\bullet}OH$. Thus, the generation of

FRs is important in AD because these have been related to its development, and Aβ and NADPH oxidase may be key targets for the treatment of this disease.

In this chapter, we describe the important implications of FRs in the development and progression of AD. First, we discuss some of the principal biomolecules involved in the production of FRs in AD, emphasizing the role of $A\beta_{1-42}$ due to its aggregation and its consequent implication in the formation of senile plaques when it reacts with metals to produce ROS. In addition, we explain how Aβ participates in microglial activation to produce more FRs due to the activity of NADPH oxidase. Subsequently, the reactions in which the ROS produced by Aβ and NADPH oxidase participate are described, and the relationship between FR production and the neuronal damage that occurs during AD is explained. Finally, we discuss how $^{\bullet}OH$ and H_2O_2 production can be determined using various experimental techniques *in vitro* and *in vivo*.

2. Biomolecules involved in free radical production in Alzheimer's disease

2.1. Amyloid beta formation

Aβ is the principal component of extracellular deposits called amyloid plaques that are present in the brains of patients with AD. According to the amyloid cascade hypothesis, which was first established in 1991, Aβ accumulation represents the critical step in the pathophysiology of AD [6]. Aβ originates from the processing of a large transmembrane glycoprotein, amyloid precursor protein (APP). APP is a single-pass transmembrane protein with a large extracellular domain. Alternate splicing of the APP transcript generates eight isoforms, the three most common of which are the 695-amino acid form, which is expressed predominantly in the central nervous system (CNS), and the 751- and 770-amino acid forms, which are more ubiquitously expressed [7].

The precise physiological function of APP is not known and remains one of the vexing issues in the field. In most studies, APP overexpression shows a positive effect on cell health and growth [8]. APP can be hydrolyzed following both the non-amyloidogenic and the amyloidogenic pathways, depending on the enzymes involved. In the non-amyloidogenic pathway, APP is hydrolyzed at amino acid residue 83 from the C-terminus by α-secretase (**Figure 1**). This cleavage produces a fragment of 83 amino acids (C83) and a large N-terminal ectodomain (sAPPα). C83 remains in the membrane, where it is hydrolyzed by the γ-secretase complex to produce p3, a short fragment, and the APP intracellular domain (AICD). In the amyloidogenic pathway, APP is hydrolyzed at amino acid residue 99 from the C-terminus by β-secretase to produce a fragment of 99 amino acids (C99) and an sAPPβ fragment. C99 remains in the membrane, where it is hydrolyzed by the γ-secretase complex, releasing the Aβ peptide, which consists of 42 amino acid residues ($A\beta_{1-42}$), and other peptides (**Figure 1**) [9]. The principal difference between these two pathways is that α-secretase cleavage occurs within the Aβ region, avoiding the formation of Aβ peptide, whereas β-secretase cleavage permits Aβ formation from APP.

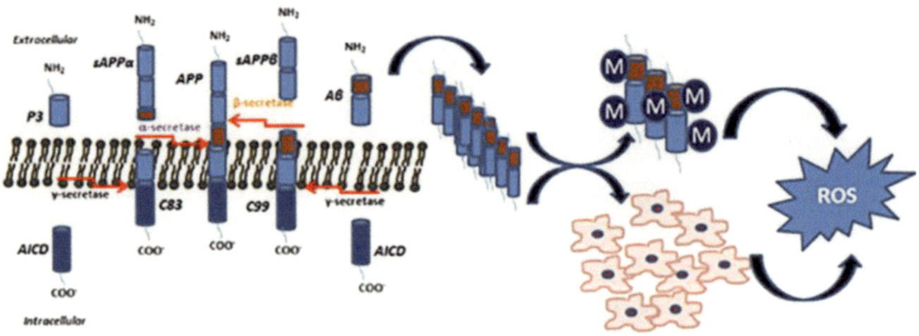

Figure 1. Hydrolysis of APP to produce the Aβ peptide. When $A\beta_{1-42}$ is released, it tends to aggregate to form oligomers and fibrils; these subsequently react with metals or with microglial cells and produce a large amount of ROS.

It is important to mention that under physiological conditions, both of these pathways occur; in fact, it has been demonstrated that Aβ is an enhancer of learning and memory and that low doses of Aβ produce presynaptic enhancement [10]. It was shown that concentrations of Aβ peptides in the picomolar-nanomolar range decrease the synthesis and release of ACh without causing neurotoxicity. The potency and reversible nature of this effect and the low concentrations of Aβ peptides found in normal brain cells suggest that Aβ-related peptides may act as modulators of cholinergic function under normal conditions [11]. However, during AD, the increase in the concentration of Aβ may be the result of an overproduction and/or a deficiency in its elimination, resulting in Aβ aggregation [12]. During the processing of APP by the amyloidogenic pathway, two principal Aβ species are produced: Aβ of 40 amino acid residues and Aβ of 42 amino acid residues ($A\beta_{1-40}$ and $A\beta_{1-42}$, respectively). Despite the difference of only two amino acids, the latter is more prone to aggregate; the additional amino acids give $A\beta_{1-42}$ distinct thermodynamic properties [13].

Two distinct mechanisms have been proposed to explain the formation of Aβ fibrils. The first invokes nucleated polymerization in which Aβ polymerization creates a nucleus to which monomers are added in an elongation process (**Figure 2**).

The second proposed mechanism is based on a nucleated conformational conversion in which oligomers are formed as intermediates; these intermediates then form protofibrils that subsequently assemble into fibrils [14]. Because Aβ oligomers have been implied in the pathophysiology of AD, it has been proposed that the second mechanism contributes more to the progression of the disease. However, although enormous efforts have been made to understand how Aβ aggregates, principally in the form of $A\beta_{1-42,}$ which is more cytotoxic than $A\beta_{1-40}$ [15], the mechanism by which $A\beta_{1-42}$ undergoes conformational changes to form oligomers and protofibrils remains unknown (**Figure 2**).

Recently, several experimental techniques such as nuclear magnetic resonance (NMR) (solid state), Fourier transform infrared spectroscopy (FTIR), cryo-electron microscopy (cryo-EM), single-touch atomic force microscopy (AFM), and fluorescence have allowed investigators to study the $A\beta_{1-42}$ fibril formation process in detail. The results suggest that a nucleated conformational conversion occurs when $A\beta_{1-42}$ is present at high concentrations (>20–30 μM). The

http://dx.doi.org/10.5772/64708

predominant oligomers formed in the early step of aggregation are dimers, tetramers, pentamers, and hexamers, but their formation is temperature- and concentration dependent. At approximately 15°C and high Aβ_{1-42} concentration, the formation of protofibrils from oligomers occurs more rapidly. The principal conformational change is observed in the lateral association of oligomers to yield protofibrils; this conformation involves conversion from a random coil structure to a β-sheet via an antiparallel β-hairpin intermediate [16]. The antiparallel β-hairpin has intramolecular hydrogen bonds between two hydrophobic β-strands, one with an LVFF sequence and another with a GLMVG sequence at the C-terminus. However, conversion to a β-sheet involves the rotation of β-strands to form intermolecular hydrogen bonds with other monomers in the Aβ_{1-42} structure. It is known that the β-strands adopt a parallel orientation in the Aβ_{1-42} fibrils. The β-sheet is stabilized by intermolecular hydrogen bonds as well as by intramolecular and intermolecular interactions between the residue side chains in the β-strands. It has been confirmed that the formation of the antiparallel β-hairpin is a rate-determining step in fibril formation, with the interaction between aspartate 23 (Asp23) and lysine 28 (Lys28) being the most important.

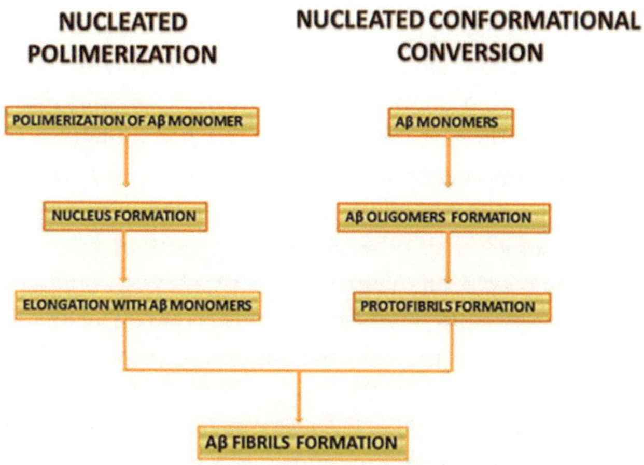

Figure 2. Proposed mechanisms of Aβ fibril formation. Left: nucleated polymerization at low Aβ concentrations. Right: nucleated conformational conversion at high Aβ concentrations. The latter mechanism is considered to be more related to the progression of AD because it produces a large amount of oligomers, which, together with the fibrils, are cytotoxic.

Other recent studies show that there are differences in Aβ_{1-42} and Aβ_{1-40} fibril formation [17]. One of these differences is that the Aβ_{1-42} fibril has a triple β-motif that consists of three β-sheets (β_1: 12–18; β_2: 24–33; β_3: 36–40); thus, this structure differs from the proposed β-loop-β motif structure for Aβ_{1-40} fibrils. Additionally, the reported structure of Aβ_{1-42} fibrils differs from that of Aβ_{1-40} fibrils from the brain, which have a U-shaped topology with Asp 23-Lys 28 forming a salt bridge and fewer β-regions [18]. Furthermore, in Aβ_{1-42} fibrils a salt bridge between Lys28 and the carboxylate of the C-terminal alanine (Ala42) was identified; this is important because it shows that Ala42 and not Asp 23, as had been proposed, stabilizes the salt-bridge interaction.

Although several models of $A\beta_{1-42}$ fibrils have been described, to date no $A\beta_{1-42}$ fibril structure has been obtained from the brain, and all that is known about the conformational structure of $A\beta_{1-42}$ fibrils has been obtained from synthetic $A\beta_{1-42}$. Therefore, all $A\beta_{1-42}$ models and observations are approximations that should be accepted with caution because $A\beta_{1-42}$ fibril formation may be influenced by temperature, pH, and other biochemical parameters that are not considered when the fibrils are formed *in vitro*. For example, it was recently reported that calcium (Ca^{2+}) interacts with glutamate 22 (Glu22) and the phospholipid bilayer to accelerate $A\beta_{1-42}$ aggregation [19]. Furthermore, this type of interaction between a cation and Glu22 could also be important in interactions of the peptide with metals such as Cu^{2+}, which at some concentrations favors $A\beta_{1-42}$ aggregation. Therefore, it is difficult to propose a definite and unique $A\beta_{1-42}$ fibril structure that could provide a basis for elucidating the steps involved in $A\beta_{1-42}$ aggregation.

As mentioned previously, the mechanism of $A\beta_{1-42}$ aggregation that has been proposed to contribute principally to the pathogenesis of AD is nucleated conformational change due to the formation of oligomers of $A\beta_{1-42}$ [20]. When the amyloid hypothesis was first proposed, it was postulated that only $A\beta_{1-42}$ fibrils were the toxic form of Aβ; however, it is now known that both oligomers and protofibrils are toxic species and that oligomers are more toxic than fibrils [21]. This has been generally accepted due to the finding that cognitive deficits are better correlated with the amount of soluble Aβ than with the number of amyloid plaques; thus, neurodegeneration is not a consequence of amyloid deposition [22]. This is consistent with the oxidative damage produced by the $A\beta_{1-42}$ oligomers. There are several hypotheses related to $A\beta_{1-42}$ aggregation and ROS production during AD development and progression. The results of a number of studies support the hypothesis that $A\beta_{1-42}$ genesis depends on ROS production, whereas other reports suggest that $A\beta_{1-42}$ is capable of forming ROS [23]. In addition, some previous evidence clearly shows an association between AD and the ROS produced by $A\beta_{1-42}$ oligomers and metals (**Figure 1**). Hence, some studies have focused on searching for strategies to avoid the oligomerization of $A\beta_{1-42}$ by inhibiting it or by decreasing ROS production through the design of multi-targeted compounds; this has resulted in a promising approach [8]. By targeting at this molecular level, it is possible to avoid $A\beta_{1-42}$ aggregate formation, which functions as a signal that activates microglial cells and initiates an innate immune response that results in the production of high levels of cytokines and ROS.

2.2. Microglial activation enhances NADPH oxidase activity

Due to their phagocytic activity, microglial cells represent the macrophages of the brain; for this reason, they are regarded as the predominant immune cells in the brain. In the healthy brain, these cells act as resting microglia, maintaining their ramified morphology and protecting the brain from pathogens by removing them by phagocytosis [24]. However, when microglial cells detect a sign such as a pathogen associated with molecular patterns (PAMPs) or damage associated with molecular patterns (DAMPs), the microglia are activated to acquire a wide range of phenotypes. Two classical phenotypes are the pro-inflammatory M1 phenotype (induced by pro-inflammatory cytokines and/or TLR activation (Toll-like receptor)) and the non-inflammatory M2 phenotype (induced by interleukin (IL)-4), according to the classification for macrophages outside the brain [25]. $A\beta_{1-42}$ oligomers and fibrils interact with SCARA1, CD36, CD14, a6β1 integrin, CD47, TLR2, TLR4, TLR6, and TLR9 receptors on the microglia; when $A\beta_{1-42}$ interacts with TLR or CD receptors, the expression of inducible nitric oxide synthase (iNOS), cyclooxygenase 2 (COX2), tumor necrosis factor (TNF)-alpha, IL-1β, IL-6, etc. is induced, resulting in a dysregulated immune response that contributes to neurodegeneration [26].

Furthermore, it was found that low concentrations of $A\beta_{1-42}$ induce microglial proliferation and cause release of H_2O_2 and $O_2^{\bullet-}$ to the extracellular space due to the activation of NADPH oxidase (**Figure 3A**) [27]. The fact that NADPH oxidase 2 (NOX2) is widely distributed in microglial cells and neurons has been corroborated in *in vitro* and *in vivo* models using microglia derived from NOX2 knockout mice and the NOX2 inhibitors diphenyleneiodonium (DPI) and apocynin [28]. In microglial cells, NOX2 is activated only after the binding of Aβ oligomers to the Mac receptor (Mac-1), an integrin receptor also known as CD11b/CD18, complement receptor 3 or aMβ2 that is important during reactive microgliosis and in neurodegeneration (**Figure 3B**) [29, 30].

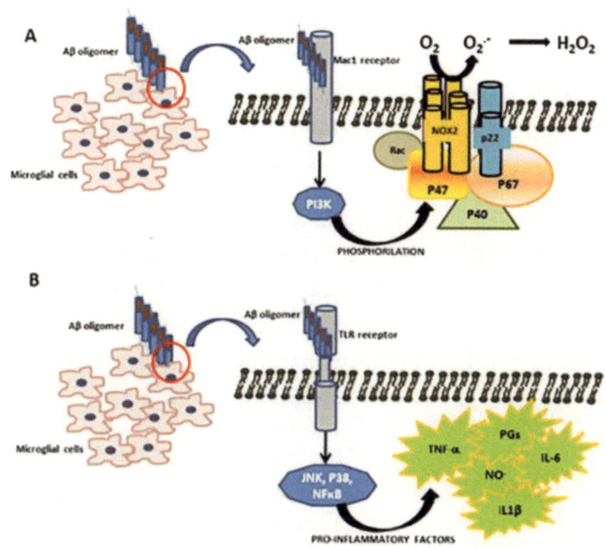

Figure 3. Pro-inflammatory factors produced by the interaction of $A\beta_{1-42}$ oligomers with TLR or Mac-1 receptors. (A) $A\beta_{1-42}$ oligomers induce the activation of NADPH oxidase. (B) Production of cytokines induced by the interaction of $A\beta_{1-42}$ oligomers with the TLR receptor.

It is currently known that unique NADPH oxidase activity is associated with the generation of $O_2^{\bullet-}$ or H_2O_2, depending on the isoform. The confirmation of NADPH oxidase participation in microglial activation and the consequent production of ROS were obtained using cells from patients with chronic granulomatous disease (CGD). Because this disease is characterized by the inability of cells to produce H_2O_2 due to mutations in the genes that encode the subunits of NADPH oxidase, monocytes and neutrophils from CGD patients fail to produce ROS in response to fibrillary Aβ peptides [31, 32].

Park et al. assessed ROS production in the neocortex using hydroethidine fluoromicrography [29]. Fibrillar Aβ superfused through a cranial window increased ROS production in the neocortex. This effect could be abolished by the addition of a peptide inhibitor of the gp91phox subunit. These authors further demonstrated that ROS levels were increased in the Tg2576 mouse model of AD; however, no signs of ROS production were evident in a mouse model in which Tg2576 mice lacked the gp91phox gene.

NOX2 is an oligomeric protein composed of three cytosolic subunits (p60phox, p47phox, and p40phox) and two transmembrane subunits (p91phox and p22phox). For the production of $O_2^{\bullet-}$ by NOX2, p22phox must form a complex with p47phox. It has been demonstrated that, in primary microglial cells and monocytes exposed to fibrillar Aβ, p47phox and p67phox subunits are translocated from the cytosol to the membrane, favoring the enhanced activity of NADPH oxidase [33].

The production of $O_2^{\bullet-}$ together with the neurotoxic factors PGE2, IL-β1, TNF-alpha, H_2O_2, nitric oxide (NO), and peroxynitrite ($ONOO^-$) can result in neuronal death [34]. Subsequently, the $O_2^{\bullet-}$ produced by NOX2 reacts with NO generated by iNOS to form $ONOO^-$. In the presence of excessive amounts of NO, nitration and S-nitrosylation of several proteins, as well as dityrosine formation, occur. Tyrosine 10 of Aβ can undergo nitration, which in turn increases the probability of Aβ aggregation; this is shown by the fact that Aβ nitrotyrosine has been found in amyloid plaques [35].

During chronic neuroinflammation, microglia maintain the transcription of mRNAs coding for pro-inflammatory factors such as NOX2, iNOS, TNF-alpha, IL-1β, and COX2. The interaction between $A\beta_{1-42}$ oligomers and TLR receptors begins the phase of neurodegeneration (**Figure 3B**); as neuroinflammation progresses, the interaction between $A\beta_{1-42}$ oligomers and Mac-1 receptors results in the production of large amounts of FRs such as $O_2^{\bullet-}$, which is converted to H_2O_2 to maintain the neuroinflammation (**Figure 3A**).

$O_2^{\bullet-}$ dismutates spontaneously or by an enzymatic reaction catalyzed by superoxide dismutase (SOD), an enzyme that can scavenge $O_2^{\bullet-}$ and convert it into H_2O_2 [36]. Because $O_2^{\bullet-}$ is the primary ROS produced during the neuroinflammatory process, this is considered to play a key role in the activation of microglia and the activation of NADPH oxidase. However, $O_2^{\bullet-}$ can also be produced by xanthine oxidase and during mitochondrial respiration. The $O_2^{\bullet-}$ can reduce and liberate ferric ion (Fe^{3+}) from ferritin or ferrous ion (Fe^{2+}) from iron-sulfur clusters. This reaction is of great importance because Fe^{2+} participates in the Fenton reaction and produces $^{\bullet}OH$. $O_2^{\bullet-}$ contributes to the Fenton reaction via the Haber-Weiss reaction, in which $O_2^{\bullet-}$ reduces Fe^{3+} produced in the Fenton reaction to Fe^{2+} and maintains iron (II), thereby facilitating the Fenton reaction. The net Haber-Weiss reaction is as follows (1-3):

$$Fe^{3+} / Cu^{2+} + O_2^{\bullet-} \rightarrow Fe^{2+} / Cu^{+} + O_2 \quad (1)$$

http://dx.doi.org/10.5772/64708

$$Fe^{2+} / Cu^{+} + H_2O_2 \rightarrow Fe^{3+} / Cu^{2+} + OH^{\bullet} + OH^{-} \quad (2)$$

$$O_2^{\bullet -} + H_2O_2 \rightarrow O_2 + OH^{\bullet} + OH^{-} \quad (3)$$

Numerous experimental studies have shown that Aβ oligomers are more toxic than Aβ fibrils, and that ROS are produced from the beginning of AD, playing a crucial role in neuroinflammation.

3. Biochemical and chemical reactions in Alzheimer's disease that yield free radicals

3.1. Metal dyshomeostasis during Alzheimer's disease

It is well known that certain transition metals are essential for neural function. The levels and transport of these metals are strictly regulated by the blood-brain barrier (BBB), and disruption of metal homeostasis in the brain is thought to play an important role in the pathogenesis of AD [37]. The principal areas of the brain in which metals tend to accumulate are the hippocampus, the amygdala, and the cerebrospinal fluid (CSF); in some of these areas, both senile plaques and neurofibrillary tangles are found (**Table 1**).

The mammalian brain contains an intrinsically high concentration of copper (Cu^{2+}), zinc (Zn^{2+}), and iron (Fe^{2+}) ions compared to other tissues due to its high requirement for numerous metal-dependent enzymes and metal-dependent metabolic processes [38]. Not only has dyshomeostasis of Cu^{2+}, Zn^{2+}, and Fe^{2+} been linked with AD but it has also been reported that senile plaques are related to high concentrations of these metals as well as of chrome (Cr^{3+}) and cadmium (Cd^{2+}) (**Table 1**) [39–41]. Furthermore, these metals are involved in FR production by their participation in the Fenton and Fenton-like reactions; importantly, it has been suggested that they may interact with biomolecules implicated in AD such as Aβ, AChE, and ACh [1], with deleterious results.

To clarify the functions and toxicities of various metals and their relationship to AD, specific information on each metal is provided as follows:

Iron: Divalent iron (Fe^{2+}) is the most abundant transition metal in the human brain. Iron is present *in vivo* in both the ferrous (Fe^{2+}) and ferric (Fe^{3+}) valence states. Fe^{2+} is crucial for neuronal processes such as myelination, synaptogenesis, and synaptic plasticity (SP). It has been well documented that Fe^{2+} deficiency can induce a series of neurochemical alterations that may eventually lead to cognitive deficits [42]. While essential for the maintenance of a healthy brain, Fe^{2+} can also play a toxic role. It exacerbates damage to brain tissue following processes such as stroke or trauma. A regional increase in Fe^{2+} within AD brains, compared with healthy controls, is considered a key factor in neuronal atrophy. Accumulations of Fe^{2+} occur in the cerebral cortex, the hippocampus, and the basal nucleus of Meynert, where they co-localize with lesions, neurofibrillary tangles, and plaques. These are particularly important areas in the clinical picture of AD because they are associated with the centers of memory and thought that are gradually lost as AD progresses [42]. Given that Fe^{2+} is highly reactive, an excess of this metal ion may result in the overproduction of reactive chemical species such as •OH. Thus, FRs are responsible for oxidative stress, which is considered a primary contributing factor in neurodegeneration [43].

Metal and concentration in AD brains (μM)	Physiological functions in the brain	Brain areas where metal is accumulated	Relationship with AD
Fe^{2+}, 669, 694	Formation and maintenance of the neuronal network and neurotransmitter synthesis.	Hippocampus (wet tissue), amygdala	Generation of an excess of reactive radical species leading to cell and tissue damage.
Cu^{2+}, 57.7, 53.2, 10–100	Cofactor and structural component of enzymes. Regulate synaptic function myelination, synaptogenesis, and synaptic plasticity.	Hippocampus (wet tissue), amygdala, cerebrospinal fluid	Copper in redox-active can catalyze the production of hydroxyl radicals (•OH) in a Fenton-like reaction. May influence clearance of Aβ from the brain at the level of the interface between the blood and cerebrovasculature in AD.
Zn^{2+}, 1000, 300	It is released from presynaptic nerve terminals into the synaptic cleft upon neuronal activation and has been shown to inhibit excitatory NMDA receptors.	Amyloid plaques, synaptic cleft (during neurotransmission)	Aggregation of the Aβ peptides to form oligomers and fibrils can be rapidly induced in the presence of zinc ions.
Cr^{3+}, 0.3, 0.4, 6.6	Carbohydrate metabolism and normal insulin sensitivity. Brain insulin signal transduction system.	Hippocampus (wet tissue), amygdala, cerebrospinal fluid	Reduction of the neuronal glucose and energy metabolism.
Cd^{2+}, 0.25–250, 50–500	It has not demonstrated a function of brain metabolism.	Parenchyma, cortical neurons	Increase of the blood-brain barrier permeability and oxidative damage.

Physiological functions, concentrations, brain areas of accumulation, and their relationship to AD.

Table 1. Principal metals involved in the development and progression of AD.

Copper: Copper in its divalent form (Cu^{2+}) is found in several enzymes involved in important biochemical pathways in neuronal and nonneuronal cells; these enzymes include SOD, cytochrome-C oxidase, ceruloplasmin, and tyrosinase. Following NMDA receptor activation, Cu^{2+} is released from neurons; the released Cu^{2+} regulates neuronal activation by limiting Ca^{2+} entry into cells [44]. Astrocytes express several Cu^{2+}-containing enzymes; however, excess Cu^{2+} in astrocytes results in damage due to the binding of Cu^{2+} to Aβ. This can catalyze the production of •OH in a Fenton-like reaction, favoring the establishment of oxidative stress and cell damage [45]. For these reasons, the increase in the distribution of brain Cu^{2+} that occurs in AD, producing concentrations ranging from 10 to 100 μM, could result in the establishment of oxidative stress in areas that are important for memory and learning such as the hippocampus and amygdala (**Table 1**).

The diet is the principal source of Cu^{2+}; in fact, studies by Sparks et al. show that the administration of trace amounts of this metal in drinking water may drive the accumulation of Aβ levels in the brain by altering the level of the interface between the blood and the cerebrovasculature in an AD rabbit model [46]. This suggests that dietary metals may promote Aβ accumulation [47].

Zinc: Under normal conditions, divalent zinc (Zn^{2+}) is concentrated in the neocortex; its concentration is closely regulated due to the potentially neurotoxic effects that occur under conditions of Zn^{2+} excess or deficiency. Zn^{2+} also has a neuromodulatory role in that it inhibits excitatory NMDA receptors, reaching concentrations of up to 300 μM [48, 49]. Religa et al. demonstrated that Zn^{2+} levels increase in parallel with tissue amyloid levels. Zn^{2+} levels were significantly elevated in the brains of the most severely demented patients with AD and in cases that displayed an amyloid burden. In fact, high concentrations of this metal ion (up to 1 mM) have also been found within amyloid plaques [50]. The formation of Aβ aggregates occurs rapidly in the presence of Zn^{2+} ions under physiological conditions *in vitro* [51]. Studies with synthetic Aβ show that chelation chemistry helps solubilize amyloid plaques and that it has a more marked effect on the extraction of Aβ than on the depletion of Cu^{2+} [52]. In addition, elevated Zn^{2+} levels have been found in AD postmortem neocortical samples (**Table 1**) [53].

Chromium: Trivalent chromium (Cr^{3+}) is essential for normal carbohydrate metabolism and normal insulin sensitivity. It has been reported that Cr^{3+} and Zn^{2+} are of importance to the brain's insulin signal transduction system. A Cr^{3+}-binding oligopeptide, which has been named chromodulin, has been reported. In the presence of insulin, chromodulin causes an eightfold stimulation of protein tyrosine kinase activity. Cr^{3+} ions increase insulin-stimulated tyrosine phosphorylation and thereby modulate cellular insulin signaling. Within the pathogenesis of AD, a reduction in neuronal glucose and energy metabolism is assumed. At the center of this lies the disruption of insulin-signaling mechanisms. The results of current biochemical studies indicate that Cr^{3+} and Zn^{2+} are important in the brain's insulin signal transduction system [54].

Cadmium: Divalent cadmium (Cd^{2+}) is a nonessential transition metal that is classified as a carcinogen due to its long biological half-life. Prolonged exposure to Cd^{2+} has toxic effects due to the accumulation of the metal in a variety of tissues, including the CNS. The principal effect of Cd^{2+} in the CNS is the induction of oxidative damage in cells. Increasing evidence has demonstrated that Cd^{2+} is a possible etiological factor for neurodegenerative diseases such as AD. Cerebral cortical neurons have been identified as targets of Cd^{2+}-mediated toxicity and Cd^{2+}-induced cell apoptosis [55].

3.2. Interaction of metals with amyloid beta and hydrogen peroxide production

Senile plaques are composed primarily of extraneuronal-aggregated Aβ, microglia, degenerated neurons, and relatively high amounts of redox-active metals such as Cu^{2+}, Fe^{2+}, and Zn^{2+}. Accurate determination of the redox potentials of Aβ and its metal complexes will certainly help unravel their roles in oxidative stress, metal homeostasis, detoxification, and Aβ aggregation/fibril formation. For these reasons, a number of techniques have been employed to determine the amino acids involved in the recognition of metals by Aβ. It is generally accepted that metal ions are bound to the histidine residues at positions 6, 13, and 14 [56]. Several studies have demonstrated that the interaction of Cu^{2+}, Zn^{2+}, Fe^{3+}, and Al^{3+} with Aβ is maintained by their coordination with His13-His14 of the peptide. The interaction is also maintained by a fourth element represented by a donor atom that can come from the aspartate at position 1 or the tyrosine at position 10, thus forming a tetragonal complex. In fact, marked inhibition of cortical amyloid accumulation by DP-109, a lipophilic metal chelator, has been shown [57].

An important aspect of the binding of Cu^{2+} to Aβ is that the complex retains its redox activity and is able to produce H_2O_2. As the principal ROS in living organisms, H_2O_2 acts as a second messenger in cellular signal transduction under physiological conditions. However, the overproduction of H_2O_2 results in the formation of high levels of $^{\bullet}OH$ and consequent oxidation of the peptide, which can be detected by the formation of carbonyl groups. It was demonstrated that this oxidation increases as the Cu^{2+}:peptide ratio increases and that it is accompanied by changes in the morphology of the aggregates as determined by AFM [58].

It has been shown that the coordination of Zn^{2+} with His13 of Aβ is critical to the metal ion-induced aggregation of Aβ [59]. NMR and circular dichroism (CD) studies of metal-Aβ complexes show that Zn^{2+} binding is dominated by intermolecular coordination and by the formation of polymeric species, including monomeric Zn^{2+}-Aβ and various Zn^{2+}-Aβ oligomeric complexes and aggregates. However, Zn^{2+}-Aβ complex formation is high only in brain areas containing synapses. There, the initial binding of Zn^{2+} to Aβ induces transformation of the peptide to an oligomeric or polymeric complex with increased Zn^{2+}-binding affinity, potentiating the effect of the metal on Aβ and possibly enabling Zn^{2+} to act as a seeding factor in amyloid plaque formation [60]. When aggregates are prepared with Cu^{2+} and Zn^{2+} ions, the ratio of Cu^{2+}:Zn^{2+} becomes an important factor in H_2O_2 generation, the formation of carbonyl groups in the peptide, and aggregate morphology. In fact, Aβ fibrils can hydrolyze H_2O_2 and generate damage by $^{\bullet}OH$ production [61].

Fe^{2+} is able to bind to Aβ, and increased amounts of redox-active iron that can generate an elevated amount of ROS have been found in the brains of AD patients; however, it is not clear how this redox-active Fe^{2+} is produced. It was postulated that Aβ may act by binding the Fe^{3+} and reducing it to pathological Fe^{2+} that is capable of inducing oxidative stress; this would suggest that Aβ possesses a strong reducing capacity for iron and that it acts as a metalloprotein capable of binding the metal ion. The interactions between iron and Aβ are governed by histidines 6, 13, and 14. These amino acid residues could coordinate a shared metal ion and generate a redox-active complex. An alternative explanation might be that an oxidative reaction that uses histidine as a substrate occurs in the presence of Aβ, thereby generating toxic oxygen species [62]. The contribution of each histidine residue to Aβ oligomerization and toxicity is different; it is thought that the His6 residue is important for beginning the Aβ dimerization process and that His13 and His14 are not. However, the latter residues could be important in producing the peptide conformations responsible for the Aβ-iron effects [63].

The reduction of metals (principally Cu^{2+}) by Aβ causes the oxidation of Met35, resulting in the production of H_2O_2 [64]. In addition, during the catalytic production of H_2O_2 by $A\beta_{1-42}$ and Cu^{2+}, the participation of Tyr10 is important because when this amino acid is substituted by alanine (Y10A) there is a significant decrease in the ability of Aβ to reduce Cu^{2+}. Here, it is important to note that the reduction of the metal and H_2O_2 production allow the formation of the $^{\bullet}OH$ radical by a Fenton-like reaction.

3.3. Fenton reaction

All the available evidence indicates that the Fenton reaction is important during Aβ aggregation and during metal dyshomeostasis in AD. This reaction was first described by H.J.H. Fenton as the strong oxidation effect of Fe^{2+}-H_2O_2 mixtures on organic compounds in a work entitled "Oxidation of tartaric acid in the presence of iron" [65]. Currently, the combination of Fe^{2+}-H_2O_2 is known as Fenton chemistry, the Fenton reaction, or Fenton reagent.

The Fenton reaction can be written as follows (4):

$$Fe^{2+} + H_2O_2 \rightarrow Fe^{3+} + HO^{\bullet} + HO^{-} \tag{4}$$

During AD, the Fenton reaction occurs due to the presence of excessive levels of active redox metals and the generation of H_2O_2 by the reaction of $A\beta_{1-42}$ with the metals. Subsequently, $^{\bullet}OH$ are formed by the interaction of $A\beta_{1-42}$ and Fe^{3+} or Cu^{2+}. Several years ago, a speculative mechanism was proposed by which Aβ interaction with metals could produce ROS. In that mechanism, the binding of the metal is followed by the binding of oxygen to the metal via a peroxo bridge and $O_2^{\bullet-}$ production; the $O_2^{\bullet-}$ are then converted to H_2O_2, which reacts with metals and produces $^{\bullet}OH$ [66].

Furthermore, it has been proposed that during the Fenton reaction an intermediate such as ferryl ion $[Fe(IV)=O]^{2+}$, a highly reactive oxidant that is able to undergo a reaction involving single-electron hydrogen abstraction and two-electron oxidation, is formed; however, this intermediate is not produced during $A\beta_{1-42}$ aggregation because it is formed during the reaction of Fe^{2+} complexes with H_2O_2 in the presence of organic substrates and a porphyrin complex. Therefore, $^{\bullet}OH$ are produced when aggregated $A\beta_{1-42}$ interacts with metals. However, several *in vitro* studies have shown that $^{\bullet}OH$ can be generated when Fe^{3+} is reduced in the presence of reducing agents such as ascorbic acid (5) or in the absence of redox agents in a reaction in which one electron from ^{-}OH (from the water self-ionization reaction) is transferred to Fe^{3+}, yielding Fe^{2+} and $^{\bullet}OH$ (6) [67]. This reaction also occurs in AD due to the presence of high levels of metals and the consequent production of $^{\bullet}OH$; this promotes $A\beta_{1-42}$ aggregation and consequently increases ROS production, creating a vicious cycle.

$$Fe^{3+} + Asc^{-} \rightarrow Fe^{2+} + Asc^{\bullet -} \quad (5)$$

$$Fe^{3+} + HO^{-} \rightarrow Fe^{2+} + HO^{\bullet} \quad (6)$$

The Fenton reaction can also occur in the presence of other metals via a Fenton reaction or a Fenton like-reaction, as shown below (7):

$$M^{n+} + H_2O_2 \rightarrow M^{(n+1)+} + HO^{\bullet} + HO^{-} \quad (7)$$

where M is the metal (such as copper, which can also be reduced by $A\beta_{1-42}$) that is oxidized in the reaction. When M = Fe^{2+}, the reaction above is known as Fenton reaction; when M = any other metal, the reaction is known as Fenton-like reaction.

In AD, it has been suggested that $^{\bullet}OH$ formation damages biomolecules such as lipids, proteins, and nucleic acids due to the ability of $^{\bullet}OH$ to catalyze reactions such as hydrogen abstraction, addition reactions, and oxidation reactions. Hydrogen abstraction is one of the most important mechanisms because in this reaction the $^{\bullet}OH$ damages lipids in the brain and, as was mentioned previously, the brain has a high content of lipids. Lipoperoxidation (LPO) is the process by which $^{\bullet}OH$ abstract hydrogen from unsaturated fatty acids, forming alkyl radicals. The principal products of LPO are aldehydes as malondialdehyde (MDA) and propanal, hexanal and 4-hydroxynonenal (4-HNE). LPO of oleic acid in the brain occurs by abstraction of the hydrogens in the ninth and tenth positions; secondary reactions include hydrogen abstraction by alkoxy radicals ($RO^{\bullet}$) and peroxyl radicals ($ROO^{\bullet}$) at the tertiary carbon atoms. Then, alkyl radicals ($R^{\bullet}$) and $ROO^{\bullet}$ are produced by ROS.

4. Damage produced by FRs during Alzheimer's disease

The brain is particularly vulnerable to oxidative stress because of its high metabolic rate, which utilizes 20% of the body's basal oxygen consumption. In addition, the brain has limited antioxidant defenses compared with other organs and high levels of transition metals, principally redox-active Cu^{2+} and Fe^{2+}; defective regulation of the levels of these metals can lead to reaction with O_2 and the production of ROS, resulting in cellular toxicity. Neurons are vulnerable to attack by FRs due to their lower glutathione content in comparison with other cells, their high proportion of polyunsaturated fatty acids susceptible to oxidation, and the fact that their metabolism requires substantial quantities of oxygen. The oxidation of biomolecules such as proteins, lipids, and DNA, and mitochondrial damage have consequences that are deleterious to neurons, including the loss of cell potential, the accumulation of excitotoxic glutamate, decreased glucose availability, decreased intracellular communication, and increased neurotoxicity [68].

http://dx.doi.org/10.5772/64708

A large number of biological sources are thought to play important roles in FR production in AD. As mentioned above, some transition metals are increased in AD brains and are present in a redox-active state [69]. Fe^{2+} catalyzes the formation of $^{\bullet}OH$ from H_2O_2 by the Fenton reaction in the brains of patients with AD due to the imbalance in metal concentrations, and together with the H_2O_2 produced by Aβ aggregation it is possible to generate $^{\bullet}OH$, which results in the oxidation of lipids, proteins, and DNA [70]. Recent histochemical studies have demonstrated that the detection of redox activity in AD lesions is inhibited by prior exposure of tissue sections to Fe^{2+}- and Cu^{2+}-selective chelators. The activity can be reinstated following reexposure of the chelator-treated sections to either copper or iron salts, suggesting that the redox imbalance in AD is dependent on these metals. It is probable that the accumulation of Fe^{2+} and Cu^{2+} is a major source of the production of reactive oxygen, which is in turn responsible not only for the numerous oxidative stress markers that appear on senile plaques but also for the more global oxidative stress parameters observed in AD [71].

Activated microglia, such as those that surround most senile plaques [72] are a source of the reactive nitrogen species (RNS) NO and the ROS $O_2^{\bullet-}$, which can react to form $ONOO^-$, leaving nitrotyrosine as an identifiable marker [73], as shown in **Figure 4**.

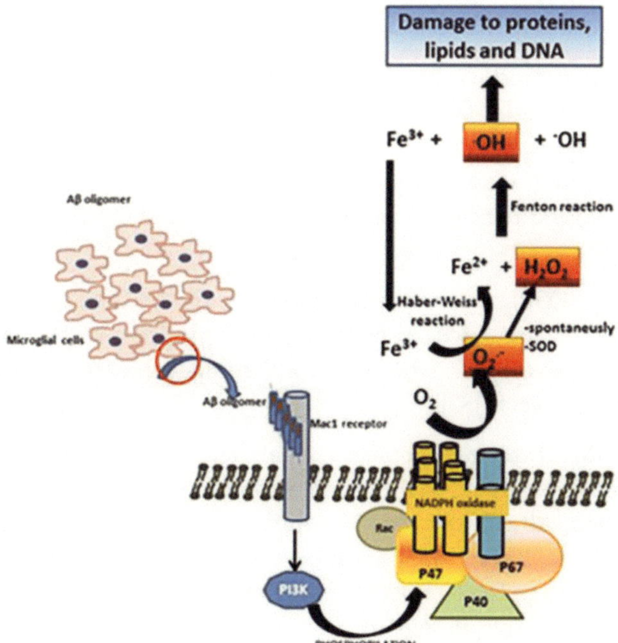

Figure 4. ROS and RNS produced after the activation of microglial cells by $A\beta_{1-42}$. ROS have effects on biomolecules such as lipids, proteins, and nucleic acids.

Several studies have reported that pro-inflammatory molecules and ROS secreted from fibrillar Aβ-stimulated microglia lead to neuronal apoptosis [74]. In addition, neurons, microglia, and astrocytes are capable of generating substantial amounts of NO through the iNOS [75]. Fibrillar

Aβ peptides stimulate iNOS and NO production through the NADPH-dependent oxidative deamination of L-arginine [76]. Microglial/neuronal coculture studies reveal that the NO released from Aβ-stimulated microglia causes neuronal cell death. In addition, iNOS has been reported to act synergistically to kill neurons through the formation of $ONOO^-$. This RNS is a potent oxidant with biological reactivity similar to that of •OH. $ONOO^-$ promotes the tyrosine nitration and nitrosylation of cysteines within cellular proteins. The addition of nitrite (NO_2^-) to tyrosine residues is extremely detrimental because it leads to protein and enzyme dysfunction and the eventual death of cultured neurons [77]. Taken together, these data suggest that Aβ-stimulated production of $ONOO^-$ plays an important role in the pathogenesis of oxidative damage in the AD brain.

The damage to lipids caused by FRs is evidenced by LPO, which has been demonstrated widely in all areas of the brain and shown to be higher in the hippocampus, the piriform cortex, the frontal lobe, and the occipital cortex [78]. Furthermore, LPO markers have been found in the cerebrospinal fluid (CSF) and urine of patients with AD, and their levels tend to increase with the progression of the disease [79]. Analysis of transgenic mice (Tg2576) that display oxidative damage similar to that found in the brains of AD patients revealed an elevation in oxidative stress markers preceding amyloid formation and increasing amyloid pathology [80]. Data from humans and transgenic mice indicate that elevated oxidative stress is an early event in AD pathogenesis.

Advanced glycation end products (AGEs) are involved in AD through several mechanisms. AGEs, which are produced by the interaction of carbohydrates and proteins, stimulate the production of ROS in the presence of transition metals by the establishment of redox cycling. In addition, both Aβ and AGEs activate receptors such as the receptor for advanced glycation end products (RAGEs) and the class A scavenger receptor and thereby increase ROS production [81].

Proteins damaged by ROS can be measured in plasma, serum, CSF, and brain tissue. Studies by Smith et al. have demonstrated an increase in the products of protein oxidation in the hippocampus of patients with AD, which showed neurodegenerative changes in comparison with normal and aged subjects [82].

The production of ROS through peptidyl radicals associated with Aβ contributes to Aβ aggregation; it was demonstrated that protein oxidation promotes the formation of protein aggregates. In addition, Aβ causes alterations in several transmembrane proteins present in neurons and glial cells, including ATPases, glutamate transporters, glucose transporters and guanosine triphosphate (GTP)-coupled transmembrane-signaling proteins, resulting in multiple changes in cellular physiology [83].

The type of damage found in macromolecules such as lipids, proteins, and carbohydrates in patients with AD has also been observed in DNA. Mecoccin et al. showed a 10-fold increase in the oxidation of mitochondria and nuclear DNA in brain samples from AD patients [84].

The formation of ROS by any of several possible mechanisms results in damage to neurons. The cholinergic system is the principal neurotransmission system that is affected by the production of oxidative stress. It was postulated that •OH may decrease the activity of AChE by modifying the amino acid residues, which form the anionic site that recognizes the natural substrate, ACh [85].

A large body of evidence implicates compromised antioxidant defense systems as a contributing factor in AD pathogenesis; however, studies of antioxidant enzymes in AD have not shown a consistent pattern. Glutathione (c-glutamyl-cysteinyl-glycine; GSH) is an abundant cellular antioxidant. Thiol-reduced GSH normally accounts for the majority (>98%) of total cellular glutathione, but it can also exist as oxidized glutathione disulfide (GSSG) or glutathione adducts. Glutathione peroxidase (GPx) catalyzes the oxidation of GSH to GSSG, whereas the reverse reaction is carried out by glutathione reductase (GR), which requires NADPH. Coupled to the oxidation of GSH, GPx can reduce H_2O_2, highlighting the importance of both GPx and GR in maintaining the cellular redox state. Indeed, the measurement of erythrocyte levels of GSH, expressed as the ratio of GSH/GSSG, provides a dynamic marker of oxidative stress *in vivo* [86, 87]. Lovell et al. found significantly elevated activity of GPx in the hippocampus, of GR in the hippocampus and amygdala, and of catalase (CAT) activity in the hippocampus and superior and middle temporal gyri in AD subjects compared with normal control subjects [88]. These changes were present in the medial temporal lobe structures where LPO was significantly increased, suggesting a compensatory rise in antioxidant activity in response to increased FR generation in these regions in AD. SOD levels were elevated in all brain regions in AD. CAT was elevated in the amygdala in AD in one study [88]. Marcus et al. demonstrated modifications in the activities of antioxidant enzymes in AD brains. The results showed a decrease in SOD activity in AD frontal and AD temporal cortex, whereas CAT activity decreased in AD temporal cortex. By contrast, these investigators found no differences in GPx activity. The results obtained in these studies show that alterations in the antioxidant enzymes in the brains of patients with AD are most significant in the temporal cortex [89]. For these reasons, the use of antioxidants represents a logical approach to the treatment of AD. This hypothesis is very attractive because most antioxidant compounds have a wide safety margin. The hypothesis has been evaluated under experimental and clinical conditions. Crapper McLachlan et al. [90] showed that the prolonged administration of an iron-chelating agent, desferrioxamine, slowed the development of the disease. Vitamin E, selegiline, and *Ginkgo biloba* extract were evaluated in clinical studies of AD and produced beneficial results [91]. These findings provide important evidence supporting the hypothesis that antioxidants may be capable of slowing the pathogenic process of AD. In addition, a decrease in the incidence of AD in patients treated chronically with non-steroidal anti-inflammatory drugs (NSAIDs) has been demonstrated; this could slow the progress of the disease by decreasing the production of prostaglandins [92].

5. Determination of free radicals in *in vivo* and *in vitro* models of Alzheimer's disease

As previously mentioned, the production of high levels of ROS is related to the establishment and progression of AD. Among these ROS are $O_2^{\bullet-}$, H_2O_2, $^{\bullet}OH$, NO, and $ONOO^-$, which can be produced by several mechanisms (direct ROS production by $A\beta_{1-42}$ oligomers, interaction of Aβ with metals, microglial activation, etc.). For these reasons, a variety of techniques have been employed to determine the species and amounts of ROS in biological samples of patients with AD and in samples from animal models.

5.1. Electronic paramagnetic resonance

Among ROS, $O_2^{\bullet-}$ and $^{\bullet}OH$ are molecules with unpaired electrons that react rapidly with various biomolecules. To quantify these molecules by electron paramagnetic resonance (EPR), it is necessary to employ compounds that increase the half-lives of the unpaired electrons. The most common compounds employed for this purpose are 5,5-dimethyl-1-pyrroline *N*-oxide (DMPO), N-tertiary-butyl-nitrone (PBN), and 2,2,6,6-tetramethyl-1-piperidinyloxy (TEMPO), all of which react with the unpaired electron of a specific FR and form a complex that is sufficiently stable to be detected by EPR. This technique allows the quantification of FRs in a wide variety of samples obtained in *in vivo* and *in vitro* studies. The nitroxide MCP (3-methoxidecarnonyl-2,2,5,5,-tetramethylpyrrolidine-1-yloxy), which permeates the blood-brain barrier, has been used as a spin probe to noninvasively evaluate redox status in the brains of AD transgenic model mice (APdE9), allowing the measurement of the generation of FRs during the development of the disease [93]. In addition, with the use of DMPO an increase in the production of $^{\bullet}OH$ radicals in activated microglial cells in *in vitro* studies was demonstrated [94].

Although the EPR technique is of great help in identifying and quantifying FRs, its use is limited due to the fact that it requires an EPR spectrometer, which is expensive. If an EPR is not available, other techniques can be used to determine the amount of ROS produced; however, one disadvantage of these techniques is that they require samples from animals that must therefore be sacrificed.

5.2. Superoxide anion determinations

There are several techniques that permit the quantification of $O_2^{\bullet-}$ in biological samples; these include cytochrome C, WST-1 [2-(4-iodophenyl)-3-(4-nitrophenyl-5-(2,4-disulfophenyl)-2H-tetrazolium monosodium salt], lucigenin, luminol, and others. Several of these techniques are described below.

Cytochrome C. This technique has been used to quantify extracellular $O_2^{\bullet-}$ in cultures of microglial cells obtained from neonatal rats stimulated with lipopolysaccharide (LPS). The principle of the method is based on the reducing properties of $O_2^{\bullet-}$. $O_2^{\bullet-}$ donates an electron to ferricytochrome C, reducing ferrocytochrome C and increasing its absorbance at 550 nm. This method presents some limitations if the sample contains high amounts of $O_2^{\bullet-}$ because the cytochrome can be reduced by various molecules such as ascorbate, glutathione, and several reductases that are able to produce ferrocytochrome C [95].

Tetrazolium salt (WST-1). The reduction of WST-1 to a water-soluble yellow formazan by $O_2^{\bullet-}$ can be measured by spectrophotometry (**Figure 5A**). This method has been compared with the ferricytochrome C reduction method in which xanthine/xanthine oxidases are used to generate $O_2^{\bullet-}$; it was demonstrated that WST-1 generated an approximately twofold greater increase in absorbance than ferricytochrome C at their respective wavelengths [96].

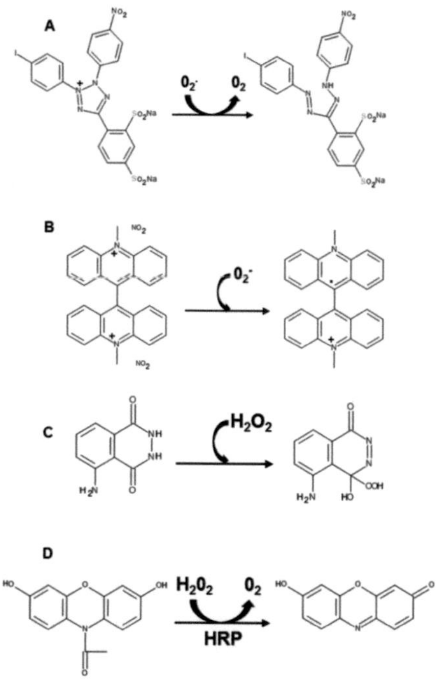

Figure 5. Reactions for the determination of $O_2^{\bullet-}$ and H_2O_2. (A) Reduction of WST-1 by $O_2^{\bullet-}$ to a water-soluble yellow formazan. (B) Reduction of lucigenin by $O_2^{\bullet-}$ to a lucigenin cation radical. (C) Oxidation of luminol by H_2O_2. (D) Oxidation of Amplex red by H_2O_2 in the presence of HRP to produce resorufin.

Lucigenin and luminol. These substances are selectively employed to determine the amounts of extracellular $O_2^{\bullet-}$ and intracellular $O_2^{\bullet-}$ and H_2O_2 by chemiluminescence. Lucigenin is selective for $O_2^{\bullet-}$, and luminol is selective for $O_2^{\bullet-}$ and H_2O_2. Lucigenin is reduced by $O_2^{\bullet-}$ to a lucigenin cation radical independently of peroxidase activity (**Figure 5B**), and luminol is oxidized using a peroxidase such as myeloperoxidase (MPO) or horseradish peroxidase (HRP) (**Figure 5C**).

5.3. Hydrogen peroxide determination

To determine the amount of H_2O_2, electrodes can be used, and the amount of H_2O_2 can then be determined polarigraphically. The sensitivity of the electrode allows precise and rapid measurement of extracellular H_2O_2. Other probes include the use of targets and are based on the ability of H_2O_2 to oxidize molecules such as Amplex red (N-acetyl-3,7-dihydroxyphenoxazine), scopoletin, and homovanillic acid in the presence of HRP. There are also many other techniques that allow the determination of the amount of H_2O_2, such as aryl-borate-based probes, peroxy Lucifer, and others; however, Amplex red is one of the most used. Amplex red is a non-fluorescent compound that is oxidized by H_2O_2 in the presence of HRP to produce resorufin, which is colored and highly fluorescent at 587 nm (**Figure 5D**). Amplex red has been used to measure H_2O_2 production by microglial cells and also directly *in vitro* to measure H_2O_2 production by Aβ during its interaction with metals such as copper [97].

6. Conclusion

It has been demonstrated that $A\beta_{1-42}$ is one of the principal biomolecules that contributes to the development and progression of AD due to its ability to generate ROS by its interaction with metals and also due to its ability to activate specific cells, producing neuroinflammation and consequently neurodegeneration. Therefore, therapeutic treatments to avoid Aβ production should be developed by the design of selective inhibitors of the β-secretase BACE-1.

Acknowledgements

This research was financially supported by COFAA-SIP/IPN [Project: 20161374; 20161383; 20161399], and CONACYT [Project: CB254600, I010/0532/2014]; [Project: PDCPN782].

Author details

Martha C. Rosales Hernández[1*], Maricarmen Hernández Rodríguez[1], Jessica E. Mendieta Wejebe[1] and José Correa Basurto[2]

*Address all correspondence to: marcrh2002@yahoo.com.mx

1 Laboratorio de Biofísica y Biocatálisis, Escuela Superior de Medicina, Instituto Politécnico Nacional Distrito Federal, México

2 Laboratorio de Modelado Molecular y Diseño de Fármacos, Escuela Superior de Medicina, Instituto Politécnico Nacional Distrito Federal, México

References

[1] Méndez-Garrido A, Hernández-Rodríguez M, Zamorano-Ulloa R, Correa-Basurto J, Mendieta-Wejebe JE, Ramírez-Rosales D, Rosales-Hernández MC. In vitro effect of H_2O_2, some transition metals and hydroxyl radical produced via Fenton and Fenton-like reactions, on the catalytic activity of AChE and the hydrolysis of ACh. Neurochemical Research. 2014;39:2093–2104. DOI: 10.1007/s11064-014-1400-5.

[2] Tariot PN, Federoff HJ. Current treatment for Alzheimer disease and future prospects. Alzheimer's Disease and Associated Disorders. 2003;17:S105–S113. DOI: 10.1097/00002093-200307004-00005.

[3] Dröge W. Free radicals in the physiological control of cell function. Physiological Reviews. 2002;82:47–95. DOI: 10.1152/physrev.00018.2001.

[4] Perry G, Cash ADD, Smith MA. Alzheimer disease and oxidative stress. Journal of Biomedicine and Biotechnology. 2002;2:120–123. DOI: 10.1155/S1110724302203010.

[5] Murphy MP, LeVine H. Alzheimer´s disease and the b-amyloid peptide. Journal of Alzheimer's Disease. 2010;19:311–323. DOI: 10.3233/JAD-2010-1221.

[6] Selkoe DJ. The molecular pathology of Alzheimer's disease. Neuron. 1991;6:487–498. DOI: http://dx.doi.org/10.1016/0896-6273(91)90052-2.

[7] Bayer TA, Cappai R, Masters CL, Beyreuther K, Multhaup G. It all sticks together—the APP-related family of proteins and Alzheimer's disease. Molecular Psychiatry. 1999;4:524–528. DOI: 10.1038/sj.mp.4000552.

[8] Young-Pearse TL, Bai J, Chang R, Zheng JB, LoTurco JJ, Selkoe DJ. A critical function for beta-amyloid precursor protein in neuronal migration revealed by in utero RNA interference. The Journal of Neuroscience. 2007;27:14459–14469. DOI: 10.1523/JNEUROSCI.4701-07.2007.

[9] Sun X, Chen WD, Wang YD. β-Amyloid: the key peptide in the pathogenesis of Alzheimer's disease. Frontiers in Pharmacology. 2015;6:221(1–9). DOI: 10.3389/fphar.2015.00221.

[10] Rajasekhar K, Chakrabarti M, Govindaraju T. Function and toxicity of amyloid beta and recent therapeutic interventions targeting amyloid beta in Alzheimer's disease. Chemical Communications (Cambridge, England). 2015;51:13434–13450. DOI: 10.1039/C5CC05264E.

[11] Kar S. Role of amyloid β peptides in the regulation of central cholinergic function and its relevance to Alzheimer's disease pathology. Drug Development Research. 2002;56:248–263. DOI: 10.1002/ddr.10080.

[12] Martorana A, Di Lorenzo F, Belli L, Sancesario G, Toniolo S, Sallustio F, Sancesario GM, Koch G. Cerebrospinal fluid Aβ42 levels: when physiological become pathological state. CNS Neuroscience and Therapeutics. 2015;21:921–925. DOI: 10.1111/cns.12476.

[13] Barz B, Urbanc B. Dimer formation enhances structural differences between amyloid β-protein (1–40) and (1–42): an explicit-solvent molecular dynamics study. PLoS One. 2012;7:e34345(1–17). DOI: 10.1371/journal.pone.0034345.

[14] Kahler A, Sticht H, Horn AH. Conformational stability of fibrillar amyloid-beta oligomers via protofilament pair formation—a systematic computational study. PLoS One. 2013;8:e70521(1–12). DOI: 10.1371/journal.pone.0070521.

[15] Tiwari MK, Kepp KP. Modeling the aggregation propensity and toxicity of amyloid-β variants. Journal of Alzheimer's Disease. 2015;47:215–229. DOI: 10.3233/JAD-150046.

[16] Fu Z, Aucoin D, Davis J, Van Nostrand WE, Smith SO. Mechanism of nucleated conformational conversion of Aβ42. Biochemistry. 2015;54:4197–4207. DOI: 10.1021/acs.biochem.5b00467.

[17] Schmidt M, Rohou A, Lasker K, Yadav JK, Schiene-Fischer C, Fändrich M, Grigorieff N. Peptide dimer structure in an Aβ(1–42) fibril visualized with cryo-EM. Proceedings of the National Academy of Sciences of the United States of America. 2015;112:11858–11863. DOI: 10.1073/pnas.1503455112.

[18] Sciarretta KL, Gordon DJ, Petkova AT, Tycko R, Meredith SC. Abeta40-Lactam (D23/K28) models a conformation highly favorable for nucleation of amyloid. Biochemistry. 2005;44:6003–6014. DOI: 10.1021/bi0474867.

[19] Yi X, Zhang Y, Gong M, Yu X, Darabedian N, Zheng J, Zhou F. Ca^{2+} interacts with Glu-22 of Aβ(1–42) and phospholipid bilayers to accelerate the Aβ(1–42) aggregation below the critical micelle concentration. Biochemistry. 2015;54:6323–6332. DOI: 10.1021/acs.biochem.5b00719

[20] Carballo-Pacheco M, Ismail AE, Strodel B. Oligomer formation of toxic and functional amyloid peptides studied with atomistic simulations. The Journal of Physical Chemistry B. 2015;119:9696–9705. DOI: 10.1021/acs.jpcb.5b04822.

[21] Viola KL, Klein WL. Amyloid β oligomers in Alzheimer's disease pathogenesis, treatment, and diagnosis. Acta Neuropathologica. 2015;129:183–206. DOI: 10.1007/s00401-015-1386-3.

[22] Zhang W, Hao J, Liu R, Zhang Z, Lei G, Su C, Miao J, Li Z. Soluble Aβ levels correlate with cognitive deficits in the 12-month-old APPswe/PS1dE9 mouse model of Alzheimer's disease. Behavioural Brain Research. 2011;222:342–350. DOI: 10.1016/j.bbr.2011.03.072.

[23] Du XT, Wang L, Wang YJ, Andreasen M, Zhan DW, Feng Y, Li M, Zhao M, Otzen D, Xue D, Yang Y, Liu RT. Aβ1–16 can aggregate and induce the production of reactive oxygen species, nitric oxide, and inflammatory cytokines. The Journal of Alzheimer's Disease. 2011;27:401–413. DOI: 10.3233/JAD-2011-110476.

[24] Matt SM, Johnson RW. Neuro-immune dysfunction during brain aging: new insights in microglial cell regulation. Current Opinion in Pharmacology. 2015;26:96–101. DOI: 10.1016/j.coph.2015.10.009.

[25] Jha MK, Lee WH, Suk K. Functional polarization of neuroglia: implications in neuroinflammation and neurological disorders. Biochemical Pharmacology. 2015; pii:S0006–2952(15)00712-1. DOI: 10.1016/j.bcp.2015.11.003.

[26] Minter MR, Taylor JM, Crack PJ. The contribution of neuro-inflammation to amyloid toxicity in Alzheimer's disease. Journal of Neurochemistry. 2015:1–18 DOI: 10.1111/jnc. 13411.

[27] Block ML, Zecca L, Hong JS. Microglia-mediated neurotoxicity: uncovering the molecular mechanisms. Nature Reviews Neuroscience. 2007;8:57–69. DOI: 10.1038/ nrn2038.

[28] Alokam R, Singhal S, Srivathsav GS, Garigipati S, Puppala S, Sriram D, Perumal Y. Design of dual inhibitors of ROCK-I and NOX2 as potential leads for the treatment of neuroinflammation associated with various neurological diseases including autism spectrum disorder. Molecular Biosystems. 2015;11:607–17. DOI: 10.1039/C4MB00570H.

[29] Park L, Anrather J, Zhou P, Frys K, Pitstick R, Younkin S, Carlson GA, Iadecola C. NADPH-oxidase-derived reactive oxygen species mediate the cerebrovascular dysfunction induced by the amyloid beta peptide. The Journal of Neuroscience. 2005;25:1769–1777. DOI: 10.1523/JNEUROSCI.5207-04.2005.

[30] Chen SH, Oyarzabal EA, Hong JS. Critical role of the Mac1/NOX2 pathway in mediating reactive microgliosis-generated chronic neuroinflammation and progressive neurodegeneration. Current Opinion in Pharmacology. 2016;26:54–60 DOI: 10.1016/j.coph. 2015.10.001.

[31] Qian L, Gao X, Pei Z, Wu X, Block M, Wilson B, Hong JS, Flood PM. NADPH oxidase inhibitor DPI is neuroprotective at femtomolar concentrations through inhibition of microglia over-activation. Parkinsonism and Related Disorders. 2007;13:S316–320. DOI: 10.1016/S1353-8020(08)70023-3.

[32] Bianca VD, Dusi S, Bianchini E, Dal Pra I, Rossi F. Beta-amyloid activates the O-2 forming NADPH oxidase in microglia, monocytes, and neutrophils. A possible inflammatory mechanism of neuronal damage in Alzheimer's disease. The Journal of Biological Chemistry. 1999;274:15493–15499. DOI: 10.1074/jbc.274.22.15493.

[33] Groemping Y, Lapouge K, Smerdon SJ, Rittinger K. Molecular basis of phosphorylation-induced activation of the NADPH oxidase. Cell. 2003;113:343–355. DOI: 10.1016/ S0092-8674(03)00314-3.

[34] Meda L, Baron P, Prat E, Scarpini E, Scarlato G, Cassatella MA, Rossi F. Proinflammatory profile of cytokine production by human monocytes and murine microglia stimulated with beta-amyloid[25–35]. Journal of Neuroimmunology. 1999;93:45–52. DOI: 10.1016/ S0165-5728(98)00188-X.

[35] Kummer MP, Hermes M, Delekarte A, Hammerschmidt T, Kumar S, Terwel D, Walter J, Pape HC, König S, Roeber S, Jessen F, Klockgether T, Korte M, Heneka MT. Nitration of tyrosine 10 critically enhances amyloid β aggregation and plaque formation. Neuron. 2011;71:833–844. DOI: 10.1016/j.neuron.2011.07.001.

[36] Bogdanova AY, Nikinmaa M. Reactive oxygen species regulate oxygen-sensitive potassium flux in rainbow trout erythrocytes. The Journal of General Physiology. 2001;117:181–190. DOI: 10.1085/jgp.117.2.181.

[37] Zheng W, Monnot AD. Regulation of brain iron and copper homeostasis by brain barrier systems: implication in neurodegenerative diseases. Pharmacology and Therapeutics. 2012;133:177–188. DOI: 10.1016/j.pharmthera.2011.10.006.

[38] Popescu BF, Nichol H. Mapping brain metals to evaluate therapies for neurodegenerative disease. CNS Neuroscience and Therapeutics. 2011;17:256–268. DOI: 10.1111/j.1755-5949.2010.00149.x.

[39] Akatsu H, Hori A, Yamamoto T, Yoshida M, Mimuro M, Hashizume Y, Tooyama I, Yezdimer EM. Transition metal abnormalities in progressive dementias. Biometals. 2012;25:337–350. DOI: 10.1007/s10534-011-9504-8.

[40] Hureau Ch. Coordination of redox active metal ions to the amyloid precursor protein and to amyloid-beta peptides involved in Alzheimer disease. Part 1: an overview. Coordination Chemistry Reviews. 2012;256:2164–2174. DOI: 10.1016/j.ccr.2012.03.037.

[41] Panayi AE, Spyrou NM, Iversen BS, White MA, Part P. Determination of cadmium and zinc in Alzheimer's brain tissue using inductively coupled plasma mass spectrometry. Journal of the Neurological Sciences. 2002;195:1–10. DOI: 10.1016/S0022-510X(01)00672-4.

[42] Muñoz P, Humeres A. Iron deficiency on neuronal function. Biometals. 2012;25:825–835. DOI: 10.1007/S10534-012-9550-X.

[43] Connor JR, Snyder BS, Arosio P, Loeffler DA, LeWitt P. A quantitative analysis of isoferritins in select regions of aged, Parkinsonian, and Alzheimer's diseased brains. Journal of Neurochemistry. 1995;65:717–724. DOI: 10.1046/j.1471-4159.1995.65020717.x.

[44] Scheiber IF, Dringen R. Astrocyte functions in the copper homeostasis of the brain. Neurochemistry International. 2013;62:556–565.

[45] Baum L, Chan IH, Cheung SK, Goggins WB, Mok V, Lam L, Leung V, Hui E, Ng C, Woo J, Chiu HF, Zee BC, Cheng W, Chan MH, Szeto S, Lui V, Tsoh J, Bush AI, Lam CW, Kwok T. Serum zinc is decreased in Alzheimer's disease and serum arsenic correlates positively with cognitive ability. Biometals 2010;23:173–179. DOI: 10.1007/s10534-009-9277-5.

[46] Dringen R, Scheiber IF, Mercer JF. Copper metabolism of astrocytes. Frontiers in Aging Neuroscience. 2013;5:9(1–4). DOI: 10.3389/fnagi.2013.00009.

[47] Atwood CS, Scarpa RC, Huang X, Moir Robert D, Jones WD, Fairlie DP, Tanzi RE, Bush AI. Characterization of copper interactions with Alzheimer amyloid-β peptides: identification of an attomolar-affinity copper binding site on amyloid β1–42. Journal of Neurochemistry. 2000;75:1219–1233. DOI: 10.1046/j.1471-4159.2000.0751219.x.

[48] Smart TG, Hosie AM, Miller PS. Zn^{2+} ions: modulators of excitatory and inhibitory synaptic activity. Neuroscientist. 2004;10:432–442. DOI: 10.1177/1073858404263463.

[49] Howell GA, Welch MG, Frederickson CJ. Stimulation-induced uptake and release of zinc in hippocampal slices. Nature. 1984;308:736–738. DOI: 10.1038/308736a0.

[50] Friedlich AL, Lee JY, van Groen T, et al. Neuronal zinc exchange with the blood vessel wall promotes cerebral amyloid angiopathy in an animal model of Alzheimer's disease. The Journal of Neuroscience. 2004;24:3453–3459. DOI: 10.1523/JNEUROSCI. 0297-04.2004.

[51] Lovell MA, Robertson JD, Teesdale WJ, Campbell JL, Markesbery WR. Copper, iron and zinc in Alzheimer's disease senile plaques. Journal of the Neurological Sciences. 1998;158:47–52. DOI:10.1016/S0022-510X(98)00092-6.

[52] Bush AI, Pettingell WH, Multhaup G, Tanzi R. Rapid induction of Alzheimer Aβ amyloid formation by zinc. Science. 1994;265:1464–1467. DOI: 10.1126/science. 8073293.

[53] Cherny RA, Legg JT, McLean CA. Aqueous dissolution of Alzheimer's disease Aβ amyloid deposits by biometal depletion. The Journal of Biological Chemistry. 1999; 274:23223–23228. DOI: 10.1074/jbc.274.33.23223.

[54] Wada, Wu GY, Yamamoto A. Purification and chromium binding substances from dog liver. Environmental Research. 2000;33:503–510. DOI: 10.1016/0013-9351(83)90210-4.

[55] Wang Y, Fang J, Leonard SS, Rao KM. Cadmium inhibits the electron transfer chain and induces reactive oxygen species. Free Radical Biology and Medicine. 2004;36:1434–1443. DOI: 10.1016/j.freeradbiomed.2004.03.010.

[56] Kong X, Zhao Z, Lei X, Zhang B, Dai D, Jiang L. Interaction of metal ions with the His13-His14 sequence relevant to Alzheimer's disease. The Journal of Physical Chemistry A. 2015;119:3528–3534. DOI: 10.1021/acs.jpca.5b01443.

[57] Lee JY, Friedman JE, Angel I, Kozak A, Koh JY. The lipophilic metal chelator DP-109 reduces amyloid pathology in brains of human beta-amyloid precursor protein transgenic mice. Neurobiology of Aging. 2004;25:1315–1321. DOI:10.1016/j.neurobiolaging.2004.01.005.

[58] Berti V, Murray J, Davies M, Spector N, Tsui WH, Li Y, Williams S, Pirraglia E, Vallabhajosula S, Mchugh P, Pupi A, De Leon MJ, Mosconi L. Nutrient patterns and brain biomarkers of Alzheimer's disease in cognitively normal individuals. The Journal of Nutrition Health and Aging. 2015;19:413–423. DOI: 10.1007/s12603-014-0534-0.

[59] Mayes J, Tinker-Mill C, Kolosov O, Zhang H, Tabner BJ, Allsop D. β-Amyloid fibrils in Alzheimer disease are not inert when bound to copper ions but can degrade hydrogen peroxide and generate reactive oxygen species. The Journal of Biological Chemistry. 2014;289:12052–12062. DOI: 10.1074/jbc.M113.525212.

[60] Liu ST, Howlett G, Barrow CJ. Histidine-13 is a crucial residue in the zinc ion-induced aggregation of the A beta peptide of Alzheimer's disease. Biochemistry. 1999;38:9373–9378. DOI: 10.1021/bi990205o.

[61] Ott S, Dziadulewicz N, Crowther DC. Iron is a specific cofactor for distinct oxidation- and aggregation-dependent Aβ toxicity mechanisms in a Drosophila model. Disease Models and Mechanism. 2015;8:657–667. DOI: 10.1242/dmm.019042.

[62] Kozin SA, Kulikova AA, Istrate AN, Tsvetkov PO, Zhokhov SS, Mezentsev YV, Kechko OI, Ivanov AS, Polshakov VI, Makarov AA. The English (H6R) familial Alzheimer's disease mutation facilitates zinc-induced dimerization of the amyloid-β metal-binding domain. Metallomics. 2015;7:422–425. DOI: 10.1039/c4mt00259h.

[63] Frederickson CJ, Koh JY, Bush AI. The neurobiology of zinc in health and disease. Nature Reviews Neuroscience. 2015;6:449–4462. DOI: 10.1038/nrn1671.

[64] Barnham KJ, Haeffner F, Ciccotosto GD, Curtain CC, Tew D, Mavros C, Beyreuther K, Carrington D, Masters CL, Cherny RA, Cappai R, Bush AI. Tyrosine gated electron transfer is key to the toxic mechanism of Alzheimer's disease beta-amyloid. The FASEB Journal. 2004;18:1427. DOI: 10.1096/fj.04-1890fje.

[65] Dunford HB. Oxidations of iron(II)/(III) by hydrogen peroxide: from aquo to enzyme. Coordination Chemistry Reviews. 2002;233–234:311–318. DOI: 10.1016/S0010-8545(02)00024-3.

[66] Tabner BJ, Turnbull S, El-Agnaf OM, Allsop D. Formation of hydrogen peroxide and hydroxyl radicals from A(beta) and alpha-synuclein as a possible mechanism of cell death in Alzheimer's disease and Parkinson's disease. Free Radical Biology & Medicine. 2002;32:1076–1083. DOI: 10.1016/S0891-5849(02)00801-8.

[67] Prousek J. Fenton chemistry in biology and medicine. Pure Applied Chemistry. 2007;79:2325–2338. DOI: 10.1351/pac200779122325.

[68] Varadarajan S, Yatin S, Aksenova M, Butterfield DA. Review: Alzheimer's amyloid β-peptide-associated free radical oxidative stress and neurotoxicity. Journal of Structural Biology. 2000;130:184–208. DOI: 10.1006/jsbi.2000.4274.

[69] Good PF, Perl DP, Bierer LM, Schmeidler J. Selective accumulation of aluminum and iron in the neurofibrillary tangles of Alzheimer's disease: a laser microprobe (LAMMA) study. Annals of Neurology. 1992;31:286–292. DOI: 10.1002/ana.410310310.

[70] Tabner BJ, Turnbull S, King JE, Benson FE, El-Agnaf OMA, Allsop D. A spectroscopic study of some of the peptidyl radicals formed following hydroxyl radical attack on beta-amyloid and alpha-synuclein. Free Radical Research. 2006;40:731–739. DOI: 10.1080/10715760600632545.

[71] Sayre LM, Perry G, Harris PL, Liu Y, Schubert KA, Smith MA. In situ oxidative catalysis by neurofibrillary tangles and senile plaques in Alzheimer's disease: a central role for

bound transition metals. Journal of Neurochemistry. 2000;74:270–279. DOI: 10.1046/j.1471-4159.2000.0740270.x.

[72] Cras P, Kawai M, Siedlak S, Mulvihill P, Gambetti P, Lowery D, Gonzalez-DeWhitt P, Greenberg B, Perry G. Neuronal and microglial involvement in β-amyloid protein deposition in Alzheimer's disease. American Journal of Pathology. 1990:137:241–246.

[73] Smith MA, Harris PLR, Sayre LM, Beckman JS, Perry G. Widespread peroxynitrite mediated damage in Alzheimer's disease. The Journal of Neuroscience. 1997;17:2653–2657.

[74] Combs CK, Karlo JC, Kao SC, Landreth GE. Beta-amyloid stimulation of microglia and monocytes results in TNF alpha dependent expression of inducible nitric oxide synthase and neuronal apoptosis. The Journal of Neuroscience. 2001;21:1179–1188.

[75] Heneka MT, Feinstein DL, Galea E, Gleichmann M, Wullner U, Klockgether T. Peroxisome proliferator-activated receptor gamma agonists protect cerebellar granule cells from cytokine induced apoptotic cell death by inhibition of inducible nitric oxide synthase. Journal of Neuroimmunology. 1999;100:156–168. DOI: 10.1016/S0165-5728(99)00192-7.

[76] Ishii K, Muelhauser F, Liebl U, Picard M, Kuhl S, Penke B, Bayer T, Wiessler M, Hennerici M, Beyreuther K, Hartmann T, Fassbender K. Subacute NO generation induced by Alzheimer's beta-amyloid in the living brain: reversal by inhibition of the inducible NO synthase. The FASEB Journal. 2000;14:1485–1489. DOI: 10.1096/fj.99-0786com

[77] Boje KM. Nitric oxide neurotoxicity in neurodegenerative diseases. Frontiers in Bioscience. 2004;9:763–776. DOI: 10.2741/1268.

[78] Connor JR, Tucker P, Johnson M, Snyder B. Ceruloplasmin levels in the human superior temporal gyrus in aging and Alzheimer's disease. Neuroscience Letters. 1993;159:88–90.

[79] Tuppo EE, Forman LJ, Spur BW, Chan-Ting RE, Chopra A, Cavalieri TA. Sign of lipid peroxidation as measured in the urine of patients with probable Alzheimer's disease. Brain Research Bulletin. 2001;54:565–568. DOI: 10.1016/S0361-9230(01)00450-6.

[80] Smith MA, Hirai K, Hsiao K, Pappolla MA, Harris PL, Siedlak SL, Tabaton M, Perry G. Amyloid-beta deposition in Alzheimer transgenic mice is associated with oxidative stress. Journal of Neurochemistry. 1998;70:2212–2215. DOI: 10.1046/j.1471-4159.1998.70052212.x.

[81] El Khoury J, Hickman SE, Thomas CA, Cao L, Silverstein SC, Loike JD. Scavenger receptor mediated adhesion of microglia to beta amyloid fibrils. Nature. 1996;382:716–719. DOI: 10.1007/s12640-015-9527-y.

[82] Smith CD, Carney JM, Starke-Reed PE, Oliver CN Stadtman ER, Floyd RA, Markesbery WR. Excess brain protein oxidation and enzyme dysfunction in normal aging and

Alzheimer disease. Proceedings of the National Academy of Sciences of the United States of America. 1991;88:10540–10543. DOI: 10.1073/pnas.88.23.10540.

[83] Lauderback CM, Hackett JM, Huang FF, Keller JN, Szweda LI, Markesbery WR, Butterfield DA. The glial glutamate transporter, GLT-1, is oxidatively modified by 4-hydroxy-2-nonenal in the Alzheimer's disease brain: the role of Aβ1–42. Journal of Neurochemistry. 2001;78: 413–416. DOI: 10.3233/JAD-141899.

[84] Mecocci P, MacGarvey U, Kaufman AE, Koontz D, Shoffner JM, Wallace DC, Beal MF. Oxidative damage to mitochondrial DNA shows marked age-dependent increases in human brain. Annals of Neurology. 1993;34:609–616. DOI: 10.1002/ana.410340416.

[85] Gibbons NC, Wood JM, Rokos H, Schallreuter KU. Computer simulation of native epidermal enzyme structures in the presence and absence of hydrogen peroxide (H_2O_2): potential and pitfalls. Journal of Investigative Dermatology. 2006;126:2576–2582. DOI: 10.1038/sj.jid.5700612.

[86] Ballatori N, Krance SM, Notenboom S, Shi S, Tieu K, Hammond CL. Glutathione dysregulation and the etiology and progression of human diseases. Biological Chemistry. 2009;390:191–214. DOI: 10.1515/BC.2009.033.

[87] Sohal RS, Arnold L, Orr WC. Effect of age on superoxide dismutase, catalase, glutathione reductase, inorganic peroxides, TBA-reactive material, GSH/GSSG, NADPH/NADP+ and NADH/NAD+ in *Drosophila melanogaster*. Mechanisms of Ageing and Development. 1990;56:223–235. DOI: 10.1016/0047-6374(90)90084-S.

[88] Lovell MA, Ehmann WD, Butler SM, Markesbery WR. Elevated thiobarbituric acid-reactive substances and antioxidant enzyme activity in the brain in Alzheimer's disease. Neurology. 1995;45:1594–1601. DOI: 10.1212/WNL.45.8.1594.

[89] Marcus DL, Thomas C, Rodriguez C, Simberkoff K, Tsai JS, Strafaci JA, Freedman ML. Increased peroxidation and reduced antioxidant enzyme activity in Alzheimer's Disease. Experimental Neurology. 1998;150:40–44. DOI: 10.1006/exnr.1997.6750.

[90] Crapper McLachlan DR, Dalton AJ, Kruck TPA, Andrews DF. Intramuscular desferrioxamine in patients with Alzheimer's disease. Lancet. 1991;337:1304–1308. DOI: 10.1016/0140-6736(91)92978-B.

[91] Sano M, Ernesto C, Thomas RG, et al. A controlled trial of selegiline, alpha-tocopherol, or both as treatment for Alzheimer's disease. The New England Journal of Medicine. 1997;336:1216–1222. DOI: 10.1056/NEJM199704243361704.

[92] Breitner JCS, Welsh KA, Helms MJ, et al. Delayed onset of Alzheimer's disease with nonsteroidal anti-inflammatory and histamine H2 blocking drugs. Neurobiology of Aging. 1995;16:523–530. DOI: 10.1016/0197-4580(95)00049-K

[93] Matsumura A, Emoto MC, Suzuki S, Iwahara N, Hisahara S, Kawamata J, Suzuki H, Yamauchi A, Sato-Akaba H, Fujii HG, Shimohama S. Evaluation of oxidative stress in the brain of a transgenic mouse model of Alzheimer disease by in vivo electron

paramagnetic resonance imaging. Free Radical Biology and Medicine. 2015;85:165–73. DOI:10.1016/j.freeradbiomed.2015.04.013.

[94] Chang RC, Rota C, Glover RE, Mason RP, Hong JS. A novel effect of an opioid receptor antagonist, naloxone, on the production of reactive oxygen species by microglia: a study by electron paramagnetic resonance spectroscopy. Brain Research. 2000;854:224–229. DOI: 10.1016/S0006-8993(99)02267-2.

[95] Mayer AM, Hall ML, Holland M, De Castro C, Molinaro A, Aldulescu M, Frenkel J, Ottenhoff L, Rowley D, Powell J. Vibrio vulnificus MO6-24/O lipopolysaccharide stimulates superoxide anion, thromboxane B_2, matrix metalloproteinase-9, cytokine and chemokine release by rat brain microglia in vitro. Marine Drugs. 2014;12:1732–1756. DOI: 10.3390/md12041732.

[96] Tan AS, Berridge MV. Superoxide produced by activated neutrophils efficiently reduces the tetrazolium salt, WST-1 to produce a soluble formazan: a simple colorimetric assay for measuring respiratory burst activation and for screening anti-inflammatory agents. Journal of Immunological Methods. 2000;238:59–68. DOI: 10.1016/j.aca.2013.07.027.

[97] Seo JW, Kim JH, Kim JH, Seo M, Han HS, Park J, Suk K. Time-dependent effects of hypothermia on microglial activation and migration. Journal of Neuroinflammation. 2012;9:164. DOI: 10.1186/1742-2094-9-164.

Chapter 13

Free Radicals and Biomarkers Related to the Diagnosis of Cardiorenal Syndrome

Carolina B.A. Restini, Bruna F.M. Pereira and Tufik M. Geleilete

Additional information is available at the end of the chapter

http://dx.doi.org/10.5772/63898

Abstract

The National Heart, Lung, and Blood Institute Working Group has postulated the cardiorenal syndrome (CRS) as an interaction between the kidneys and the cardiovascular system in which therapy to relieve congestive heart failure (HF) symptoms is limited by the further worsening renal function. CRS is classified from type I to V, taking into account the progression of the symptoms in terms of mechanisms, clinical conditions, and biomarkers. Experimental and clinical studies have shown the kidney as both a trigger and a target to sympathetic nervous system (SNS) overactivity. Renal damage and ischemia, activation of the renin angiotensin aldosterone system (RAAS), and dysfunction of nitric oxide (NO) system are associated with kidney adrenergic activation. Indeed, the imbalances of RAAS and/or SNS share an important common process in CRS: the activation and production of free radicals, especially reactive oxygen species (ROS). The present chapter addresses connections of the free radicals as potential biomarkers as the imbalances in the RAAS and the SNS are developed. Understanding the involvement of free radicals in CRS may bring knowledge to design studies in order to develop accurate pharmacological interventions.

Keywords: Cardiorenal syndrome, renin angiotensin aldosterone system, sympathetic nervous system, reactive oxygem species, free radicals

1. Introduction

Cardiorenal syndrome (CRS) refers to multiple abnormalities characterized by a cluster of concurring symptoms related to cardiac and renal damage. The syndrome is commonly initiated by renal insufficiency secondary to heart failure (HF) [1]. However, the term CRS is also used to describe the negative effects of reduced renal function on the heart and the circulation [2].

A lack of a precise definition to CRS has been pointed out by recognized authors [3]. Based on epidemiologic data, the primary failing organ [4] can be either the heart or the kidney. Therefore, it is accepted that CRS can begin and perpetuate due to a merge in neurohormonal feedback mechanisms involving cardiac and renal dysfunctions. This concept expanded the comprehension about its pathogenesis and treatment.

Ronco et al. and the National Kidney Foundation [5] address CRS as a heart and kidney disorder where acute or chronic dysfunction in one of these organs may induce acute or chronic dysfunction in the other. In addition, Ronco et al. [6] presented a concept that interchanges cardio and renal functions causing CRS and classified it from type I to V, as following:

- Type I (acute cardiorenal syndrome): acute decline in heart function causing kidney dysfunction.
- Type II (chronic cardiorenal syndrome): chronic abnormalities in heart function causing kidney dysfunction.
- Type III (acute renocardiac syndrome): acute decline in kidney function causing heart dysfunction.
- Type IV (chronic renocardiac syndrome): chronic abnormalities in kidney function causing heart dysfunction.
- Type V (secondary cardiorenal syndromes): coinciding heart and kidney dysfunction secondary to systemic conditions.

In the next paragraphs each type of CRS will be described, whose injuries are linked to inflammation and to other deleterious processes connected to free radicals generators. Giving its main classification, the key-systems involved in CRS are the sympathetic nervous system (SNS) and the renin-angiotensin-aldosterone system (RAAS).

Type I—acute CRS characterized by a rapid worsening of cardiac function that leads to acute kidney injury (AKI). Sudden worsening of cardiac function (due to, e.g., acute cardiogenic shock, acute decompensation of chronic heart failure, procedures like coronary angiography, or cardiac surgery) triggers acute renal dysfunction, which consequently leads to humorally mediated damages that involves the activation of both SNS and RAAS systems, as well as to sodium and water retention, and to vasoconstriction. This process enhances the initial impairment in cardiac function, creating, therefore, a snowball effect.

The acute decline in renal function in CRS type I presents a diagnostic challenge since the activation of inflammatory pathways is involved in the acute impairment and acceleration in cardiovascular pathobiology [4, 7].

Diuretic responsiveness is decreased in CRS type I. In a congestive state, decreased response to diuretics may result from the physiological phenomenon of diuretic braking (diminished diuretic effectiveness secondary to postdiuretic sodium retention) [8].

http://dx.doi.org/10.5772/63898

Type II—chronic CRS. The progressive chronic kidney disease (CKD) is linked to chronic cardiac abnormalities; the main example is congestive heart failure. In fact, reduced renal perfusion is related to the mechanism underlying the long-term aggravation of the renal function in chronic heart failure, which has micro-and macrovascular disease as predisposing factors [9, 10].

Frequently, there can be excessive production of vasoconstrictive mediators (epinephrine, angiotensin, and endothelin) and altered sensitivity and/or release of endogenous vasodilators (natriuretic peptides and nitric oxide—NO) [2].

Among the causes of chronic heart disease that increase susceptibility to kidney impairments toward CKD is low cardiac output, an important cause of chronic kidney hypoperfusion and of apoptosis. Initially, kidney damage begins with the development of sclerosis and fibrosis, related to the low cardiac output, subclinical inflammation, endothelial dysfunction, and accelerated atherosclerosis; these main changes, then, progress to CKD. The most important features of chronic heart disease involved are chronic hypoperfusion, increased renovascular resistance, increased venous pressure, and embolisms.

Regarding the kidney, the main alterations that feed chronic heart disease are anemia, sodium and water retention, calcium and phosphates abnormalities, uremic solute retention, left ventricular hypertrophy, hypertension, and activation of SNS and RAAS.

Type III—acute renocardiac syndrome, which has the abrupt worsening of kidney function as the primary cause (e.g., AKI, ischemia, or glomerulonephritis), being responsible for acute cardiac dysfunction (e.g., heart failure, arrhythmia, and ischemia). Although AKI can affect the heart [6], the cause and effect relationship has not been well established. It is known, nonetheless, that pulmonary edema occurs due to fluid overload, that elevated serum potassium levels could culminate in arrhythmias and cardiac arrest, that uremia builds up myocardial depressant factors affecting negatively the inotropism [11] and could cause inflammatory processes in the pericardium [12], and that high hydrogen ion serum concentration leads to pulmonary vasoconstriction [13], a strong contributor to right-sided heart failure. In addition, low blood pH (acidemia) decreases myocardial contractility [14], and when combined with electrolyte imbalance, heightens the risk of irregular heart rhythms [15]. Ultimately, compromised kidney perfusion alone can initiate inflammatory and apoptotic processes in the heart [3].

Type IV—chronic renocardiac syndrome, in which primary CKD, is the main condition (e.g., chronic glomerular disease) that decreases cardiac function and causes ventricular hypertrophy, diastolic dysfunction, and/or increases the risk of adverse cardiovascular events. According to the National Kidney Foundation [5], CKD is subdivided in five stages based on the severity of kidney damage and glomerular filtration rate.

Type V—secondary CRS characterized by the presence of both cardiac and renal dysfunction is due to acute or chronic systemic disorders. Although systematic information on CRS type V is limited, there is a notorious increase in mortality as more organs fail. Comprehension is limited in terms of how simultaneous renal and cardiovascular failure may affect differently an outcome when compared to simultaneous pulmonary and renal failure, for example.

Nonetheless, it is clear that several acute and chronic diseases can affect both organs concurrently and that once started, one organ can affect the other. An example of a very common and serious condition affecting the heart and the kidney is severe sepsis. Other examples include diabetes, amyloidosis, systemic lupus erythematosus, and sarcoidosis. Several chronic conditions such as diabetes and hypertension may contribute to CRS types II and IV.

As seen earlier, an imbalance in the components of the SNS and the RAAS contributes to CRS. Generally, a reduced cardiac output in cardiac heart failure resulting in decreased renal perfusion is thought to be an easy explanation for the worsening renal function [16]. Interestingly though, worsening renal function has been demonstrated in patients with acute decompensated heart failure with preserved left ventricular ejection fraction [17, 18]. This decline in renal function, despite presumed blood flow preservation, has led to an investigation for other mechanisms of CRS, including the role of the renin-angiotensin-aldosterone system (RAAS), of various chemicals (nitric oxide [NO], prostaglandins, natriuretic peptides, endothelins, etc.), of oxidative stress, and of sympathetic overactivity.

The following sections in this chapter aim to conclude that the lack of balance between the RAAS and the SNS triggers deleterious effects in CRS due to processes associated with free radicals production and excessive oxidative stress. Before reaching this conclusion, however, free radical concepts must be addressed.

2. Biomarkers, free radicals, and oxidative stress: basic concepts

A *Biomarker* is a biological marker that reveals medical signs, in other words, it is an objective indicator of a medical state that can be measured accurately and reproducibly without being invasive [19]. The National Institute of Health Biomarkers Definitions Working Group [20], as well as heads in the field of clinical trials and biostatistics from the US National Institute of Health and the US Food and Drug Administration, developed consistent and comprehensive definitions of terms relating to the use of biomarkers. According to them, a biomarker is *objectively measured and evaluated as an indicator of normal biological and pathogenic processes, or pharmacologic responses to a therapeutic intervention.* The use of biomarkers in basic and clinical research as well as in clinical practice has become so conventional that it is now accepted almost without question.

A free radical is a molecular species that contains an unpaired electron in an atomic orbital resulting in high reactivity and instability, yet it is capable of independent existence. These molecules can either donate or accept electrons, therefore, behaving as oxidizing or reducing agents [21]. Among the most important free radicals in cardiovascular disease, especially in CRS, are the reactive oxygen species (ROS) composed of: hydroxyl radical ($OH\bullet$), superoxide anion radical ($O\bullet^-$), hydrogen peroxide (H_2O_2), oxygen singlet ($^1O_2$), hypochlorite (ClO^-), NO radical ($NO\bullet$), and peroxynitrite radical ($ONOO^-$). As other highly reactive species, they are potentially capable of disrupting homeostasis in the nucleus and in the cellular membrane by damaging DNA, proteins, carbohydrates, and lipids [22].

ROS are derived either from normal essential metabolic processes in the human body or from external sources such as exposure to X-rays, ozone, cigarette smoke, air pollutants, and industrial chemicals [23]. Free radical formation occurs continuously in the cells due to enzymatic and nonenzymatic oxygen reactions with organic compounds. Enzymatic reactions that produce free radicals include those involved in the respiratory chain, in phagocytosis, in prostaglandin synthesis, and in the cytochrome P450 system [24].

The term "oxidative stress" describes the oxidative damage resulting from unfavorable antioxidant defenses against free radical generation [25, 26]. Short-term oxidative stress may occur in tissues injured by trauma, infection, heat, hypertonia, toxins, or excessive exercise. Injured tissues produce higher levels of radical generating enzymes (e.g., xanthine oxidase, lipogenase, and cyclooxygenase), increase phagocyte activation and free iron and copper release, and produce an excess of ROS by disrupting the electron transport and oxidative phosphorylation. The initial mutation and progression of cancer, as well as the side effects of radiation and chemotherapy, have all been linked to the imbalance between ROS and the antioxidant defense system.

In addition, ROS has been implicated in the induction and in the complications of cardiac and renal [27] dysfunctions related to CRS [28] through the SNS and the RAAS [29].

3. RAAS and SNS: renal and cardiovascular systems

This section attempts to explain basic concepts about the signaling transductions of the RAAS and the SNS involved in CRS progression.

The RAAS plays an important role in systemic blood pressure regulation as well as in fluid and in electrolyte balance [30]. Angiotensin II (Ang II), the main effector peptide, is involved in cardiovascular and renal physiological and pathological effects, with inflammatory aspects [31] of different diseases present in CRS.

3.1. Ang II and its main signaling pathways to produce cardio and renal injuries

AT1 and AT2 are the main receptors activated by Ang II, being the first prominent receptor involved in harmful consequences of RAAS activation.

The main effect of Ang II is vasoconstriction by [32–34] increasing sympathetic tone [35] and arginine vasopressin (AVP) release [36–38] through stimulation of AT1 receptors mainly present in the vasculature. Activation of Ang II receptors and even nonreceptor pathways has been presented in a review by Touyz and Berry [39]. Briefly, ligand-receptor binding leads to activation of G proteins through an exchange of guanosine triphosphate (GTP) for guanosine diphosphate (GDP), releasing α and β-γ complexes, which mediate downstream actions. AT1 receptors can be interacted with various heterotrimeric G proteins including Gq/11, Gi, Gα12, and Gα13. Different G protein isoforms lead to distinct signaling cascades. Gq activation results in the activation of phospholipase C (PLC), whereas GαI leads to cGMP formation. Although G protein-coupled receptors do not contain intrinsic kinase activity, the members of the G protein receptor kinase family phosphorylate the G protein-coupled receptors on serine and threonine residues. AT1 receptors are phosphorylated in response to Ang II stimulation. Several tyrosine kinases, including Janus kinases (JAK and TYK), Src family kinases, and focal adhesion kinase (FAK) can phosphorylate AT1 receptors [40].

Angiotensin II has a long-term control over blood pressure through various mechanisms: direct stimulation of AT1 kidney receptors [10] and indirect adrenal gland aldosterone releasing regulate renal reabsorption of sodium and water [41], and acts on the hypothalamus causing thirst [36, 37].

The renin activity on the α2-globulin angiotensinogen produces the decapeptide angiotensin I (Ang I), which is then cleaved by an angiotensin-converting enzyme (ACE) to produce the octapeptide Ang II [42].

In mammals, there are two isoforms of ACE: somatic ACE, abundant on the surface of pulmonary endothelial cells, and testicular ACE. Both isoforms are found as soluble enzymes in the plasma and in seminal fluid [43]. Production of Ang II from Ang I also occurs through an ACE-independent way by the activity of other enzymes such as cathepsin G, a chymostatin-sensitive Ang II-generating enzyme, and chymase [36].

Besides its primary vasoconstrictor effects, Ang II also presents growth factor and cytokine-like properties [44]. The different forms of intracellular signaling processes explain its varied effects. In VSMC and also in renal cells, including glomerular endothelial and mesangial cells, Ang II induces chemokines such as monocyte chemoattractant protein-1 (MCP-1) [45–48].

AT1 signaling through phospholipids involves phospholipase C (PLC), phospholipase D (PLD), and phospholipase A_2 (PLA_2).

PLC signaling results in rapid production of the second messengers 1,4,5-inositol triphosphate (IP_3) and diacylglycerol (DAG). While IP_3 stimulates Ca^{2+} mobilization from the sarcoplasmic reticulum, DAG causes Ca^{2+} influx from extracellular space after protein kinase C (PKC) stimulation [49]. The increased cytoplasmic calcium concentration ($[Ca^{2+}]$ c) leads to Ca^{2+}-dependent, calmodulin-activated phosphorylation of the myosin light chain, which, in turn, leads to cellular contraction. This is the main mechanism involved in the vascular smooth muscle cell (VSMC) contraction. PKC activation by this process regulates intracellular pH through the Na+/H+ exchanger [49, 50] and also activates both the nicotinamide adenine dinucleotide phosphate-oxidase (NADPH oxidase) signaling as well as the ROS production.

PLD signaling is related to the phosphatidylcholine hydrolysis. The AT1 receptors mediating PLD activation involve Gβ-γ, Gα12, Src, and RhoA [51]. The pathways associated with Ang II-induced activation of PLD in VSMC are PKC independent, but involve intracellular Ca^{2+} mobilization and Ca^{2+} influx that is tyrosine kinase-dependent. Ang II-induced PLD signaling has been implicated in cardiac hypertrophy, VSMC proliferation, and vascular contractility [52, 53]. Among the PLD-mediated responses, there are vascular generation of superoxide anions by stimulating NADPH oxidase, and, under long-term stimulation of AT1 receptors, growth and remodeling in the cardiovascular system [54].

The PLA2 activation due to Ang II binding on AT1 receptors is responsible for arachidonic acid release from cell membrane phospholipids [55], and its consequent metabolism by cyclooxygenases, lipoxygenases, or cytochrome P450 oxygenases results in various different eicosanoids influencing vascular and renal mechanisms that are important in blood pressure regulation. The main PLA2-derived eicosanoids resultants from cyclooxygenases include prostaglandin (PG) H2, which is then converted to thromboxane (Tx), PGI2 (prostacyclin), or to PGE2, PGD2, or PGF2α, by different enzymes (22). Lipoxygenases-derived molecules are the leukotrienes [55]. Cytochrome P450 oxygenases leads to the production of the hydroxy-eicosatetraenoic acids (HETE)—acids derived from epoxidation and allylic oxidation.

In VSMC, AT1 receptor stimulation by Ang II interconnects all phospholipases (PLA_2, PLD, and PKC) activation to initiate NADPH oxidase activity. DAG and Ca^{2+}, from the sarcoplasmic reticulum by IP3, activate PKC, which leads to phosphorylation of p47phox and initial activation of the NADPH oxidase [56, 57]. PLD also mediates PKC activation; phosphatic acid (PA) is produced, serving as a source of DAG [58–60]. Furthermore, PLA2 is activated by calcium cleaving phosphatidylcholine to products that heightens NADPH oxidase action, lysophosphatidylcholine (LPC) and arachidonic acid (AA) [61].

AT1-mediated tyrosine phosphorylation leads to mitogen-activated protein kinase (MAPK) activation associated with growth factors and cytokine activity, which corroborate to mitogenic and inflammatory consequences of Ang II. Moreover, AT1 receptor activation may be mediated by the activation of receptor tyrosine kinases (RTK) to bring about the Ang II stimuli on epidermal growth factor receptor (EGFR), platelet-derived growth factor receptor (PDGFR), and insulin growth factor receptor (IGFR) [62, 63].

Furthermore, Ang II stimulates phosphorylation of several nonreceptor tyrosine kinases such as PLC-γ, Src family kinases, Janus kinase (JAK), focal adhesion kinase (FAK), Ca^{2+}-dependent tyrosine kinases, p130Cas, and phosphatidylinositol 3-kinase (PI3K) [64]. Altered VSMC function in hypertension is associated with increased activation of c-Src by Ang II. Vascular and cardiac growth, remodeling, and repair are assumed to involve Janus kinase, and the signal transducers and activators of transcription from early growth response genes mediated by Ang II [65]. FAK-dependent signaling pathways triggered by Ang II are related to cell migration and changes in cell shape and volume [66]. p130Cas mediated-Ang II effects regulate α-actin expression, cellular proliferation and migration, and cell adhesion, playing a relevant role in cardiovascular disease and actin filament assembly [67]. PI3K in Ang II signaling in VSMC may control the balance between mitogenesis and apoptosis [68].

Ang II activates the three major members of the mitogen-activated protein kinases (MAPK) family [69, 70]: ERK1/2 (related to enhanced proto-oncogene expression, and activation of the transcription factor, cell cycle progression, and protein synthesis in VSMC [71]), JNKs (regulation of cell growth, and vascular damage associated with cardiovascular disease [72]), and p38 MAPK (inflammatory responses, apoptosis, and inhibition of cell growth [73]).

Finally, by signaling through heterotrimeric G proteins, AT1 receptors activate monomeric small (21 kDa) guanine nucleotide-binding proteins (small G proteins) in VSMC. Activation of Ang II via AT1 receptor is coupled with Rho subfamily (RhoA, Rac1, and Cdc42), whose

Ang II effects are associated with increased Ca^{2+} sensitization, VSMC contraction, cytoskeletal organization, cell growth, inflammation, and regulation of NADPH oxidase [74]. In general Ang II, as other Gq coupled receptors, effectively activates NADPH oxidase in the cardiovascular system, enhancing production of ROS, whose effects majorly contribute to the pathogenesis of cardiovascular and kidney disease [75].

The integration of all the concepts above leads to the comprehension that important deleterious effects of Ang II could contribute to features observed in the CRS. This is supported by therapeutic involvement of angiotensin-converting enzyme inhibitors (ACEi) and of angiotensin receptor inhibitor, which have proven to be effective in the CRS therapy (for pharmacotherapy guidance we suggest reading the guideline organized by Dickstein et al. [76]). The activation of the RAAS determines renal hypoxia, vasoconstriction, intraglomerular hypertension, glomerulosclerosis, tubulointerstitial fibrosis, and proteinuria [77]. Similarly, the activation of the SNS involves proliferation of smooth muscle cells and adventitial fibroblasts in the intrarenal vascular walls [78]. Ang II increases renal vascular resistance in animal models, and the addition of an α_2-adrenoceptors agonist enhances this response. NADPH oxidase inhibition, as well as Rho kinase inhibition, or the presence of a superoxide dismutase (SOD) mimetic attenuates this interaction between Ang II and α_2-adrenoceptors agonist. Furthermore, in preglomerular VSMCs, the α_2-adrenoceptors agonist enhanced Ang II-induced intracellular O_2^- production and activation of RhoA, responses which were prevented by inhibition of phospholipase C (PLC), PKC, c-Src, NADPH oxidase, and by a SOD mimetic.

3.2. Free radicals: key biomarkers in experimental models to explain RAAS and SNS in CRS

Excessive and inappropriate activation of the RAAS [79] is directly implicated in many ways in the progression of renal disease due to heart failure. In parallel to the heart failure, the ongoing, uncontrolled activation of the RAAS is indicative of renal failure.

The model proposed by Guyton [80] describes a heart–kidney connection regarding extracellular fluid volume (ECFV), cardiac output, and mean arterial pressure. In this arrangement, the pathophysiological basis of CRS is structured on the combined renal and cardiac disease invoking a number of specific factors that synergistically aggravate the disease.

In Guyton's model [80], the kidney is placed as a regulator of extracellular fluid volume and the RAAS is placed with its corresponding extensions (aldosterone and endothelin) and its antagonists (natriuretic peptides and NO). The model explains changes in extracellular fluid volume, blood pressure, and cardiac output in merged heart and renal failure. An extension to this model, however, was projected by Bongartz et al. [29] to explain the accelerated atherosclerosis, the cardiac remodeling and hypertrophy, and the progression of renal disease observed in the severe CRS. When the heart or the kidney fails, a vicious cycle, called the cardiorenal connection [81, 82] in a scheme depicted by Bongartz et al. [29], progresses: the RAAS, the NO-ROS balance, the sympathetic nervous system, and inflammation interact and synergize.

The reduction in circulating arterial blood volume triggers arterial baroreceptors and activates neurohormonal pathways resulting in compensatory mechanisms in order to restore physiological tissue perfusion to correct the relative hypovolemia, such as in hemorrhage [83].

Indeed, not only the RAAS is activated but also the SNS. The endothelin and arginine-vasopressin systems are triggered by low renal function as protection mechanisms. Additionally, sodium-retentive vasoconstriction can counterbalance the activation of vasodilatory natriuretic hormone (natriuretic peptide) systems and cytokines (prostaglandins, bradykinin, and NO) [84].

These pathways lead to an outcome of heart failure, an impairment involving volume retention due to hemodynamics and reabsorptive actions of angiotensin II (Ang II) [86].

In addition to the imbalance of extracellular fluid volume (ECFV) and vasoconstriction, the activation of NADPH-oxidase by Ang II harms the cardiorenal connection by generating ROS [87].

Ang II not only stimulates NADPH oxidase-dependent O_2^- production in VSMCs but also in endothelial cells and adventitial fibroblasts [88, 89]. Additionally, stretch of the vasculature could enhance O_2^- and hydrogen peroxide (H_2O_2) production by NADPH oxidase during a relatively short period of time [90, 91].

Mohazzab and Wolin [92] and Rajagopalan et al. [93] have identified NADPH oxidase as a major site of O_2^- generation in intact arteries (endothelial cells and vascular smooth muscle cells [94]) besides renal tubular cells [95] and cardiomyocytes [96]. Interestingly, constituents of phagocyte NADPH oxidase were found in many different tissues, like in mesangial cells [97], vascular smooth muscle cells [98, 99], endothelial cells [100], glomerular epithelial podocytes [101], kidney proximal tubular epithelial cells [102], and fibroblasts [103].

The multimolecular enzyme NADPH oxidase has the following components: a membrane-associated 22-kDa α-subunit (p22phox) and a 91-kDa β-subunit (gp91phox) with cytoplasmic constituents (p47phox, p67phox, and p40phox) [104].

The severity of CRS is positively associated with oxidative damage to renal tubular or interstitial cells due to interference with feedback systems involved in renin secretion and angiotensin formation. Chronic inhibition of NO synthesis causes upregulation of cardiac ACE and Ang II receptors, possibly mediating inflammatory changes [105]. It has been demonstrated [105] a complete NADPH oxidase system along the luminal membrane of the macula densa, suggesting that O_2- generated at this site forms a barrier and limits the actions of NO locally generated to reach targets on the luminal membrane. Thus, local NADPH oxidase impairs the bioavailability of NO, which is implicated by the regulation of sodium reabsorption in distal nephrons and activation of macula densa cells of hypertensive rats.

Renal blood flow reduction due to activation of the RAS leads to stimulation of the macula densa and subsequent secretion of renin; in critical kidney impairment (such as in hypoxia), this vicious cycle of RAAS starts or maintains the development of CRS [27].

Ang II may produce cell changes in the glomerular epithelium [106]. Local expression of the RAS in podocytes has been recently confirmed in human podocytes [107, 108]. Direct injury to podocytes of transgenic rat models with overexpression of the human Ang II Type 1 receptor, developed substantial selective proteinuria (albuminuria) without an increase in blood pressure. This model's glomerular injury led to nephron loss through the classic pathway present in focal segmental glomerulosclerosis [109]. Also, aldosterone, an end product of Ang II, directly injures podocytes [110, 111].

Therefore, added to these direct consequences of tubulointerstitial damages, present mainly in CRS type II, activation of this system can induce glomerulosclerosis and anatomical damage to glomerular tufts, with a subsequent decrease in postglomerular capillary perfusion.

Beswick et al. [112] identified ROS production in a model of mineralocorticoid (deoxycorticosterone acetate [DOCA]-salt) hypertensive rats. NADPH oxidase activity is increased in the aortic wall of the DOCA-salt rat, and such an increase is associated with elevated O_2^- production; long-term inhibition of NADPH oxidase significantly decreased O_2^- production and systolic blood pressure, but treatment of DOCA-salt rats with the losartan (Ang II inhibitor) does not significantly alter blood pressure, suggesting that locally produced Ang II does not contribute to the elevated peripheral vascular resistance. This calls into question the role of Ang II in O_2^- generation in this model. On the other hand, NADPH-oxidase mediated ROS release in glomeruli of Dahl [113] salt-sensitive rats with heart failure, which was attenuated by ACEi [114]. In human beings, similarly, NADPH-oxidase is active in the hearts of patients with end-stage heart failure [115]. Inhibition of ACE possibly decreases vascular oxidative stress and/or improves extracellular SOD activity in patients with coronary artery disease due to higher NO bioavailability [116].

Ang II has a role in vascular inflammation via the nuclear factor kappa B (NF-kB) pathway, responsible for producing chemotactic and adhesion molecules [117, 118].

Complicated mechanisms link the RAS to the SNS [119]. The rise of sympathetic hyperactivity detected in kidney failure has been attributed to the failing organ [120], and ACEi could control this outflow in chronic failure [121, 122]. Blocking Ang II signaling transduction causes reduced SNS hyperactivity after myocardial infarction in rats, attenuating ensuing development of heart failure [123].

Oxidative stress induced by hydrogen peroxide presented higher activation of preganglionic sympathetic neurons both in vivo and in vitro in rats, culminating in a greater mean blood pressure and pulse [124]. Moreover, spontaneously hypertensive rats were found to have sympathetic renal activity controlled by vascular superoxide concentrations [125].

4. Oxidative stress in target CRS organs

Considering the RAAS and the SNS and that the impaired functions of the target organs (kidney and heart) can conjointly trigger and intensify diseases related to the syndrome's development, this section aims to provide the reader with molecular/cellular explanations about why free radicals and consequent oxidative stress are feasible to act as CRS biomarkers.

4.1. Heart and oxidative stress

ATP is constantly demanded in physiologic cardiac functioning. So mitochondria organelles, as major sources of ATP, must be in prompt activity to keep homeostasis [126]. When the balance between cardiac cells and mitochondria is lost, there is cardiac damage due to increased oxidative stress as can be observed in heart failure.

In a normal heart, most of the ATP is produced by fatty acid oxidation, while the remaining part is due to oxidizing pyruvate, an end product of glycolysis or derived from lactate [127]. On the other hand, with decreasing ATP concentrations, there is a metabolic shift from fatty acid oxidation to glycolysis in cardiomyocytes under heart failure progression [128–130]. Indeed, the decrease in mitochondrial oxidative metabolism is reduced by a compensatory increase in glucose uptake and glycolysis [131, 132].

The main cause of the damage affecting the cardiomyocytes is the self-perpetuation of the oxidative stress as the reduced oxidative metabolism leads to an accumulation of free fatty acid in cardiomyocytes.

The PKC activation and consequent sarcoplasmic reticulum stress are the main intracellular mechanisms explaining both contributors to mitochondrial oxidative stress: lipotoxicity of circulating fatty acid and intracellular lipid accumulation [133].

Independent of the heart failure stage, changes in mitochondrial electron transport chain components were described [134–137]. Indeed, the progressive decrease of ATP production is linked to both a decrease of fatty acid oxidation and a reduction of mitochondrial respiration due to electron transport chain defects [138].

The disruption of the mitochondrial electron transport chain homeostasis is a well-established source of ROS that forms a vicious cycle by amplifying the electron transport chain dysfunctions. In heart failure, the decreased mitochondrial respiratory activity leads to a further drop in oxidative phosphorylation, associated with an increased electron leakage and superoxide generation.

As already mentioned, ROS are produced by nicotinamide adenine dinucleotide phosphate (NADPH) oxidases (NOX). There are seven NOX isoforms that function primarily as ROS-generating enzymes, being important sources of O_2^- and H_2O_2 in the cardiovascular system [139]. When physiological functioning of NOXs is disrupted, the production of ROS increases.

Overactivation of the RAAS and the SNS are essential to maintain and amplify the oxidative stress in heart failure, as previously explained. NADPH oxidase activated by Ang II is the primary source of ROS that produces mitochondrial dysfunction [140]. The effects are due to both NOX4 and NOX2, which are upregulated by Ang II in a mitochondrial ROS-independent and dependent manner, respectively [141].

ROS accounts for the damage observed in heart failure, such as cardiac remodeling, cardiomyocyte contractility, ion transport, and Ca^{2+} handling. ROS act on multiple intracellular signaling pathways for transcriptional activation of selected nuclear genes and finally eliciting transcriptional reprogramming [142]. In response, the most prominent adaptive processes accompanying HF are an increase in sympathetic tone. Increased adrenergic activity causes a reduction on the physiological role of respirasomes, and consequently mitochondrial dysfunction, and a gradual decrease in the cardiac performance [28]. The excessive sympathetic activity can induce cardiomyocyte apoptosis, hypertrophy, and focal myocardial necrosis [85].

The lack of energy in cardiomyocytes is an important result of the oxidative stress observed in decompensated HF, explained by reduced Ca^{2+} sensitivity in response to oxidative impairment of myofibrillar proteins [143].

ROS were shown to activate matrix metalloproteinase (MMP) in cardiac fibroblasts [144]. MMP are a large family of Ca^{2+}-dependent zinc-containing endopeptidases that are responsible for tissue remodeling and degradation of extracellular matrix (ECM), including collagens, elastins, gelatin, matrix glycoproteins, and proteoglycan. Overexpression of MMPs results in imbalance between its activity and the activity of TIMPs and can lead to a variety of disorders [145–149]. Since MMP plays a central role in organ development and subsequent tissue remodeling in inflammation and in injury, they are relevant HF biomarkers, especially in CRS [150].

4.2. Kidney and oxidative stress

Oxidative stress and inflammation are progressively enhanced in progressing stages of kidney diseases directly related to CRS such as CKD [151–153]. This section describes mechanisms that link RAAS and its components to the increased oxidative stress and inflammation within the kidneys [154–156].

Ang II acts preferentially in tubular epithelial cells, whereas aldosterone acts in podocyte injury [157]. As previously said, NOX enzymes (NADPH oxidases) are the primary source of ROS. Under Ang II and aldosterone stimuli, cytosolic subunits of NADPH oxidase can translocate into the mitochondrial membrane and increase ROS production and affect the NO function. It is the balance between NO and Ang II rather than their absolute concentration that determines the physiological/pathophysiological effects on multiple organ systems including cardiovascular and renal systems. Ang II systematically decreases regional blood flows, impairs renal function, and causes cardiac hypertrophy [158].

In the kidney, NOX are active in vascular smooth cells in both cortex and medulla [159, 160]. NOX4, NOX2, and NOX1 are expressed in the kidney cortex, being NOX4 the most abundantly expressed renal isoform, primarily not only located in renal tubular cell [161–163] but also found in glomerular mesangial cells [164, 165].

A critical role played by NOX-produced ROS is the uncoupling of NO synthase (NOS). Considering its physiological role, NO produced by endothelial cells causes vasodilatation of the afferent arteriole, consequently increasing renal blood flow, attenuating tubuloglomerular feedback, and promoting pressure natriuresis [166]. NO stimulates soluble guanylyl cyclase (sGC) and increases cGMP production that triggers cGMP-dependent protein kinases, phosphodiesterases, and ion channels [167]. On the other hand, NO is activated in a non-cGMP-dependent process and causes covalent proteins changes [168]. NO reacts with O_2^- to form $ONOO^-$ [169], therefore, limiting its physiological activity of afferent arteriole relaxation [170,

171], which leads to reduced renal blood flow. Vasoconstriction, inflammation, and impaired vascular and renal functions [172] are the main results of $ONOO^-$ accumulation.

O_2^- and $ONOO^-$ are the main free radicals that start proinflammatory and profibrotic cascades [55]. In the absence of or in a low concentration of NO, the cyclooxygenases (COX) activity is amplified, so vasoconstriction is enhanced due to TxA2, yet the vascular relaxation is impaired due to reduced PGI2 production [172, 173].

Mesangial cell apoptosis [174] and cellular hypertrophy, respectively, due to MAP kinase and ERK1/ERK2 pathways [175], explain the development of epithelial-mesenchymal transition (EMT) [176, 177] caused by NOX-derived ROS. EMT of tubular epithelial cells is characterized by loss of epithelial properties and gain of excessive deposition of extracellular matrix-producing characteristics of myofibroblast [178, 179]. The transforming growth factor β (TGF-β) induces EMT and is assumed to be one of the major causes of renal fibrosis [180–182].

According to Yang and Liu [183], and to Rubattu et al. [28], EMT regulates the loss of epithelial cell adhesion, the *de novo* α-smooth muscle actin (α-SMA) expression and reorganization, the disruption of tubular basement membrane, and the enhanced cell migration and invasion into the interstitium. Increased expressions of PLA2, MCP-1, CSF-1, and COX-2 promote fibrosis and inflammation on renal interstitium, all due to NOX activation under oxidative stress progression [184–187]. The main transcription factors involved are NF-kB [74] and c-jun [188].

Second, free radicals' inflammatory effects can be related to uncoupling proteins (UCPs) [189, 190]. UCPs are mitochondrial transporters present in the inner membrane; they belong to the family of anion mitochondrial carriers including adenine nucleotide transporters. There are three UCPs (1–3). In comparison to the established uncoupling and thermogenic activities of UCP1, UCP2, and UCP3 appear to be involved in the limitation of free radical levels in cells rather than in physiological uncoupling and thermogenesis.

UCP2 gene variants are positively associated with kidney diseases, being considered as a predictor of genetic risk for CKD [191, 192].

5. Oxidative stress: biomarkers and therapeutic strategies in CRS

The main proposal of biomarkers is an early diagnosis of CRS allowing early therapeutic intervention. The continuance of mitochondrial biogenesis against cardiac insult and the reduction of mitochondrial ROS production are the two most promising approaches that may soon yield effective treatments for HF [193].

The action of ROS and their products in organs, such as heart, kidney, and the entire cardiovascular system, turn them into promising biomarkers for predicting cardiovascular risk in CRS and also for therapeutic responses. Important investigations have characterized new oxidation byproducts in specific circumstances, however, oxidized lipoproteins, including low-density lipoproteins (LDL) have a long track record as biomarkers and appear to be among the most promising oxidation markers to potentially impact clinical practice in the near future

[194]. Nonetheless, this biomarker is more appropriate for atherosclerosis than for HF related to CRS. Biomarkers such as MMP and mitochondrial function may be more adequate.

Concerning clinical evaluation of cardiovascular and renal dysfunctions, ROS is examined due to the association between plasma and urine markers of oxidative stress. There are several clinical studies where biomarkers were and are being tested [195]. The following sections attempt to cover potential biomarkers related to oxidative stress.

5.1. Heart biomarkers of oxidative stress

The main molecules approached in this section are the ones involved in HF since this is the main cardiac disease in CRS linked to kidney dysfunction.

The molecules are matrix metalloproteinase (MMP), myeloperoxidases (MPO), and mid-regional proadrenomedullin (MR-proADM).

Although HF, but not myocardial infarction, is the main cardiac disease related to CRS, studies have shown that increased MMP production is a biomarker related to both. Since dramatic reduction in the incidence of rupture and reduction in heart size and development of heart failure is observed when MMP activation is reduced, it can predict CKD present in CRS [196].

Considering the role of MMP in stem cell mobilization following cardiac injury, in the very active field of cell-based therapy following myocardial infarction, MMP-9 was found in bone marrow; its function is to release mononuclear cells into the blood flow. After ischemic injury, there seems there to be local formation of inflammatory cytokines, such as tumor necrosis factor (TNF), platelet-derived growth factor, and vascular endothelial growth factor [197]. A significant component of regulation of MMP production following myocardial infarction is induced by the local inflammatory cytokines, which is practically what is observed in HF. Excess TNF in the myocardium has direct relation to an elevated formation of local MMP-9 and MMP-2, and this is associated with modifications in integrin isoform transition [196]. The consequence is aggressive collagen dissolution with possible acute myocardial rupture. If the dissolution goes on without rupture, the heart becomes expressively dilated, with decreased function and poor survival [196]. On the other hand, if the gene for TNF is removed, there is a significant reduction in the levels of the inflammatory cytokines associated with the reduction in MMP activation.

Once MMP are formed, they stay as proenzymes in the ground substance of the extracellular space. However, if met by other activation signals like oxygen free radicals and ischemic triggers such as thrombin or chymase or angiotensin-converting enzyme (ACE) from mast cells, then propeptides are unconfined, liberating the enzyme's active site [198]. A membrane type MMP can also catalyze this process or other proteolytic agents such as plasminogen activators (urokinase-type plasminogen activator) or plasmin. Plasmin's activation is due to inflammation and coagulation cascades. Reduction in cardiac rupture after myocardial infarction could be reached by inhibiting MMPs, plasminogen activators, or cytokines [196, 198].

Taking into account the kidney and the heart to explain the role of the free radicals, Rubattu et al. [28] published a review about pathogenesis of CRS and oxidative stress. The information is addressed briefly in the next paragraphs. Myocardial MMP activity is also increased in the failing heart [199]. Sustained MMP activation causes structural changes due to an abnormal extracellular environment for myocytes. Dimethylthiourea, a hydroxyl radical scavenger, inhibits matrix metalloproteinase 2 (MMP2) activation parallel to left ventricular remodeling and failure [200]. Additionally, release of mitochondrial intermembrane proteins crucially triggers apoptotic pathways: cytochrome c, endonuclease G (EndoG), apoptosis-inducing factor (AIF), and second mitochondria-derived activator of caspase (Smac) lead to caspase activation, nuclear DNA fragmentation, and cell death [201]. Release and nuclear translocation of EndoG and AIF stimulate DNA degeneration, independent of caspase activation [202]. Stress kinases, such as c-Jun N-terminal kinase (JNK) and p38-mitogen activated protein kinase (MAPK), are activated by increase in ROS levels [203]. The link between hypertrophy mitochondrial dysfunction seen in HF could be due to JNK. Actually, in addition to the induction of hypertrophic cardiomyocytes, JNK promotes autophagy through Bcl-2 and 19-KDa interacting protein-3 (BNIP3), eventually leading to mitophagy [204, 205]. In turn, higher mitophagy rates ends in MMP activation [206].

Besides the MMP, there are the myeloperoxidases (MPO) considered a key player in the initiation and maintenance of chronic heart failure (CHF) by contributing to intracellular NO depletion. NO consumption through MPO activity may lead to protein chlorination or nitration and to tissue damage.

As revised by Anatoliotakis et al. [207], the principal mechanism by which MPO exerts its effects on the human heart and vessels is thought to be by direct effects of oxidative products on the arterial wall causing endothelial dysfunction, as well as by affecting the function and distribution of cholesterol in the form of LDL and HDL. MPO is the main molecule responsible for lipid peroxidation and conversion of LDL to an atherogenic form that is subsequently taken up by macrophages, a step crucial for the formation of foam cells [208]. Additionally, MPO acts as an enzymatic sink for NO, thus impairing NO-dependent blood vessel relaxation and guanylate cyclase activation [209].

La Rocca et al. [210] demonstrated that human endocardial endothelial cells can express MPO after oxidative stress through the buildup of the end product, 3-chlorotyrosine. Abnormalities in endothelial functions may lead to many cardiovascular issues, including CHF. The authors concluded that the endothelium suffers the consequences as well as plays an important role in cardiovascular stress due to oxidation.

Considering what was the earlier approach about CRS, a positive association can be made with an MPO increase and disease progression. MPO, a marker of oxidative stress [211, 212], maintained a modest association with HF in this cohort when combined with each of the established and emerging biomarkers.

MR-proADM shows great promise as an independent prognostic tool for cardiac diseases. Although it has been shown as a strong predictive marker for a variety of cardiac disease, it is also a biomarker for other diseases including chronic obstructive pulmonary disorder, pneumonia, and pulmonary embolism [213, 214]. Since MR-proADM levels have been shown to differ based on New York Heart Association (NYHA) class and severity of HF, it has the potential to help identify those patients who may benefit from more invasive therapy [215].

Adrenomedullin (ADM), a 52-amino-acid peptide, was first discovered from a pheochromocytoma. It is expressed by many endothelial tissues throughout the body including the adrenal medulla, lungs, kidneys, gastrointestinal organs, and heart [216–219]. ADM is secreted as an inactive precursor (pro-ADM) and subsequently cleaved into the active form where it acts as a potent vasodilator through the nitric oxide pathway and increases diuresis and natriuresis [220–222].

Considering emerging biomarkers of hemodynamic stress that are strongly predictive of poor outcomes in patients with heart failure (HF), MR-proADM is the main molecule related to CRS [223]; others include copeptin and midregional proatrial natriuretic peptide [MR-proANP].

5.2. Kidney biomarkers of oxidative stress

Considering renal biomarkers of oxidative stress as part of the pathophysiology, the pool includes oxidized low-density lipoproteins (Ox-LDL), advanced oxidation protein products (AOPP), thiobarbituric acid reactive substances (TBARS), plasma and urinary F2-isoprostanes, malondialdehyde (MDA), protein reduced thiols, total antioxidant status (TAS), protein carbonyls, advanced glycation end products (AGE), rinary 8-hydroxydeoxy guanosine (8-OHdG), 4-hydroxy-nonenal, antioxidant enzyme activities (e.g., superoxide dismutase, glutathione peroxidase, and catalase) [195, 224–229]. It is important to highlight that these biomarkers could indicate the possible correlated diseases, and not strictly renal injuries from CRS. Studies that involve cardiovascular and kidney disease, such as hypertension and CRS, try to correlate oxidative stress to the absence of antioxidant defenses (extrinsic and intrinsic). In general oxidized phospholipids (OxPL) have been associated with cardiovascular disease and new cardiovascular events [230]. OX-LDL, a particle derived from circulating LDL, may have peroxides or their degradation products generated within the LDL molecule or elsewhere in the body. This includes minimally oxidized LDL, but not apoprotein changes, and malondialdehyde (MDA) modified particles with MDA arising from platelets or elsewhere. However, LDL particles with oxidized apo B amino acids without lipid changes have not been described [231]. In kidney diseases, Ox-LDL has been studied as a biomarker to assess end-stage renal failure. Nonetheless, as a CRS biomarker, Ox-LDL needs correlational studies [232].

According to Witko-Sarsat et al. [233], AOPP is a biomarker of phagocyte-derived oxidative stress. The authors point out the role of AOPP in the pathophysiology of chronic renal failure and dialysis-related complications. Considering AOPP production, they describe that myeloperoxidase (MPO) has a significant role in the consequent formation of chlorinated oxidants, contrary to the prior belief of its sole microbicidal action. Undeniably, AOPP seems to mediate inflammation because they can initiate the oxidative burst and the production of cytokines in leucocytes. Therefore, it can be inferred that by the uremia-associated defect in anti-oxidant systems that the AOPP, from the reaction between chlorinated oxidants and plasma proteins, constitute new uremic toxins with proinflammatory effects. Specific plasma proteins are

http://dx.doi.org/10.5772/63898

critical targets for oxidants that can be evaluated by spectrophotometric assays, which allows AOPP detection in uremic plasma [234], mainly from patients under hemodialysis [235].

F2-isoprostanes are a series of active compounds like prostaglandin F2. They are produced regardless of the route of the COX in the peroxidation of AA. F2-isoprostanes are formed in situ on the membrane phospholipid chains and subsequently released. Their concentrations in the plasma and urine of healthy adults are 10–100 times greater than those of prostanoid formed by way of the cyclooxygenase. They significantly increase oxidative stress. The F2 isoprostanes are potential markers of lipid peroxidation, but their measurement requires sophisticated equipment (mass spectrometer). Recently, Elisa methods have become available [236].

Biomarkers of cell damage due to systemic oxidative stress, such as plasma thiobarbituric acid-reactive substances (TBARS) and 8-epi-isoprostanes, are elevated in patients with hypertension [237, 238] who mainly present kidney injury. Antioxidant capacity and the levels of antioxidant vitamins and enzymes were reduced in patients with hypertension [239, 240] with renal insufficiency.

6. Conclusion

The Acute Decompensated Heart Failure National Registry (ADHERE) database has pointed out that renal dysfunction in patients with heart failure is complex and often multifactorial in origin. Along these lines, CRS is conceived as a moderate or a greater renal dysfunction existing or developing in a patient with decompensated heart failure during treatment [241]. Important works present a common agreement: concurrent kidney and heart failure has a bad prognosis [242–244]. The literature, on the other hand, is not homogeneous in relation to the damages and their mechanisms due to a number of factors, causes, and on the processes that makes CRS reversable in some cases. Since both the RAAS and the SNS are related to the processes leading to inflammation and are tightly involved in production and/or activation of free radicals, this chapter's rationale is that the diagnosis and progression of CRS could be evaluated through oxidative stress. Some CRS pharmacotherapeutics approaches are deficient, although mainly involving the primary condition linking renal dysfunction to heart failure, like in volume-loaded patients with diuretic braking [245]. There is a gap in clinical trials composed of patients with heart failure and with substantial kidney dysfunction, because most patients are recruited from a population with relatively preserved kidney function [246]. Further studies are needed to better define renal function in patients with heart failure or vice-versa. Attention must be taken to drugs that may impair kidney function, and specially evaluated regarding populations selected for clinical trials, who have already had their kidney functions compromised or put at risk. Understanding the involvement of free radicals in the Cardiorenal Syndrome could lead to accurate pharmacological studies and future interventions.

Author details

Carolina B.A. Restini*, Bruna F.M. Pereira and Tufik M. Geleilete

*Address all correspondence to: carolbaraldi@hotmail.com

School of Medicine, University of Ribeirão Preto, SP, Brazil

References

[1] Liang KV, Williams AW, Greene EL, Redfield MM. Acute decompensated heart failure and the cardiorenal syndrome. Crit Care Med. 2008;36:S75–S88. DOI: 10.1097/01.CCM.0000296270.41256.5C.

[2] Ronco C, House AA, Haapio M. Cardiorenal syndrome: refining the definition of a complex symbiosis gone wrong. Intensive Care Med. 2008;34:957–962. DOi: 10.1016/j.jacc.2008.07.051

[3] Patel J, Heywood JT. Management of the cardiorenal syndrome in heart failure. Curr Cardiol Rep. 2006;8:211–216. DOI: 10.1007/s11886-006-0036-8.

[4] Berl T, Henrich W. Kidney-heart interactions: epidemiology, patho-genesis, and treatment. Clin J Am Soc Nephrol. 2006;1:8–18. DOI: 10.2215/CJN.00730805.

[5] National Kidney Foundation. K/DOQI clinical practice guidelines for chronic kidney disease: evaluation, classification, and stratification. Am J Kidney Dis. 2002;39:S1–S266. DOI: 10.7326/0003-4819-139-2-200307150-00013.

[6] Ronco C, Haapio M, House AA, Anavekar N, Bellomo R. Cardiorenal syndrome. J Am Coll Cardiol. 2008;52:1527–1539. DOI: 10.1016/j.jacc.2008.07.051.

[7] Tokuyama H, Kelly DJ, Zhang Y, Gow RM, Gilbert RE. Macrophage infiltration and cellular proliferation in the non-ischemic kidney and heart following prolonged unilateral renal ischemia. Nephron Physiol. 2007;106:54–62. DOI: 10.1159/000103910.

[8] Ellison DH. Diuretic resistance: physiology and therapeutics. Semin Nephrol. 1999;19:581–597. <http://europepmc.org/abstract/med/10598546>.

[9] Butler J, Forman DE, Abraham WT, Gottlieb SS, Loh E, Massie BM, O'Connor CM, Rich MW, Stevenson LW, Wang Y, Young JB, Krumholz HM. Relationship between heart failure treatment and development of worsening renal function among hospitalized patients. Am Heart J. 2004;147:331–338. DOI: 10.1016/j.ahj.2003.08.012.

[10] Bhatia RS, Tu JV, Lee DS, Austin PC, Fang J, Haouzi A, Gong Y, Liu PP. Outcome of heart failure with preserved ejection fraction in a

population-based study. N Engl J Med. 2006;355:260–269. DOI: 10.1056/NEJMoa051530.

[11] Blake P, Hasegawa Y, Khosla MC, Fouad-Tarazi F, Sakura N, Paganini EP. Isolation of "myocardial depressant factor(s)" from the ultrafiltrate of heart failure patients with acute renal failure. ASAIO J. 1996;42:M911–M915. PMID: 8945020 [PubMed—indexed for MEDLINE]

[12] Meyer TW, Hostetter TH. Uremia. N Engl J Med. 2007;357:1316–1325. DOI: 10.1056/NEJMra071313.

[13] Figueras J, Stein L, Diez V, Weil MH, Shubin H. Relationship between pulmonary hemodynamics and arterial pH and carbon dioxide tension in critically ill patients. Chest. 1976;70:466–472. DOI: 10.1378/chest.70.4.466

[14] Brady JP, Hasbargen JA. Acid-base in renal failure: a review of the effects of correction of acidosis on nutrition in dialysis patients. Semin Dial. 2000;13:252–255. DOI: 10.1046/j.1525-139x.2000.00068.x.

[15] McCullough PA, Sandberg KR. Chronic kidney disease and sudden death: strategies for prevention. Blood Purif 2004;22:136–142. DOI: 10.1159/000074934.

[16] Pokhrel N, Maharjan N, Dhakal B, RR. Cardiorenal syndrome: A literature review. Exp Clin Cardiol. 2008;13:165–170. PMCID: PMC2663478

[17] Mahon NG, Blackstone EH, Francis GS, Starling RC 3rd, Young JB, Lauer MS. The prognostic value of estimated creatinine clearance alongside functional capacity in ambulatory patients with chronic congestive heart failure. J Am Coll Cardiol. 2002;40:1106–1113. DOI: 10.1016/S0735-1097(02)02125-3.

[18] Yancy CW, Lopatin M, Stevenson LW, De Marco T, Fonarow GC. ADHERE Scientific Advisory Committee and Investigators. Clinical presentation, management, and in-hospital outcomes of patients admitted with acute decompensated heart failure with preserved systolic function: a report from the Acute Decompensated Heart Failure National Registry (ADHERE) Database. J Am Coll Cardiol. 2006;47:76–84. DOI: 10.1016/j.jacc.2005.09.022.

[19] Strimbu K, Tavel JA. What are Biomarkers? Curr Opin HIV AIDS. 2010;5:463–466. DOI: 10.1097/COH.0b013e32833ed177.

[20] Biomarkers Definition Working Group. Biomarkers and surrogate endpoints: preferred definitions and conceptual framework. Clin Pharmacol Therapeutics. 2001;69:89–95. DOI: 10.1067/mcp.2001.113989

[21] Cheeseman KH, Slater TF. An introduction to free radicals chemistry. Br Med Bull. 1993;49:481–493. PMID: 8221017 [PubMed—indexed for MEDLINE].

[22] Young IS, Woodside JV. Antioxidants in health and disease. J Clin Pathol. 2001;54:176–186. DOI: 10.1136/jcp.54.3.176.

[23] Bagchi K, Puri S. Free radicals and antioxidants in health and disease. East Mediterranean Health J. 1998;4:350–360. http://applications.emro.who.int/emhj/0402/emhj_1998_4_2_350_360.pdf?ua=1.

[24] Liu T, Stern A, Roberts LJ, Morrow JD. The isoprostanes: novel prostanglandinlike products of the free radical catalyzed peroxidation of arachidonic acid. J Biomed Sci. 1999;6:226–235. DOI: 10.1159/000025391.

[25] Rock CL, Jacob RA, Bowen PE. Update o biological characteristics of the antioxidant micronutrients—Vitamin C, Vitamin E and the carotenoids. J Am Diet Assoc. 1996;96:693–702. DOI: 10.1016/S0002-8223(96)00190-3.

[26] Mc Cord JM. The evolution of free radicals and oxidative stress. Am J Med. 2000;108:652–659. DOI: 10.1016/S0002-9343(00)00412-5.

[27] Nangaku M, Fujita T. Activation of the renin-angiotensin system and chronic hypoxia of the kidney. Hypertens Res. 2008;31:175–184. DOI: 10.1291/hypres.31.175

[28] Rubattu S, Mennuni S, Testa M, Mennuni M, Pierelli G, Pagliaro B, Gabriele E, Coluccia R, Autore C, Volpe M. Pathogenesis of chronic cardiorenal syndrome: is there a role for oxidative stress? Int J Mol Sci. 2013;14:23011–23032. DOI: 10.3390/ijms141123011.

[29] Bongartz LG, Cramer JM, Doevendans PA, Joles JA, Braam B. The severe cardiorenal syndrome: "Guyton revisited." Eur Heart Jour. 2005;26:11–17.DOI: 10.1093/eurheartj/ehi020.

[30] Donato V, Lacquaniti A, Cernaro V, Lorenzano G, Trimboli D, Buemi A, Lupica R, Buemi M. From Water to aquaretics: a legendary route. Cell Physiol Biochem. 2014; 33:1369–1388. DOI: 10.1159/000358704.

[31] Wolf G, Wenzel U, Burns KD, Harris RC, Stahl RAK, Thaiss F. Angiotensin II activates nuclear transcription factor-kappaB through AT1 and AT2 receptors. Kidney Int. 2002;61:1986–1995. DOI: 10.1046/j.1523-1755.2002.00365.x.

[32] Wakui H, Dejima T, Tamura K, Uneda K, Azuma K, Maeda A, Ohsawa M, Kanaoka T, Azushima K, Kobayashi R, Matsuda M, Yamashita A, Umemura S. Activation of angiotensin II type 1 receptor-associated protein exerts an inhibitory effect on vascular hypertrophy and oxidative stress in angiotensin II-mediated hypertension. Cardiovasc Res. 2013; 100:511–519. DOI: 10.1093/cvr/cvt225.

[33] Schinzari F, Tesauro M, Rovella V, Adamo A, Mores N, Cardillo C. Co-existence of functional angiotensin II type 2 receptors mediating both vasoconstriction and vasodilation in humans. J Hypertension. 2011;29:1743–1748. DOI: 10.1097/HJH.0b013e328349ae0d.

[34] Pernomian L, Gomes MS, Restini CBA, Ramalho LNZ, Tirapelli CR, Oliveira AM. The role of reactive oxygen species in the modulation of the contraction induced by angiotensin II in carotid artery from diabetic rat. Eur Jour of Pharmacol. 2012;678:15–25. DOI: 10.1016/j.ejphar.2011.12.036.

[35] Patel KP, Mayhan WG, Bidasee KR, Zheng H. Enhanced angiotensin II-mediated central sympathoexcitation in streptozotocin-induced diabetes: role of superoxide anion. Am J Physiol Regul Integr Comp Physiol. 2011;300:311–320. DOI: 10.1152/ajpregu.00246.2010.

[36] Lavoie J, Sigmund CD. Minireview: overview of the renin-angiotensin system—endocrine and paracrine system. Endocrinology. 2003;144:2179–2183. DOI: 10.1210/en.2003-0150.

[37] Rahimi Z. The role of renin angiotensin aldosterone system genes in diabetic nephropathy. Can J Diabetes. 2015; pii:S1499-2671(15)00627-9. DOI: 10.1016/j.jcjd.2015.08.016.

[38] Reis WL, Saad WA, Camargo LA, Elias LLK, Rodrigues JA. Central nitrergic system regulation of neuroendocrine secretion, fluid intake and blood pressure induced by angiotensin-II. Behav Brain Funct. 2010;6:64–72. DOI: 10.1186/1744-9081-6-64.

[39] Touyz RM, Berry C. Recent advances in angiotensin II signaling. Braz J Med Biol Res. 2002;35:1001–1015. DOI: 10.1590/S0100-879X2002000900001.

[40] Berk BC, Corson MA. Angiotensin II signal transduction in vascular smooth muscle. Role of tyrosine kinases. Circ Res. 1997;80:607–616. DOI: 10.1161/01.RES.80.5.607.

[41] Calò LA, Schiavo S, Davis PA, Pagnin E, Mormino P, D'Angelo A, Pessina AC. Angiotensin II signaling via type 2 receptors in a human model of vascular hyporeactivity: implications for hypertension. J Hypertension 2010; 28:111–118. DOI: 10.1097/HJH.0b013e328332b738.

[42] Herichova I, Szantoova K. Renin-angiotensin system: upgrade of recent knowledge and perspectives. Endocr Regul. 2014;47:39–52. DOI: 10.4149/endo_2013_01_39

[43] Guimarães PB, Alvarenga EC, Siqueira PD, Paredes-Gamero EJ, Sabatini RA, Morais RLT, Reis RI, Santos EL, Teixeira LGD, Casarini DE, Martin RP, Shimuta SI, Carmona AK, Nakaie CR, Jasiulionis MG, Ferreira AT, Pesquero JL, Oliveira SM, Bader M, Costa-Neto CM, Pesquero JB. Angiotensin II binding to angiotensin I-converting enzyme triggers calcium signaling. Hypertension. 2011;57:965–972. DOI: 10.1161/HYPERTENSIONAHA.110.167171.

[44] Kim S, Iwao H. Molecular and cellular mechanisms of angiotensin II-mediated cardiovascular and renal diseases. Pharmacol Rev. 2000;52:11–34. http://intl.pharmrev.org/content/52/1/11.full.pdf. DOI: 0031-6997/11/5201-0011$03.00/0.

[45] Wolf G, Schneider A, Helmchen UM, Stahl RAK. AT1-receptor antagonists abolish glomerular MCP-1 expression in a model of mesangial proliferative glomerulonephritis. Exp Nephrol. 1998;6:112–120. DOI: 10.1159/000020513.

[46] Ruiz-Ortega M, Rupérez M, Esteban V, Sánchez-López E, Rodríguez-Vita J, Carvajal G, Egido J. Inflammation and chronic disease, 2006:1–25 ISBN: 81-7895-199-1. Editors: P. Esbrit and Mª. V. Alvarez-Arroyo. Transworld Research Network 37/661 (2), Fort P.O.,

Trivandrum-695 023, Kerala, India. http://www.trnres.com/ebook/uploads/esbritcontent/T_1231403182Esbrit%201.pdf.

[47] Chen XL, Tummala PE, Olbrych MT, Alexander RW, Medford RM. AngiotensinII induces monocyte chemo attractant protein-1 gene expression in rat vascular smooth muscle cells. Cir Res. 1998;83:952–959. DOI: 10.1161/01.RES.83.9.952.

[48] Wolf G, Ziyadeh FN, Thaiss F, Tomaszewski J, Caron RJ, Wenzel U, Zahner G, Helmchen U, Stahl RAK. Angiotensin II stimulates expression of the chemokine RANTES in rat glomerular endothelial cells. Role of the angiotensin type 2 receptor. J Clin Invest. 1997;100:1047–1058. DOI: 0021-9738/97/09/1047/12.

[49] Ushio-Fukai M, Griendling KK, Akers M, Lyons PR, Alexander RW. Temporal dispersion of activation of phospholipase C-beta 1 and -gamma isoforms by angiotensin II in vascular smooth muscle cells. Role of alphaq/11, alpha12, and beta gamma G protein subunits. J Biol Chem. 1998;273:19772–19777. DOI: 10.1074/jbc.273.31.19772.

[50] Alexander RW, Brock TA, Gimbrone-Jr MA, Rittenhouse SE. Angiotensin increases inositol trisphosphate and calcium in vascular smooth muscle. Hypertension. 1985;7:447–451. DOI: 10.1161/01.HYP.7.3.447

[51] Ushio-Fukai M, Alexander RW, Akers M, Lyons PR, Lassègue B & Griendling KK. Angiotensin II receptor coupling to phospholipase D is mediated by the ßg subunits of heterotrimeric G proteins in vascular smooth muscle cells. Mol Pharmacol. 1999;55:142–149. DOI: 10.1124/mol.55.1.142.

[52] Dhalla NS, Xu Y-J, Sheu S-S, Tappia PS, Panagia V. Phosphatidic acid: a potential signal transducer for cardiac hypertrophy. J Mol Cell Cardiol. 1997;29:2865–2871. DOI: 10.1006/jmcc.1997.0522.

[53] Touyz RM, Schiffrin EL. Ang II–stimulated superoxide production is mediated via phospholipase d in human vascular smooth muscle cells. Hypertension. 1999;34:976–982. DOI: 10.1161/01.HYP.34.4.976.

[54] Billah MM. Phospholipase D and cell signaling. Curr Opin Immunol. 1993;5:114–123. DOI: 10.1016/0952-7915(93)90090-F.

[55] Bonventre JV. Phospholipase A2 and signal transduction. J Am Soc Nephrol. 1992;3:128–150. http://jasn.asnjournals.org/content/3/2/128.full.pdf.

[56] Seshiah PN, Weber DS, Rocic P, Valppu L, Taniyama Y, and Griendling KK. Angiotensin II stimulation of NAD(P)H oxidase activity: upstream mediators. Circ Res. 2002;91:406 —413. DOI: 10.1161/01.RES.0000033523.08033.16.

[57] Touyz RM, Chen X, Tabet F, Yao G, He G, Quinn MT, Pagano PJ, Schiffrin EL. Expression of a functionally active gp91phox-containing neutrophil-type NAD(P)H oxidase in smooth muscle cells from human resistance arteries: regulation by angiotensin II. Circ Res. 2002; 90:1205—1213. DOI: 10.1161/01.RES.0000020404.01971.2F.

[58] Lassegue B, Alexander RW, Clark M, Griendling KK. Angiotensin II-induced phosphatidylcholine hydrolysis in cultured vascular smooth-muscle cells. Regulation and localization. Biochem J. 1991;276: 19–25. http://www.ncbi.nlm.nih.gov/pmc/articles/PMC1151137/pdf/biochemj00159-0028.pdf.

[59] Lassegue B, Clempus RE. Vascular NAD(P)H oxidases: specific features, expression, and regulation. Am J Physiol Regul Integr Comp Physiol. 2003;285:R277—R297. DOI: 10.1152/ajpregu.00758.2002.

[60] Touyz RM, Schiffrin EL. Increased generation of superoxide by angiotensin II in smooth muscle cells from resistance arteries of hypertensive patients: role of phospholipase D-dependent NAD(P)H oxidase-sensitive pathways. J Hypertens. 2001;19:1245–1254. PMID: 11446714 [PubMed—indexed for MEDLINE].

[61] Zafari AM, Ushio-Fukai M, Minieri CA, Akers M, Lassegue B, Griendling KK. Arachidonic acid metabolites mediate angiotensin II-induced NADH/NADPH oxidase activity and hypertrophy in vascular smooth muscle cells. Antioxid Redox Signal. 1999;1:167–179. PMID: 11228745 [PubMed—indexed for MEDLINE].

[62] Matsusaka T, Ichikawa I. Biological functions of angiotensin and its receptors. Annu Rev Physiol. 1997;59:395–412. DOI: 10.1146/annurev.physiol.59.1.395.

[63] Berk BC, Corson M. Angiotensin II signal transduction in vascular smooth muscle. Role of tyrosine kinases. Circul Res. 1997;80:607–616. DOI: 10.1161/01.RES.80.5.607.

[64] Sayeski PP, Ali MS, Harp JB, Marrero MB, Bernstein KE. Phosphorylation of p130Cas by angiotensin II is dependent on c-Src, intracellular Ca2+, and protein kinase C. Circul Res. 1998;82:1279–1288. DOI: 10.1161/01.RES.82.12.1279.

[65] Marrero MB, Schieffer B, Li B, Sun J, Harp JB, Ling BN. Role of Janus kinase/signal transducer and activator of transcription and mitogen-activated protein kinase cascades in angiotensin II and platelet-derived growth factor-induced vascular smooth muscle cell proliferation. J Biol Chem. 1997;272:24684–24690. DOI: 10.1074/jbc.272.39.24684.

[66] Leduc I, Meloche S. Angiotensin II stimulates tyrosine phosphorylation of the focal adhesion protein paxillin in aortic smooth muscle cells. J Biol Chem. 1995;270:4401–4404. DOI: 10.1074/jbc.270.9.4401.

[67] Takahashi T, Kawahara Y, Taniguchi T, Yokoyama M. Tyrosine phosphorylation and association of p130Cas and c-Crk II by Ang II in vascular smooth muscle cells. Am J Physiol. 1998;274:H1059–H1065. http://ajpheart.physiology.org/content/ajpheart/274/4/H1059.full.pdf.

[68] Takahashi T, Taniguchi T, Konishi H, Kikkawa U, Ishikawa Y, Yokoyama M. Activation of Akt/PKB after stimulation with Ang II in vascular smooth muscle cells. Am J Physiol. 1999;276:H1927–H1934. http://ajpheart.physiology.org/content/276/6/H1927.full-text.pdf+html.

[69] Touyz RM, He G, Deng LY, Schiffrin EL. Role of extracellular signal-regulated kinases in angiotensin II—stimulated contraction of smooth muscle cells from human resistance arteries. Circulation. 1999;99:392–399. DOI: 10.1161/01.CIR.99.3.392.

[70] Touyz RM, He G, El Mabrouk M, Diep Q, Mardigyan V, Schiffrin EL. Differential activation of extracellular signal-regulated protein kinase 1/2 and p38 mitogen activated-protein kinase by AT1 receptors in vascular smooth muscle cells from Wistar-Kyoto rats and spontaneously hypertensive rats. J Hypertens. 2001;19:553–559. DOI: 10.1097/00004872-200103001-00006.

[71] Robinson MJ, Cobb MH. Mitogen-activated protein kinase pathways. Curr Opin Cell Biol. 1997;9:180–186. DOI: 10.1016/S0955-0674(97)80061-0.

[72] Liao DF, Monia B, Dean N, Berk BC. Protein kinase C-zeta mediates angiotensin II activation of ERK1/2 in vascular smooth muscle cells. J Biol Chem. 1997;272:6146–6150. DOI: 10.1074/jbc.272.10.6146

[73] Ushio-Fukai M, Alexander RW, Akers M, Griendling KK. Mitogen activated protein kinase is a critical component of the redox-sensitive signaling pathways activated by angiotensin II. Role in vascular smooth muscle cell hypertrophy. J Biol Chem. 1998;273:15022–15029.DOI: 10.1074/jbc.273.24.15022.

[74] Laufs U, Liao JK. Targeting Rho in cardiovascular disease. Circul Res. 2000;87:526–528. DOI: 10.1161/01.RES.87.7.526.

[75] San Martin A, Griendling KK. NADPH oxidases: progress and opportunities. Antioxid Redox Signal. 2014;20:2692–2694. DOI: 10.1089/ars.2014.5947.

[76] Dickstein K, Cohen-Solal A, Filippatos G, McMurray JJV, Ponikowski P, Poole-Wilson PA, Strömberg A, van Veldhuisen DJ, Atar D, Hoes AW, Keren A, Mebazaa A, Nieminen M, Priori SG, Swedberg K, ESC Committee for Practice Guidelines (CPG). ESC guidelines for the diagnosis and treatment of acute and chronic heart failure. The Task Force for the Diagnosis and Treatment of Acute and Chronic Heart Failure 2008 of the European Society of Cardiology. Developed in collaboration with the Heart Failure Association of the ESC (HFA) and endorsed by the European Society of Intensive Care Medicine (ESICM). Eur Heart J. 2008;29:2388–2442. DOI: 10.1093/eurheartj/ehn309.

[77] Silverberg D, Wexler D, Blum M, Schwartz D, Adrian I. The association between congestive heart failure and chronic renal disease. Curr Opin Nephrol Hypertens. 2004;13:163–170. PMID: 15202610 [PubMed—indexed for MEDLINE].

[78] Joles JA, Koomans HA. Causes and consequences of increased sympathetic activity in renal disease. Hypertension. 2004;43:699–706. DOI: 10.1161/01.HYP.0000121881.77212.b1.

[79] Schrier RW, Abraham WT. Hormones and hemodynamics in heart failure. N Engl J Med. 1999;341:577–585. DOI: 10.1056/NEJM199908193410806.

[80] Guyton AC. The surprising kidney-fluid mechanism for pressure control—its infinite gain. Hypertension. 1990;16:725–730. DOI: 10.1161/01.HYP.16.6.725.

[81] Bongartz LG, Cramer MJ, Braam B: The cardiorenal connection. Hypertension. 2004;43:e14. DOI: 10.1161/01.HYP.0000118521.06245.b8.

[82] Viswanathan G, Scott G. The cardiorenal syndrome: making the connection. Int J Nephrol. 2001; ID:283137. http://dx.doi.org/10.4061/2011/283137.

[83] Brewster UC, Perazella MA. The renin-angiotensin-aldosterone system and the kidney: effects on kidney disease. Am J Med. 2004;116:263–272. DOI: 10.1016/j.amjmed.2003.09.034.

[84] Cadnapaphornchai MA, Gurevich AK, Weinberger HD, Schrier R.W. Pathophysiology of sodium and water retention in heart failure. Cardiology. 2001;96:122–131. DOI: 10.1159/000047396.

[85] Braam B, Koomans HA. Renal responses to antagonism of the renin-angiotensin system. Curr Opin Nephrol Hypertens. 1996;5:89–96. PMID: 8834166 [PubMed—indexed for MEDLINE]

[86] Griendling KK, Minieri CA, Ollerenshaw JD, Alexander RW. Angiotensin II stimulates NADH and NADPH oxidase activity in cultured vascular smooth muscle cells. Circ Res. 1994;74:1141–1148. DOI: 10.1161/01.RES.74.6.1141.

[87] Pedruzzi E, Guichard C, Ollivier V, Driss F, Fay M, Prunet C, Marie JC, Pouzet C, Samadi M, Elbim C, O'Dowd Y, Bens M, Vandewalle A, Gougerot-Pocidalo MA, Lizard G, Ogier-Denis E. NAD(P)H oxidase Nox-4 mediates 7-ketocholesterol-induced endoplasmic reticulum stress and apoptosis in human aortic smooth muscle cells. Mol Cell Biol. 2004;24:10703–10717. DOI: 10.1128/MCB.24.24.10703-10717.2004.

[88] Zhang H, Schmeisser A, Garlichs CD, Plotze K, Damme U, Mugge A, Daniel WG. Angiotensin II-induced superoxide anion generation in human vascular endothelial cells: role of membrane-bound NADH-/NADPH-oxidases. Cardiovasc Res. 2009;44:215–222. DOI: 10.1016/S0008-6363(99)00183-2.

[89] Hishikawa K, Luscher TF. Pulsatile stretch stimulates superoxide production in human aortic endothelial cells. Circulation. 1997;96:3610–3616. DOI: 10.1161/01.CIR.96.10.3610.

[90] Hishikawa K, Oemar BS, Yang Z, Luscher TF. Pulsatile stretch stimulates superoxide production and activates nuclear factor-kB in human coronary smooth muscle cells. Circ Res. 1997;81:797–803. DOI: 10.1161/01.RES.81.5.797.

[91] Mohazzab KM, Wolin MS. Sites of superoxide anion production detected by lucigenin in calf pulmonary artery smooth muscle. Am J Physiol. 1994;267:H2568–H2572. PMID: 7810685 [PubMed—indexed for MEDLINE].

[92] Rajagopalan S, Kurz S, Munzel T, Tarpey NI, Freeman BA, Griendling KK, Harrison DG. Angiotensin II-mediated hypertension in the rat increases vascular superoxide

production via membrane NADH/NADPH oxidase activation: contribution to alterations of vasomotor tone. J Clin Invest. 1996;97:1916–1923. DOI: 10.1172/JCI118623.

[93] Ushio-Fukai M, Zafari AM, Fukui T Ishizaka N, Griendling KK. p22phox is a critical component of the superoxide-generating NADH/NADPH oxidase system and regulates angiotensin II-induced hypertrophy in vascular smooth muscle cells. J Biol Chem. 1996;271:23317–23321. DOI: 10.1074/jbc.271.38.23317

[94] Chabrashvili T, Kitiyakara C, Blau J, Karber A, Aslam S, Welch WJ, Wilcox CS. Effects of ANG II type 1 and 2 receptors on oxidative stress, renal NADPH oxidase, and SOD expression. Am J Physiol Regul Integr Comp Physiol. 2003;285:R117–R124. DOI: 10.1152/ajpregu.00476.2002.

[95] Nakagami H, Takemoto M, Liao JK. NADPH oxidase-derived superoxide anion mediates angiotensin II-induced cardiac hypertrophy. J Mol Cell Cardiol. 2003;35:851–859.DOI: 10.1016/S0022-2828(03)00145-7.

[96] Radeke HH, Cross AR, Hancock JT, Jones OT, Nakamura Ni, Kaever V, Resch K. Functional expression of NADPH oxidase components (α- and β-subunits of cytochrome b558 and 45-kDa flavoprotein) by intrinsic human glomerular mesangial cells. J Biol Chem. 1991;266:21025–21029. PMID: 1657945 [PubMed—indexed for MEDLINE] http://www.jbc.org/content/266/31/21025.full.pdf.

[97] Fukui T, Lassegue B, Kai H, Alexander RW, Griendling KK. Cytochrome b-558 α-subunit cloning and expression in rat aortic smooth muscle cells. Biochim Biophys Acta. 1995;1231:215–219. DOI: 10.1016/0005-2728(95)00098-4.

[98] Suh YA, Arnold RS, Lassegue B, Shi J, Xu X, Sorescu D, Chung AB, Griendling KK, Lambeth JD. Cell transformation by the superoxide-generating oxidase Mox1. Nature. 1999;401:79–82. DOI: 10.1038/43459.

[99] Jones SA, O'Donnell VB, Wood JD, Broughton JP, Hughes EJ, Jones OT. Expression of phagocyte NADPH oxidase components in human endothelial cells. Am J Physiol. 1996;271:H1626–H1634. PMID: 8897960 [PubMed—indexed for MEDLINE].

[100] Greiber S, Munzel T, Kastner S, Muller B, Schollmeyer P, Pavenstädt H. NAD(P)H oxidase activity in cultured human podocytes: effects of adenosine triphosphate. Kidney Int. 1998;53:654–663.DOI: 10.1046/j.1523-1755.1998.00796.x.

[101] Geiszt M, Kopp JB, Varnai P, Leto TL. Identification of renox, an NAD(P)H oxidase in kidney. Proc Natl Acad Sci U S A. 2000;9:8010–8014. DOI: 10.1073/pnas.130135897.

[102] Pagano PJ, Clark JK, Cifuentes-Pagano ME, Clark SM, Callis GM, Quinn MT. Localization of a constitutively active, phagocyte-like NADPH oxidase in rabbit aortic adventitia: enhancement by angiotensin II. Proc Natl Acad Sci U S A. 1997;94:14483–14488.

[103] Babior BM. NADPH oxidase: an update. Blood. 1999;93:1464–1476. PMID: 10029572 [PubMed—indexed for MEDLINE]. 0006-4971/99/9305-0033$3.00/0.

[104] Katoh M, Egashira K, Usui M, Ichiki T, Tomita H, Shimokawa H, Rakugi H, Takeshita A. Cardiac angiotensin II receptors are upregulated by long-term inhibition of nitric oxide synthesis in rats. Circ Res. 1998;83:743–751. DOI: 10.1161/01.RES.83.7.743.

[105] Chabrashvili T, Tojo A, Onozato ML, Kitiyakara C, Quinn MT, Fujita T, Welch WJ, Wilcox CS. Expression and cellular localization of classic NADPH oxidase subunits in the spontaneously hypertensive rat kidney. Hypertension. 2002;39:269–274. DOI: 10.1161/hy0202.103264.

[106] Racusen LC, Prozialeck DH, Solez K. Glomerular epithelial cell changes after ischemia or dehydration. Possible role of angiotensin II. Am J Pathol. 1984;114:157–163. PMCID: PMC1900389.

[107] Liebau MC, Lang D, Bohm J, Endlich N, Bek MJ, Witherden I, Mathieson PW, Saleem MA, Pavenstädt H, Fischer KG. Functional expression of the renin-angiotensin system in human podocytes. Am J Physiol Renal Physiol. 2006;290:F710–F719. DOI: 10.1152/ajprenal.00475.2004.

[108] Hoffmann S, Podlich D, Hahnel B, Kriz W, Gretz N. Angiotensin II type 1 receptor overexpression in podocytes induces glomerulosclerosis in transgenic rats. J Am Soc Nephrol. 2004;15:1475–1487. DOI: 10.1097/01.ASN.0000127988.42710.A7

[109] Shibata S, Nagase M, Yoshida S, Kawachi H, Fujita T. Podocyte as the target for aldosterone: roles of oxidative stress and Sgk1. Hypertension. 2007;49:355–364. DOI: 10.1161/01.HYP.0000255636.11931.a2.

[110] Nagase M, Yoshida S, Shibata S, Nagase T, Gotoda T, Ando K, Fujita T. Enhanced aldosterone signaling in the early nephropathy of rats with metabolic syndrome: possible contribution of fat-derived factors. J Am Soc Nephrol. 2006;17:3438–3446. DOI: 10.1681/ASN.2006080944.

[111] Beswick RA, Zhang H, Marable D, Catravas JD, Hill WD, Webb RC. Long-term antioxidant administration attenuates mineralocorticoid hypertension and renal inflammatory response. Hypertension. 2001;37:781–781. DOI: 10.1161/01.HYP.37.2.781.

[112] Rapp JP. Dahl salt-susceptible and salt-resistant rats. Hypertension. 1982;4:753–763. http://hyper.ahajournals.org/content/4/6/753.full.pdf.

[113] Tojo A, Onozato ML, Kobayashi N, Goto A, Matsuoka H, Fujita T. Angiotensin II and oxidative stress in Dahl Salt-sensitive rat with heart failure. Hypertension. 2002;40:834–839. DOI: 10.1161/01.HYP.0000039506.43589.D5.

[114] Heymes C, Bendall JK, Ratajczak P, Cave AC, Samuel JL, Hasenfuss G, Shah AM. Increased myocardial NADPH oxidase activity in human heart failure. J Am Coll Cardiol. 2003;41:2164–2171. DOI: 10.1016/S0735-1097(03)00471-6.

[115] Hornig B, Landmesser U, Kohler C, Ahlersmann D, Spiekermann S, Christoph A, Tatge H, Drexler H. Comparative effect of ace inhibition and angiotensin II type 1 receptor antagonism on bioavailability of nitric oxide in patients with coronary artery disease:

role of superoxide dismutase. Circulation. 2001;103:799–805. DOI: 10.1161/01.CIR.103.6.799.

[116] Ruiz-Ortega M, Lorenzo O, Egido J. Angiotensin III increases MCP-1 and activates NF-kappaB and AP-1 in cultured mesangial and mononuclear cells. Kidney Int. 2000;57:2285–2298. DOI: 10.1046/j.1523-1755.2000.00089.x.

[117] Pueyo ME, Gonzalez W, Nicoletti A, Savoie F, Arnal JF, Michel JB. Angiotensin II stimulates endothelial vascular cell adhesion molecule-1 via nuclear factor-kappaB activation induced by intracellular oxidative stress. Arterioscler Thromb Vasc Biol. 2000;20:645–651. DOI: 10.1161/01.ATV.20.3.645.

[118] Reid IA. Interactions between ANG II, sympathetic nervous system, and baroreceptor reflexes in regulation of blood pressure. Am J Physiol. 1992;262:E763–E778. http://ajpendo.physiology.org/content/ajpendo/262/6/E763.full.pdf.

[119] Converse RL Jr, Jacobsen TN, Toto RD, Jost CMT, Cosentino F, Fouad-Tarazi F, Victor RG. Sympathetic overactivity in patients with chronic renal failure. N Engl J Med. 1992;327:1912–1918. DOI: 10.1056/NEJM199212313272704.

[120] Ligtenberg G, Blankestijn PJ, Oey PL, Klein IHH, Dijkhorst-Oei LT, Boomsma F, Wieneke GH, van Huffelen AC, Koomans HA. Reduction of sympathetic hyperactivity by enalapril in patients with chronic renal failure. N Engl J Med. 1999;340:1321–1328. DOI: 10.1056/NEJM199904293401704.

[121] Klein IH, Ligtenberg G, Oey PL, Koomans HA, Blankestijn PJ. Enalapril and losartan reduce sympathetic hyperactivity in patients with chronic renal failure. J Am Soc Nephrol. 2003;14:425–430. DOI: 10.1097/01.ASN.0000045049.72965.B7.

[122] Zhang W, Huang BS, Leenen FH. Brain renin-angiotensin system and sympathetic hyperactivity in rats after myocardial infarction. Am J Physiol. 1999;276:H1608–H1615. PMID: 10330245 [PubMed—indexed for MEDLINE].

[123] Lin HH, Chen CH, Hsieh WK, Chiu TH, Lai CC. Hydrogen peroxide increases the activity of rat sympathetic preganglionic neurons in vivo and in vitro. Neuroscience. 2003;121:641–647. DOI: 10.1016/S0306-4522(03)00517-7.

[124] Shokoji T, Nishiyama A, Fujisawa Y, Hitomi H, Kiyomoto H, Takahashi N, Kimura S, Kohno M, Abe Y. Renal sympathetic nerve responses to tempol in spontaneously hypertensive rats. Hypertension. 2003;41:266–273. DOI: 10.1161/01.HYP.0000049621.85474.CF.

[125] Chen L, Knowlton AA. Mitochondrial dynamics in heart failure. Congest Heart Fail. 2010;17:257–261. DOI: 10.1016/j.bbamcr.2012.03.008.

[126] Stanley WC, Chandler MP. Energy metabolism in the normal and failing heart: potential for therapeutic interventions. Heart Fail Rev. 2002;7:115–130. DOI: 10.1023/A:1015320423577.

[127] Beer M, Seyfarth T, Sandstede J, Landschütz W, Lipke C, Köstler H, von Kienlin M, Harre K, Hahn D, Neubauer S. Absolute concentrations of high-energy phosphate metabolites in normal, hypertrophied, and failing human myocardium measured noninvasively with (31)P-SLOOP magnetic resonance spectroscopy. J Am Coll Cardiol. 2002;40:1267–1274. DOI: 10.1016/S0735-1097(02)02160-5.

[128] Conway MA, Allis, J. Ouwerkerk R, Niioka T, Rajagopalan B, Radda GK. Detection of low phosphocreatine to ATP ratio in failing hypertrophied human myocardium by 31P magnetic resonance spectroscopy. Lancet. 1991;338:973–976. DOI: 10.1016/0140-6736(91)91838-L.

[129] Tian R, Nascimben L, Kaddurah-Daouk R, Ingwall JS. Depletion of energy reserve via the creatine kinase reaction during the evolution of heart failure in cardiomyopathic hamsters. J Mol Cell Cardiol. 1996;28:755–765. DOI: 10.1006/jmcc.1996.0070.

[130] Kato T, Niizuma S, Inuzuka Y, Kawashima T, Okuda J, Tamaki Y, Iwanaga Y, Narazak M, Matsuda T, Soga T, Kita T, Kimura T, Shioi T. Analysis of metabolic remodeling in compensated left ventricular hypertrophy and heart failure. Circ Heart Fail. 2010;3:420–430. DOI: 10.1161/CIRCHEARTFAILURE.109.888479

[131] Lei B, Lionetti V, Young ME, Chandler MP, d'Agostino C, Kang E, Altarejos M, Matsuo K, Hintze TH, Stanley WC, Recchia FA. Paradoxical downregulation of the glucose oxidation pathway despite enhanced flux in severe heart failure. J Mol Cell Cardiol. 2004;36:567–576. DOI: 10.1016/j.yjmcc.2004.02.004.

[132] Katz AM, Konstam MA. Heart failure : pathophysiology, molecular biology, and clinical management (2nd ed.). Philadelphia: Wolters Kluwer Health/Lippincott Williams & Wilkins; 2009. ISBN 978-0781769464.

[133] Scheubel RJ, Tostlebe M, Simm A, Rohrbach S, Prondzinsky R, Gellerich FN, Silber RE, Holtz J. Dysfunction of mitochondrial respiratory chain complex I in human failing myocardium is not due to disturbed mitochondrial gene expression. J Am Coll Cardiol. 2002;40:2174–2181. DOI: 10.1016/S0735-1097(02)02600-1

[134] Lemieux H, Semsroth S, Antretter H, Höfer D, Gnaiger E. Mitochondrial respiratory control and early defects of oxidative phosphorylation in the failing human heart. Int J Biochem Cell Biol. 2011;43:1729–1738. DOI: 10.1016/j.biocel.2011.08.008.

[135] Buchwald A, Till H, Unterberg C, Oberschmidt R, Figulla HR, Wiegand V. Alterations of the mitochondrial respiratory chain in human dilated cardiomyopathy. Eur Heart J. 1990;11:509–516. http://dx.doi.org/ 509-516.

[136] Marin-Garcia J, Goldenthal J, Mo GW. Mitochondrial pathology in cardiac failure. Cardiovasc Res. 2001;49:17–26. DOI: 10.1016/S0008-6363(00)00241-8.

[137] Rosca MG, Vazquez EJ, Kerner J, Parland W, Chandler MP, Stanley W, Sabbah HN, Hoppel CL. Cardiac mitochondria in heart failure: Decrease in respirasomes and oxidative phosphorylation. Cardiovasc Res. 2008;80:30–39. DOI: 10.1093/cvr/cvn184.

[138] Touyz RM, Briones AM, Sedeek M, Burger D, Montezano AC. NOX Isoforms and reactive oxygen species in vascular health. Mol Interv. 2011;11:27–35. DOI: 10.1124/mi. 11.1.5.

[139] Kimura S, Zhang GX, Nishiyama A, Shokoji T, Yao L, Fan YY, Rahman M, Suzuki T, Maeta H, Abe Y. Role of NAD (P) H oxidase-and mitochondria-derived reactive oxygen species in cardioprotection of ischemic reperfusion injury by angiotensin II. Hypertension. 2005;45:860–866. DOI: 10.1161/01.HYP.0000163462.98381.7f.

[140] Dai DF, Johnson SC, Villarin JJ, Chin MT, Nieves-Cintrón M, Chen T, Marcinek DJ, Dorn GW, Kang YJ, Prolla TA, Santana LF, Rabinovitch PS. Mitochondrial oxidative stress mediates angiotensin II–induced cardiac hypertrophy and Gαq overexpression–induced heart failure. Novelty and significance. Circ Res. 2011;108:837–846. DOI: 10.1161/CIRCRESAHA.110.232306.

[141] Marín-García J, Akhmedov AT, Moe GW. Mitochondria in heart failure: the emerging role of mitochondrial dynamics. Heart Fail Rev. 2013;18:439–456. DOI: 10.1007/ s10741-012-9330-2.

[142] Jackson G, Gibbs CR, Davies MK, Lip GYH. ABC of heart failure: pathophysiology. BMJ. 2000;320:167–170. DOI: 10.1136/bmj.320.7228.167.

[143] Rosca MG, Hoppel CL. New aspects of impaired mitochondrial function in heart failure. J Bioenerg Biomembr. 2009;41:107–112. DOI: 10.1007/s10863-009-9215-9.

[144] Siwik DA, Pagano PJ, Colucci WS. Oxidative stress regulates collagen synthesis and matrix metalloproteinase activity in cardiac fibroblasts. Am J Physiol Cell Physiol. 2001;280:C53–C60. PMID: 11121376 [PubMed—indexed for MEDLINE].

[145] Aranapakam V, Grosu GT, Davis JM, Hu B, Ellingboe J, Baker JL, Skotnicki JS, Zask A, DiJoseph JF, Sung A, Sharr MA, Killar LM, Walter T, Jin G, Cowling RJ. Synthesis and structure-activity relationship of alpha-sulfonylhydroxamic acids as novel, orally active matrix metalloproteinase inhibitors for the treatment of osteoarthritis. Med Chem. 2003; 46:2361–2375. DOI: 10.1021/jm0205548.

[146] Engel CK, Pirard B, Schimanski S, Kirsch R, Habermann J, Klingler O, Schlotte V, Weithmann KU, Wendt KU. Structural basis for the highly selective inhibition of MMP-13. Chem Biol. 2005;12:181–189. DOI: 10.1016/j.chembiol.2004.11.014.

[147] Amin EA, Welsh WJ. Three-dimensional quantitative structure-activity relationship (3D-QSAR) models for a novel class of piperazine-based stromelysin-1 (MMP-3) inhibitors: applying a "divide and conquer" strategy. J Med Chem. 2001;44:3849–3855. DOI: CHEMBL1134678.

[148] Raspollini MR, Castiglione F, Degl'Innocenti DR, Garbini F, Coccia ME, Taddei GL. Difference in expression of matrix metalloproteinase-2 and matrix metalloproteinase-9 in patients with persistent ovarian cysts. Fertil Steril. 2005;84:1049–1052. DOI: 10.1016/ j.fertnstert.2005.02.058.

[149] Venkatesan AM, Davis JM, Grosu GT, Baker J, Zask A, Levin JI, Ellingboe J, Skotnicki JS, DiJoseph JF, Sung A, Jin G, Xu W, McCarthy DJ, Barone D. Synthesis and structure–activity relationships of 4-alkynyloxy phenyl sulfanyl, sulfinyl, and sulfonyl alkyl hydroxamates as tumor necrosis factor-α converting enzyme and matrix metalloproteinase inhibitor. J Med Chem. 2004;47:6255–6269. DOI: 10.1021/jm040086x.

[150] Woessner JF Jr. Matrix metalloproteinases and their inhibitors in connective tissue remodeling. FASEB J 1991;5:2145–2154. http://www.fasebj.org/content/5/8/2145.full.pdf.

[151] Dounousi E, Papavasiliou E, Makedou A, Ioannou K, Katopodis KP, Tselepis A, Siamopoulos KC, Tsakiris D. Oxidative stress is progressively enhanced with advancing stages of CKD. Am J Kidney Dis. 2006;48:752–760. DOI: 10.1053/j.ajkd.2006.08.015.

[152] Oberg BP, McMenamin E, Lucas FL, McMonagle E, Morrow J, Ikizler TA, Himmelfarb J. Increased prevalence of oxidant stress and inflammation in patients with moderate to severe chronic kidney disease. Kidney Int. 2004;65:1009–1016. DOI: 10.1111/j.1523-1755.2004.00465.x.

[153] Nerpin E, Helmersson-Karlqvist J, Risérus U, Sundström J, Larsson A, Jobs E, Basu S, Ingelsson E, Arnlöv. J. Inflammation, oxidative stress, glomerular filtration rate, and albuminuria in elderly men: a cross-sectional study. BMC Res. Notes 2012;5:537. DOI: 10.1186/1756-0500-5-537.

[154] Shlipak MG, Fried LF, Crump C, Bleyer AJ, Manolio TA, Tracy RP, Furberg CD, Psaty BM. Elevations of inflammatory and procoagulant biomarkers in elderly persons with renal insufficiency. Circulation 2003;107:87–92. DOI: 10.1161/01.CIR.0000042700.48769.59.

[155] Stuveling EM, Hillege HL, Bakker SJ, Gans RO, de Jong PE, de Zeeuw D. C-reactive protein is associated with renal function abnormalities in a non-diabetic population. Kidney Int. 2003;63:654–661. DOI: 10.1046/j.1523-1755.2003.00762.x.

[156] Ikizler TA, Morrow JD, Roberts LJ, Evanson JA, Becke B, Hakim RM, Shyr Y, Himmelfarb J. Plasma F2-isoprostane levels are elevated in chronic hemodialysis patients. Clin Nephrol. 2002;58:190–197. DOI: 10.5414/CNP58190.

[157] Nagase M. Activation of the aldosterone/mineralocorticoid receptor system in chronic kidney disease and metabolic syndrome. Clin Exp Nephrol. 2010;14:303–314. DOI: 10.1007/s10157-010-0298-8.

[158] Raij L. Workshop: hypertension and cardiovascular risk factors: role of the angiotensin II-nitric oxide interaction. Hypertension. 2001;37:767–773. DOI: 10.1161/01.HYP.37.2.767.

[159] Zou AP, Li N, Cowley AW. Production and actions of superoxide in the renal medulla. Hypertension 2001;37:547–553. DOI: 10.1161/01.HYP.37.2.547.

[160] Chabrashvili T, Tojo A, Onozato ML, Kitiyakara C, Quinn MT, Fujita T, Welch WJ, Wilcox CS. Expression and cellular localization of classic NADPH oxidase subunits in

the spontaneously hypertensive rat kidney. Hypertension. 2002;39:269–274. DOI: 10.1161/hy0202.103264.

[161] Geiszt M, Kopp JB, Várnai P, Leto TL. Identification of renox, an NAD (P) H oxidase in kidney. Proc Natl Acad Sci U S A. 2000;97:8010–8014. DOI: 10.1073/pnas.130135897.

[162] Shiose A, Kuroda J, Tsuruya K, Hirai M, Hirakata H, Naito S, Hattori M, Sakaki Y, Sumimoto H. A novel superoxide-producing NAD (P) H oxidase in kidney. J Biol Chem. 2001;276:1417–1423. DOI: 10.1074/jbc.M007597200.

[163] Cheng G, Cao Z, Xu X, Meir EGV, Lambeth JD. Homologs of gp91phox: cloning and tissue expression of Nox3, Nox4, and Nox5. Gene. 2001;269:131–140. DOI: 10.1016/S0378-1119(01)00449-8.

[164] Bedard K, Krause KH. The NOX family of ROS-generating NADPH oxidases: Physiology and pathophysiology. Physiol Rev. 2007;87:245–313. DOI: 10.1152/physrev.00044.2005.

[165] Gorin Y, Ricono JM, Kim NH, Bhandari B, Choudhury GG, Abboud HE. Nox4 mediates angiotensin II-induced activation of Akt/protein kinase B in mesangial cells. Am J Physiol Ren Physiol. 2003;285: F219–F229. DOI: 10.1152/ajprenal.00414.2002.

[166] Raij L. Nitric oxide and cardiovascular and renal effects. Osteoarthr Cartil. 2008;16:S21–S26. DOI: 10.1016/S1063-4584(08)60009-6.

[167] Mayer B, Pfeiffer S, Schrammel A, Koesling D, Schmidt K, Brunner F. A new pathway of nitric oxide/cyclic GMP signaling involving S-nitrosoglutathione. J Biol Chem. 1998;273:3264–3270. DOI: 10.1074/jbc.273.6.3264.

[168] Gladwin MT, Schechter AN, Kim-Shapiro DB, Patel RP, Hogg N, Shiva S, Cannon RO, Kelm M, Wink DA, Espey MG, Oldfield EH, Pluta RM, Freeman BA, Lancaster Jr JR, Feelisch M, Lundberg JO. The emerging biology of the nitrite anion. Nat Chem Biol 2005;1:308–314. DOI: 10.1038/nchembio1105-308.

[169] Kelm M, Dahmann R, Wink D, Feelisch M. The nitric oxide/superoxide assay. Insights into the biological chemistry of the NO/O-2. interaction. J Biol Chem 1997;272:9922–9932. http://www.jbc.org/content/272/15/9922.full.pdf+html.

[170] Wilcox CS. Redox regulation of the afferent arteriole and tubuloglomerular feedback. Acta Physiol Scand. 2003;179,217–223. DOI: 10.1046/j.0001-6772.2003.01205.x.

[171] López B, Salom MG, Arregui B, Valero F, Fenoy FJ. Role of superoxide in modulating the renal effects of angiotensin II. Hypertension. 2003;42:1150–1156. DOI: 10.1161/01.HYP.0000101968.09376.79.

[172] Liaudet L, Soriano FG, Szabó C. Biology of nitric oxide signaling. Crit Care Med. 2000;28:N37–N52. DOI: 10.1097/00003246-200004001-00005.

[173] Schnackenberg CG. Physiological and pathophysiological roles of oxygen radicals in the renal microvasculature. Am J Physiol Regul Integr Comp Physiol. 2002;282:R335–R342. DOI: 10.1152/ajpregu.00605.2001.

[174] Lodha S, Dani D, Mehta R, Bhaskaran M, Reddy K, Ding G, Singhal PC. Angiotensin II-induced mesangial cell apoptosis: role of oxidative stress. Mol Med. 2002;8:830–840. PMC2039960/pdf/12606818.pdf.

[175] Gorin Y, Ricono J, Wagner B, Kim N, Bhandari B, Choudhury G, Abboud H. Angiotensin II-induced ERK1/ERK2 activation and protein synthesis are redox-dependent in glomerular mesangial cells. Biochem J. 2004;381:231–239. DOI: 10.1042/BJ20031614.

[176] Rhyu DY, Yang Y, Ha H, Lee GT, Song JS, Uh ST, Lee HB. Role of reactive oxygen species in TGF-β1-induced mitogen-activated protein kinase activation and epithelial-mesenchymal transition in renal tubular epithelial cells. J Am Soc Nephrol. 2005;16:667–675. DOI: 10.1681/ASN.2004050425.

[177] Thiery JP, Sleeman JP. Complex networks orchestrate epithelial–mesenchymal transitions. Nat Rev Mol Cell Biol. 2006;7:131–142. DOI: 10.1038/nrm1835.

[178] Ng YY, Huang TP, Yang WC, Chen ZP, Yang AH, Mu W, Nikolic-Paterso DJ, Atkins RC, Lan HY. Tubular epithelial-myofibroblast transdifferentiation in progressive tubulointerstitial fibrosis in 5/6 nephrectomized rats. Kidney Int. 1998;54:864–876. DOI: 10.1046/j.1523-1755.1998.00076.x.

[179] Iwano M, Plieth D, Danoff TM, Xue C, Okada H, Neilson EG. Evidence that fibroblasts derive from epithelium during tissue fibrosis. J Clin Investig. 2002;110:341–350. DOI: 10.1172/JCI15518.

[180] Napoli C, Casamassimi A, Crudele V, Infante T, Abbondanza C. Kidney and heart interactions during cardiorenal syndrome: a molecular and clinical pathogenic framework. Future Cardiol. 2011;7:485–497. DOI: 10.2217/fca.11.24.

[181] Kalluri R, Weinberg RA. The basics of epithelial-mesenchymal transition. J Clin Investig. 2009;119:1420–1428. DOI: 10.1172/JCI39104.

[182] Yoshikawa M, Hishikawa K, Marumo T, Fujita T. Inhibition of histone deacetylase activity suppresses epithelial-to-mesenchymal transition induced by TGF-β1 in human renal epithelial cells. J Am Soc Nephrol. 2007;18:58–65. DOI: 10.1681/ASN.2005111187.

[183] Yang J, Liu Y. Dissection of key events in tubular epithelial to myofibroblast transition and its implications in renal interstitial fibrosis. Am J Pathol. 2001;159:1465–1475. DOI: 10.1016/S0002-9440(10)62533-3.

[184] Mezzano SA, Ruiz-Ortega M, Egido J. Angiotensin II and renal fibrosis. Hypertension. 2001;38:635–638. DOI: 10.1161/hy09t1.094234.

[185] Dorsam G, Tahe MM, Valerie KC, Kuemmerle NB, Chan JC, Franson RC. Diphenyleneiodium chloride blocks inflammatory cytokine-induced up-regulation of group IIA

phospholipase A2 in rat mesangial cells. J Pharmacol Exp Ther. 2000;292:271–279. http://jpet.aspetjournals.org/content/292/1/271.full.pdf

[186] Satriano JA, Shuldiner M, Hora K, Xing Y, Shan Z, Schlondorff D. Oxygen radicals as second messengers for expression of the monocyte chemoattractant protein, JE/MCP-1, and the monocyte colony-stimulating factor, CSF-1, in response to tumor necrosis factor-alpha and immunoglobulin G. Evidence for involvement of reduced nicotinamide adenine dinucleotide phosphate (NADPH)-dependent oxidase. J Clin Investig 1993;92:1564–1571. DOI: 10.1172/JCI116737.

[187] Feng L, Xia Y, Garcia GE, Hwang D, Wilson CB. Involvement of reactive oxygen intermediates in cyclooxygenase-2 expression induced by interleukin-1, tumor necrosis factor-alpha, and lipopolysaccharide. J Clin Investig. 1995;95:1669–1675. DOI: 10.1172/JCI117842

[188] Cui XL, Douglas JG. Arachidonic acid activates c-jun N-terminal kinase through NADPH oxidase in rabbit proximal tubular epithelial cells. Proc Natl Acad Sci USA. 1997;94:3771–3776. PMCID: PMC20516.

[189] Rousset S, Alves-Guerra MC, Mozo J, Miroux B, Cassard-Doulcier AM, Bouillaud F, and Ricquier D. The biology of mitochondrial uncoupling proteins. Diabetes. 2004;53:130–135. DOI: 10.2337/diabetes.53.2007.S130.

[190] Di Castro, S.; Scarpino, S.; Marchitti, S.; Bianchi, F.; Stanzione, R.; Cotugno, M.; Sironi, L.; Gelosa, P.; Duranti, E.; Ruco, L., Volpe M, Rubattu S. Differential modulation of UCP2 in kidneys of stroke-prone spontaneously hypertensive rats under high salt/low potassium diet. Hypertension 2013, 61, 534–541. DOI: 10.1161/HYPERTENSIONAHA.111.00101.

[191] Yoshida T, Kato K, Fujimak T, Yokoi K, Oguri M, Watanabe S, Metoki N, Yoshida H, Satoh K, Aoyagi Y, Nishigaki Y, Tanaka M, Nozawa Y, Kimura G, Yamada Y. Association of genetic variants with chronic kidney disease in Japanese individuals. Clin J Am Soc Nephrol. 2009;4:883–890. DOI: 10.2215/CJN.04350808.

[192] Metra M, Davison B, Bettari L, Sun H, Edwards C, Lazzarini V, Piovanelli B, Carubelli V, Bugatti S, Lombardi C, Cotter G, Dei Cas L. Is worsening renal function an ominous prognostic sign in patients with acute heart failure? The role of congestion and its interaction with renal function. Circ Heart Fail. 2012;5:54–62. DOI: 10.1161/CIRCHEARTFAILURE.111.963413.

[193] Bayeva M, Gheorghiade M, Ardehali H. Mitochondria as a therapeutic target in heart failure. J Am Coll Cardiol. 2013;61:599–610. DOI: 10.1016/j.jacc.2012.08.1021.

[194] Chen K, Keaney JF. Evolving concepts of oxidative stress and reactive oxygen species in cardiovascular disease. Curr Atheroscler Rep. 2012;14:476–483. DOI: 10.1007/s11883-012-0266-8.

[195] Fassett RG, Venuthurupalli SK, Gobe GC, Coombes JS, Cooper MA, Hoy WE. Biomarkers in chronic kidney disease: a review. Kidney Int. 2011;80:806–821; DOI: 10.1038/ki.2011.198.

[196] Sun M, Dawood F, Wen WH, Chen M, Dixon I, Kirshenbaum LA, Liu PP. Excessive tumor necrosis factor activation after infarction contributes to susceptibility of myocardial rupture and left ventricular dysfunction. Circulation. 2004;110:3221–3228. DOI: 10.1161/01.CIR.0000147233.10318.23.

[197] Liu P, Sun M, Sader S. Matrix metalloproteinases in cardiovascular disease. Can J Cardiol. 2006;22:25B–30B. PMCID: PMC2780831.

[198] Stewart JA Jr, Wei CC, Brower GL, Rynders PE, Hankes GH, Dillon AR, Lucchesi PA, Janicki JS, Dell'Italia LJ. Cardiac mast cell- and chymase-mediated matrix metalloproteinase activity and left ventricular remodeling in mitral regurgitation in the dog. J Mol Cell Cardiol. 2003;35:311–319. DOI: 10.1016/S0022-2828(03)00013-0.

[199] Spinale FG, Coker ML, Thomas CV, Walker JD, Mukherjee R, Hebbar L. Time-dependent changes in matrix metalloproteinase activity and expression during the progression of congestive heart failure relation to ventricular and myocyte function. Circ Res. 1998;82:482–495. DOI: 10.1161/01.RES.82.4.482.

[200] Matsushima S, Ide T, Yamato M, Matsusaka H, Hattori F, Ikeuchi M, Kubota T, Sunagawa K, Hasegawa Y, Kurihara T, Oikawa S, Kinugawa S, Tsutsui H. Overexpression of mitochondrial peroxiredoxin-3 prevents left ventricular remodeling and failure after myocardial infarction in mice. Circulation. 2006;113:1779–1786. DOI: 10.1161/CIRCULATIONAHA.105.582239.

[201] Danial NN, Korsmeyer SJ. Cell death: critical control points. Cell. 2004;116:205–219. DOI: 10.1016/S0092-8674(04)00046-7.

[202] Li LY, Luo X, Wang X. Endonuclease G is an apoptotic DNase when released from mitochondria. Nature. 2001;412:95–99. DOI: 10.1038/35083620.

[203] Kwon SH, Pimentel DR, Remondino A, Sawyer DB, Colucci WS. H2O2 regulates cardiac myocyte phenotype via concentration-dependent activation of distinct kinase pathways. J Mol Cell Cardiol. 2003;35:615–621. DOI: 10.1016/S0022-2828(03)00084-1

[204] Chaanine AH, Jeong D, Liang L, Chemaly ER, Fish K, Gordon RE, Hajjar RJ. JNK modulates FOXO3a for the expression of the mitochondrial death and mitophagy marker BNIP3 in pathological hypertrophy and in heart failure. Cell Death Dis. 2012;3:265. DOI: 10.1038/cddis.2012.5.

[205] Chiong M, Wang ZV, Pedrozo Z, Cao DJ, Troncoso R, Ibacache M, Criollo A, Nemchenko A, Hill JA, Lavandero S. Cardiomyocyte death: mechanisms and translational implications. Cell Death Dis. 2011;2: e244. DOI: 10.1038/cddis.2011.130.

[206] Vacek, T.P.; Vacek, J.C.; Tyagi, S.C. Mitochondrial mitophagic mechanisms of myocardial matrix metabolism and remodelling. Arch Physiol Biochem. 2012;118:31–42. DOI: 10.3109/13813455.2011.635660. Epub 2011 Dec 19.

[207] Anatoliotakis N, Deftereos S, Bouras G, Giannopoulos G, Tsounis D, Angelidis C, Kaoukis A, Stefanadis C. Myeloperoxidase: expressing inflammation and oxidative stress in cardiovascular disease. Curr Top Med Chem. 2013;13:115–138. DOI: 10.2174/1568026611313020004.

[208] Nicholls SJ, Hazen SL. Myeloperoxidase and cardiovascular disease. Arterioscler Thromb Vasc Biol. 2005; 25:1102–1111. DOI: 10.1161/01.ATV.0000163262.83456.6d.

[209] Eiserich JP1, Baldus S, Brennan ML, Ma W, Zhang C, Tousson A, Castro L, Lusis AJ, Nauseef WM, White CR, Freeman BA. Myeloperoxidase, a leukocyte-derived vascular NOoxidase. Science. 2002, 296, 2391–2394. DOI: 10.1126/science.1106830.

[210] La Rocca G, Di Stefano A, Eleuteri E, Anzalone R, Magno F, Corrao S, Loria T, Martorana A, Di Gangi C, Colombo M, Sansone F, Patanè F, Farina F, Rinaldi M, Cappello F, Giannuzzi P, Zummo G. Oxidative stress induces myeloperoxidase expression in endocardial endothelial cells from patients with chronic heart failure. Basic Res Cardiol. 2009;104:301–320. DOI: 10.1007/s00395-008-0761-9

[211] Morrow DA, Scirica BM, Karwatowska-Prokopczuk E, et al. Evaluation of a novel anti-ischemic agent in acute coronary syndromes: design and rationale for the Metabolic Efficiency with Ranolazine for Less Ischemia in Non-ST-elevation acute coronary syndromes (MERLIN)-TIMI 36 trial. Am Heart J. 2006;151:1186.e1–9. DOI: 10.1016/j.ahj.2006.01.004.

[212] Baldus S, Heeschen C, Meinertz T, Zeiher AM, Eiserich JP, Münzel T, Simoons ML, Hamm CW; CAPTURE Investigators. Myeloperoxidase serum levels predict risk in patients with acute coronary syndromes. Circulation. 2003;108:1440–1445. DOI: 10.1161/01.CIR.0000090690.67322.51.

[213] Schuetz P, Wolbers M, Christ-Crain M, Thomann R, Falconnier C, Widmer I, Neidert S, Fricker T, Blum C, Schild U, Morgenthaler NG, Schoenenberger R, Henzen C, Bregenzer T, Hoess C, Krause M, Bucher HC, Zimmerli W, Mueller B; ProHOSP Study Group. Prohormones for prediction of adverse medical outcome in community-acquired pneumonia and lower respiratory tract infections. Crit Care. 2010;14:R106. DOI: 10.1186/cc9055.

[214] Kruger S, Ewig S, Giersdorf S, Hartmann O, Suttorp N, Welte T. Cardiovascular and inflammatory biomarkers to predict short- and long-term survival in community-acquired pneumonia. Am J Respir Crit Care Med 2010;182:1426–1434. DOI: 10.1164/rccm.201003-0415OC

[215] Choudhary R, Gopal D, Kipper BA, Landa ADLP, Aramin H, Lee E, Shah S, Maisel AS. Cardiorenal biomarkers in acute heart failure. J Ger Cardiol. 2012;9:292–304. DOI: 10.3724/SP.J.1263.2012.02291.

[216] Maisel A, Neath SX, Landsberg J, Mueller C, Nowak RM, Peacock WF, Ponikowski P, Möckel M, Hogan C, Wu AH, Richards M, Clopton P, Filippatos GS, Di Somma S, Anand I, Ng LL, Daniels LB, Christenson RH, Potocki M, McCord J, Terracciano G, Hartmann O, Bergmann A, Morgenthaler NG, Anker SD. Use of Procalcitonin (PCT) for the diagnosis of pneumonia in patients presenting with a chief complaint of dyspnoea: Results from the BACH (Biomarkers in Acute Heart Failure) trial. Eur J Heart Fail. 2012;14:278–286. DOI: 10.1093/eurjhf/hfr177.

[217] Herget-Rosenthal S, Marggraf G, Pietruck F, Hüsing J, Strupat M, Philipp T, Kribben A. Procalcitonin for accurate detection of infection in hemodialysis. Nephrol Dial Transplant. 2001;16:975–979. DOI: 10.1093/ndt/16.5.975.

[218] Herget-Rosenthal S, Marggraf G, Hirsch T, Jakob HG, Philipp T, Kribben A. Modulation and source of procalcitonin in reduced renal function and renal replacement therapy. Scand J Immunol. 2005;61:180–186. DOI: 10.1111/j.0300-9475.2005.01545.x.

[219] Yamaguchi T, Baba K, Doi Y, Yano K. Effect of adrenomedullin on aldosterone secretion by dispersed rat adrenal zona glomerulosa cells. Life Sci. 1995;56:379–387. PMID: 7830499 [PubMed—indexed for MEDLINE].

[220] Yandle T, Troughton R. Improving risk stratification in heart failure: a role for new biomarkers? Eur J Heart Fail. 2010;12:315–318. DOI: 10.1093/eurjhf/hfq030.

[221] Nicholls MG1, Charles CJ, Lainchbury JG, Lewis LK, Rademaker MT, Richards AM, Yandle TG. Adrenomedullin and heart failure. Regul Pept. 2003;112:51–60. DOI: 10.1291/hypres.26.S135.

[222] Chan D, NG LL. Biomarkers in acute myocardial infarction. BMC Med 2010; 8: 34. DOI: 10.1186/1741-7015-8-34.

[223] Gaggin HK, Januzzi JL Jr. Biomarkers and diagnostics in heart failure. Biochim Biophys Acta. 2013;1832:2442–2450. DOI: 10.1016/j.bbadis.2012.12.014.

[224] D'Marco L, Bellasi A, Raggi P. Cardiovascular biomarkers in chronic kidney disease: state of current research and clinical applicability. Disease Markers. 2015;ID 586569. DOI: 10.1155/2015/586569.

[225] Junyent M, Martinez M, Borras M, Bertriu A, Coll B, Craver L, Marco MP, Sarró F, Valdivielso JM, Fernández E. Usefulness of imaging techniques and novel biomarkers in the prediction of cardiovascular risk in patients with chronic kidney disease in Spain: the NEFRONA project. Nefrologia 2010;30:119–126. DOI: 10.3265/Nefrologia.pre2010.

[226] Wheeler DC, Townend JN, Landray MJ. Cardiovascular risk factors in predialysis patients: baseline data from the Chronic Renal Impairment in Birmingham (CRIB) study. Kidney Int Suppl 2003; 84:S201–S203.

[227] Takamatsu N, Abe H, Tominaga T, Nakahara K, Ito Y, Okumoto Y, Kim J, Kitakaze M, Doi T. Risk factors for chronic kidney disease in Japan: a community-based study. BMC Nephrol. 2009;10:34. DOI: 10.1186/1471-2369-10-34.

[228] Shan Y, Zhang Q, Liu Z, Hu X, Liu D. Prevalence and risk factors associated with chronic kidney disease in adults over 40 years: a population study from Central China. Nephrology. 2010;15:354–361. DOI: 10.1111/j.1440-1797.2009.01249.x.

[229] Baumeister SE, Boger CA, Kramer BK, Döring A, Eheberg D, Fischer B, John J, Koenig W, Meisinger C. Effect of chronic kidney disease and comorbid conditions on health care costs: a 10-year observational study in a general population. Am J Nephrol. 2010;31:222–229. DOI: 10.1159/000272937.

[230] Bossola M, Tazza L, Merki E, Giungi S, Luciani G, Miller ER, Lin EB, Tortorelli A, Tsimikas S: Oxidized low-density lipoprotein biomarkers in patients with end-stage renal failure: acute effects of hemodialysis. Blood Purif. 2007;25:457–465. DOI: 10.1159/000112465.

[231] Sampath P, Achuthan R, Mahdi OG, Nalini S. Oxidized low-density lipoprotein. Methods Mol Biol. 2010;610:403–417. DOI: 10.1007/978-1-60327-029-8_24.

[232] Shoji T, Ishimura E, Inaba M, Tabata T, Nishizawa Y. Atherogenic lipoproteins in end-stage renal disease. Am J Kidney Dis. 2001;38:S30–33. DOI: 10.1053/ajkd.2001.27393.

[233] Witko-Sarsat V, Friedlander M, Nguyen Khoa T, Capeillère-Blandin C, Nguyen AT, Canteloup S, Dayer JM, Jungers P, Drüeke T, Descamps-Latscha B. Advanced oxidation protein products as novel mediators of inflammation and monocyte activation in chronic renal failure. J Immunol. 1998;161:2524–2532. http://www.jimmunol.org/content/161/5/2524.full#ref-list-1.

[234] Gonzalez E, Bajo MA, Carrero JJ, Lindholm B, Grande C, Sánchez-Villanueva R, Del Peso G, Díaz-Almirón M, Iglesias P, Díez JJ, Selgas R. An increase of plasma advanced oxidation protein products levels is associated with cardiovascular risk in incident peritoneal dialysis patients: a pilot study. Oxid Med Cell Longev. 2015; ID 219569. DOI: 10.1155/2015/219569.

[235] Witko-Sarsat V, Gausson V, Descamps-Latscha B. Are advanced oxidation protein products potential uremic toxins? Kidney Int Suppl. 2003;84:S11–14. DOI: 10.1046/j.1523-1755.63.s84.47.x.

[236] Lefèvre G, Beljean-Leymarie M, Beyerle MF, Bonnefont-Rousselot D, Cristol JP, Thérond P, Torreilles J: Evaluation de la peroxydation lipidique par le dosage des substances réagissant avec l'acide thiobarbiturique. Ann Biol Clin. 1998;56:305–319. PMID: 9754263 [PubMed—indexed for MEDLINE].

[237] Cottone S, Mule` G, Guarneri M, Palermo A, Lorito MC, Riccobene R, Arsena R, Vaccaro F, Vadala` A, Nardi E, Cusimano P, Cerasola G: Endothelin-1 and F2-isoprostane relate to and predict renal dysfunction in hypertensive patients. Nephrol Dial Transplant. 2009;24:497–503. DOI: 10.1093/ndt/gfn489.

[238] Lavi S, Yang EH, Prasad A, Mathew V, Barsness GW, Rihal CS, Lerman LO, Lerman A: The interaction between coronary endothelial dysfunction, local oxidative stress, and

endogenous nitric oxide in humans. Hypertension. 2008;51:127–133. DOI: 10.1161/HYPERTENSIONAHA.107.099986.

[239] Giustarini D, Dalle-Donne I, Tsikas D, Rossi R: Oxidative stress and human diseases: origin, link, measurement, mechanisms, and biomarkers. Crit Rev Clin Lab Sci. 2009;46:241–281. DOI: 10.3109/10408360903142326.

[240] Labio´s M, Martinez M, Gabriel F, Guiral V, Dasi F, Beltra´n B, and Muñoz A. Superoxide dismutase and catalase anti-oxidant activity in leucocyte lysates from hypertensive patients: effects of eprosartan treatment. J Renin Angiotensin Aldosterone Syst. 2009;10:24–30. DOI: 10.1177/1470320309104067.

[241] Heywood JT: The cardiorenal syndrome: lessons from the ADHERE database and treatment options. Heart Fail Rev. 2004;9:195–201. DOI: 10.1007%2Fs10741-005-6129-4.

[242] Yancy CW, Lopatin M, Stevenson LW, De Marco T, Fonarow GC. Clinical presentation, management, and in-hospital outcomes of patients admitted with acute decompensated heart failure with preserved systolic function: a report from the Acute Decompensated Heart Failure National Registry (ADHERE) Database. J Am Coll Cardiol. 2006;47:76–84. DOI: 10.1016/j.jacc.2005.09.022.

[243] Stevenson LW, Nohria A, Mielniczuk L. Torrent or torment from the tubules? Challenge of the cardiorenal connections. J Am Coll Cardiol. 2005;45:2004–2007. DOI: 10.1016/j.jacc.2005.03.028.

[244] van Kimmenade RR, Januzzi JL Jr., Baggish AL, Lainchbury JG, Bayes-Genis A, Richards AM, Pinto YM. Amino-terminal pro-brain natriuretic Peptide, renal function, and outcomes in acute heart failure: redefining the cardiorenal interaction? J Am Coll Cardiol. 2006;48:1621–1627. DOI: 10.1016/j.jacc.2006.06.056.

[245] Leier CV. Renal roadblock in managing low output heart failure. Crit Care Med. 2004;32:1228-1229. DOI: 10.1097/01.CCM.0000125510.02846.AF.

[246] Shlipak MG. Pharmacotherapy for heart failure in patients with renal insufficiency. Ann Intern Med. 2003;138:917–924. DOI: 10.7326/0003-4819-138-11-200306030-00013.

Chapter 14

Subcellular ROS Signaling in Cardiovascular Disease

M. Ruhul Abid and Frank W. Sellke

Additional information is available at the end of the chapter

http://dx.doi.org/10.5772/64570

Abstract

This review discusses recent findings that have challenged the long-held dogma in the field that reduction in reaction oxygen species (ROS) would improve clinical outcome in the patients with cardiovascular disease (CVD). Attempts will be made to shed light on the differential spatial and temporal roles of subcellular ROS in vascular endothelium in health and disease. Recent findings demonstrating that above-physiological levels of endothelial cell (EC)-specific NADPH oxidase-derived ROS *in vivo* exert beneficial effects on vascular endothelium will be discussed. The paradoxical roles of ROS in CVD suggest that subcellular sources and types of ROS may play crucial roles in the prevention, development, and progression of CVD. A better understanding of the precise mechanisms by which subcellular ROS modulate cardiovascular health and functions will certainly better prepare us with effective treatment modalities for CVD.

Keywords: reactive oxygen species, cardiovascular disease, endothelium, oxidative stress, signal transduction

1. Introduction

Cardiovascular disease (CVD) is the leading cause of death in the USA. Increased levels of reactive oxygen species (ROS) are often associated with microvascular pathology in CVD, causing endothelial dysfunction and coronary artery disease (CAD) and leading to myocardial ischemia and infarction (MI) [1–5]. However, failure of large clinical trials using antioxidants in patients with CVD [6–11], challenges the prevailing view that ROS production is damaging to the microvasculature. Indeed, findings from our laboratory and others show negative effects of ROS reduction on endothelial function and angiogenesis [12–14] and suggest that a well-regulated temporal balance of ROS production is important for normal endothelial cell (EC) function.

The paradoxical roles of ROS in CVD studied by different groups of workers also suggest that subcellular sources and types of ROS may also play crucial roles in the prevention, development, and progression of CVD. This review discusses recent findings that are challenging the long-held dogma in the field and also attempts to shed light on the differential spatial and temporal roles of subcellular ROS in vascular endothelium in CVD. A better understanding of the precise mechanisms by which subcellular ROS modulate cardiovascular health and functions will certainly better equip us with effective treatment modalities for CVD in future.

2. Cardiovascular disease (CVD)

Cardiovascular disease (CVD) is a leading cause of death and morbidity in the Western world. Recent reports suggest an increasing incidence of CVD in the developing countries too. In the USA, CVD with an annual toll of 1.2 million lives is the leading cause of deaths since 1921. At present, 85.6 million people in the country are living with CVD. In 2015, American Heart Association (AHA) reported that the prevalence of CVD among US adults is 6% with a calculated financial burden of $300 billion per year [15].

Vascular endothelium is critical for the optimal function of the heart and the vascular system, in particular due to its production of nitric oxide (NO) that regulates vascular tone and blood pressure (**Figure 1**). By regulating vascular tone including coronary vasodilation, NO plays an important role in blood supply to the myocardium (by coronary vessels) and other tissues in the body. Damage to coronary endothelium results in reduction in NO levels by reducing the level and/or activity of the enzyme, endothelial nitric oxide synthase (eNOS). This in turn contributes to the development of endothelial dysfunction (i.e. loss of vasodilation) and coronary artery disease (CAD), which may lead to ischemic insult to the heart including myocardial infarction and heart failure (HF). In myocardial ischemia, coronary vasodilation is an immediate response that may improve coronary blood flow in the heart. Another potent way myocardium employs to defend itself from ischemic insults is by preserving the existing coronary capillary vessels and/or by inducing growth of coronary vessels in the ischemic area [16–18]. Once the ischemic insult has occurred, survival of the affected cardiac tissue depends on the speed with which coronary vessels can increase blood flow. Thus, a functional coronary vascular system with endothelium-dependent NO-induced vasodilation mechanism is critical for the maintenance of coronary vascular health in the heart. Endothelial health and NO levels are also critical for the maintenance of blood pressure and prevention of hypertension that is an important risk factor for CVD.

Another major contributor to CVD is atherosclerosis, which is characterized by the accumulation of inflammatory leukocytes and lipid-laden macrophages in the vascular wall resulting in the gradual narrowing of the vascular lumens and wall thickness (**Figure 1A**). These changes, if generalized, result in arterial stiffness and can give rise to high blood pressure (hypertension); if the changes are localized, they may result in blocking of blood flow (ischemia and peripheral arterial disease), and in more severe cases, they may result in myocardial infarction, cerebrovascular disease/accident (stroke), atherosclerotic plaque rupture, and/or weakening of the vessel walls (aneurysm) (**Figure 1**).

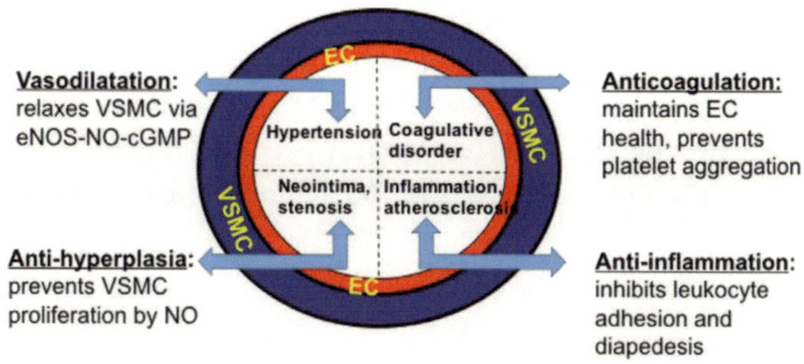

A. Protective functions of endothelium

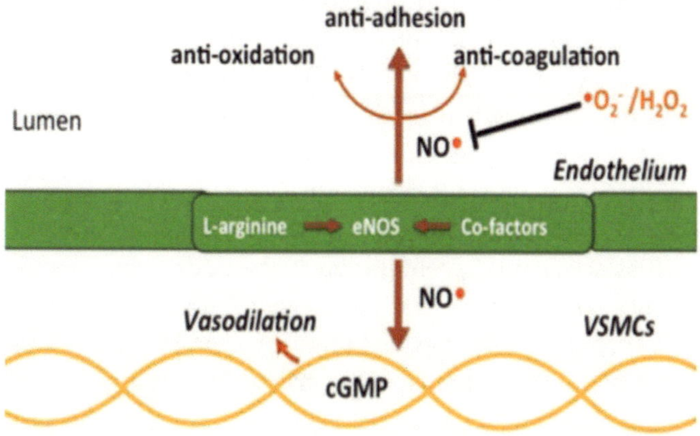

B. Vasodilatation: NO *vs* ROS

Figure 1. (A) Vascular endothelium performs critical functions in cardiovascular system, including nitric oxide (NO)-dependent vasodilation, maintenance of blood fluidity by preventing breach in the EC layer and platelet aggregation, NO-mediated inhibition of vascular smooth muscle cell (VSMC) proliferation and neointima formation, and inhibition of leukocyte adhesion to EC. Pathogenesis that may occur due to lack of specific function of EC is shown inside the circle. EC, endothelial cell; VSMC, vascular smooth muscle cell; and eNOS, endothelial nitric oxide synthase. (B) Nitric oxidase (NO)-mediated vasodilatation and other critical functions of vascular endothelium can be inhibited or blocked by excess ROS, specifically by superoxide. Endothelial nitric oxide synthase (eNOS) produces NO that acts on the luminal surface of the endothelium to prevent leukocyte adhesion and platelet aggregation/coagulation. NO diffuses to adjacent vascular smooth muscle layer (VSMC) to activate cyclic GMP (cGMP) signaling resulting in calcium ion release and relaxation of VSMC. All these NO functions can be blocked or reduced by the presence of excess ROS in the vascular wall.

Metabolic syndrome characterized by hypertension, obesity, glucose intolerance (diabetes), and hyperlipidemia is often accompanied by CVD. The endothelial dysfunction associated with metabolic syndrome has also been shown to have diminished angiogenic response and aberrant collateral vessels to chronic myocardial ischemia in large animal model [19, 20].

CVD including hypertension and heart failure (HF) are the most common cause of mortality in diabetes mellitus (DM) and usually result from DM-induced cardiomyopathy and CAD. The Framingham study showed that patients with DM are four times more likely to develop CVD. The worldwide prevalence of DM has recently been reported to be increased (total DM patients in 2015 have been projected to be over 300 millions) due to changes in lifestyle.

3. ROS and CVD cohabitation

Reactive oxygen species (ROS) has long been implicated in CVD. Increased levels of ROS are often observed in vascular tissues including coronary endothelium in CVD, and thus are believed to cause coronary endothelial dysfunction, CAD, myocardial ischemia, and infarction [1–5]. Although the mechanisms by which ROS may cause CVD has not been elucidated, increased levels of ROS, also known as oxidant stress, are believed to arise from endothelial cells (EC) resulting in loss of EC-dependent vasorelaxation and EC injury (**Figure 1B**). Oxidant-induced injury in EC in turn may result in recruitment of the inflammatory cells in the vessel wall leading to a cascade of vascular injuries. Dysfunctional EC leads to remodeling of the vascular tissues such as accelerated proliferation of the underlying vascular smooth muscle cells resulting in neointimal hyperproliferation/thickening and narrowing of the vessel lumen/stenosis (**Figure 1**). Vascular stenosis results in tissue ischemia and may also be complicated with thrombus formation. In the presence of hyperlipidemia, injury to EC may contribute to atherosclerotic changes. Remodeling of vessel wall, depending on the vascular bed affected and associated pathology/comorbidity, may result in hypertension, pulmonary hypertension, diabetic retinopathy, peripheral artery disease, myocardial ischemia, and stroke.

Interestingly, recent reports from several groups of workers demonstrated that reduction in ROS did not improve EC function and/or angiogenesis [12, 13, 21]. These findings challenged the long-held dogma that ROS are harmful and/or causative factor for developing CVD. More recently, our laboratory has shown that EC-specific increase in ROS resulted in the improvement of EC function and EC-dependent coronary vasodilation in transgenic animals [22]. All these imply that cohabitation of ROS and CVD may not be simply concluded to have deleterious effects on cardiovascular system. In addition, failure of the clinical trials (e.g. HOPE) to improve CVD using antioxidants and recent reports of beneficial effects of ROS on EC function warrant careful studies to delineate the spatial and temporal roles of ROS at the subcellular levels.

3.1. Types of ROS

ROS are reactive molecules that contain oxygen, they include molecules that have unpaired electrons, such as superoxide ($O_2^{\bullet-}$), hydroxyl anion (HO^-), and nitric oxide (NO^-) or that have the oxidizing ability but do not possess free electrons, such as hydrogen peroxide (H_2O_2), hypochlorous acid, and peroxynitrite ($ONOO^-$).

3.1.1. Superoxide

It is produced usually as part of the metabolic processes by many intracellular enzymes such as NADPH oxidases (Nox), mitochondrial electron chain transport (ETC) system, Xanthine oxidase (XO), cytochrome P450, xanthine oxidase, lipoxygenase, myeloperoxidase, and uncoupled eNOS. $O_2^{\bullet-}$ is highly reactive and thus very unstable and has a short lifespan. It cannot cross cellular membranes and thus has a limited "area of action." Superoxide is usually converted to H_2O_2 spontaneously or can be metabolized to H_2O_2 by the antioxidant enzyme superoxide dismutases (SODs).

3.1.2. Hydrogen peroxide

As aforementioned, H_2O_2 is usually produced by dismutation of $O_2^{\bullet-}$ by SOD or by metal ions spontaneously in the Fenton reaction. Recently, Nox4 has been reported to be a source for H_2O_2; it has been reported that major ROS emanates from Nox4 enzyme is most likely H_2O_2 [23]. In comparison to superoxide, H_2O_2 is stable and can cross biological membranes, the properties that make this ROS a major player in cell signal transduction mechanisms.

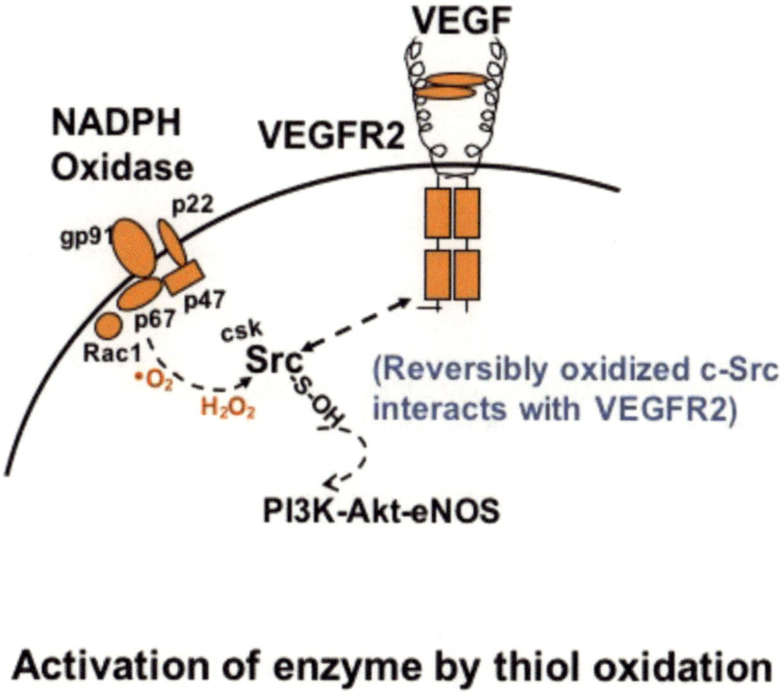

Figure 2. Reversible oxidation of thiol on cysteine residues modulate activity of the signaling molecules (kinases, phosphatases, and enzymes). NAPDH oxidase-derived ROS reversibly oxidize cysteine thiol (SH) to sulfenic acid (-SOH) on c-Src, which in turn facilitates interaction between c-Src and VEGFR2 resulting in the activation of downstream PI3K-Akt-eNOS signaling pathway in coronary endothelial cells (ECs). VEGF, vascular endothelial growth factor; VEGFR2, VEGF receptor 2; PI3K, phosphoinositol 3 kinase; Akt, protein kinase B; eNOS, endothelial nitric oxidase synthase; and Src, c-Src.

Due to its stability and membrane-crossing properties, H_2O_2 may act farther from its site of origin. H_2O_2 can react with thiol (SH) residues present on cysteine and methionine, and can catalyze the formation of the disulfide bonds (S-S) and reversible sulfenic acid (-SOH) and sulfinic acid ($-SO_2H$) moieties. All these changes can be reversed by antioxidant enzymes such as glutathione peroxidase (Gpx). However, these changes, if involves the catalytic site of the protein, can significantly modulate (activate, increase, decrease, or inhibit) the functional properties of an enzyme. It has been recently reported that c-Src oxidation by NADPH oxidase-derived ROS is crucial for c-Src and VEGF receptor 2 (VEGFR2) binding and activation of downstream c-Src-PI3K-Akt-eNOS signaling (**Figure 2**). Further oxidation of sulfinic acid to sulfonic acid ($-SO_3H$) is irreversible and does not participate in signal transduction (**Figure 2**).

3.1.3. Hydroxyl anions

HO^- is usually produced from H_2O_2 by free metals (Fenton reaction) or from the interaction between water and excited O_2. HO^- is highly reactive with a very short lifespan, is promiscuous in its interaction, and thus can cause sustained damage to DNA, amino acids, lipids, and glucose moieties mostly due to irreversibility of its interaction with biological molecules. It is thus considered a major contributor to "oxidative stress."

3.1.4. Nitric oxide

It is considered to be the "golden" molecule for cardiovascular health, which is crucial in the maintenance of the health of cardiac and vascular tissues. In EC, NO^- is produced by the enzyme eNOS and is involved in survival, growth, proliferation, and migration of vascular ECs. It is very critical for the maintenance of a continuous EC layer throughout the cardiovascular system. In fact, many of the critical functions carried out by EC are performed by NO^-, such as endothelium-dependent vasodilation (by activating cGMP pathway to decrease Ca_2^+ in vascular smooth cells, VSMC), prevention of adhesion of the anti-inflammatory cells to EC, maintenance of blood fluidity (anticoagulant, anti-thrombotic, and profibrinolytic actions), and anti-hypertrophic activity of EC through inhibition of VSMC proliferation and migration (**Figure 1**). NO, though it possess all the properties of a ROS, is often not considered as ROS by classical redox biologists. Interestingly, uncoupled eNOS may also generate superoxide.

3.1.5. Peroxynitrite

$ONOO^-$is generated by interaction between $O_2^{\bullet -}$ and NO^-. Like hydroxyl radical, peroxynitrite is also highly reactive and damaging to biological molecules including protein/enzyme due to its irreversible interaction. Thus, it is often considered as a marker for oxidative stress and/or oxidative tissue damage. In cardiovascular system, in addition to tissues damages, increase in $ONOO^-$ is considered to be an indicator of high ROS and low availability of NO^-, since $O_2^{\bullet}$ $^-$ interacts with and quenches NO^-. Decrease availability of NO^-, often marked by increase in peroxynitrite levels, is considered to be responsible for endothelial dysfunction, i.e., reduced vasorelaxation, often an initial marker for CVD.

http://dx.doi.org/10.5772/64570

3.2. Subcellular sources of ROS

Biological sources of ROS are mitochondria (produced as a by-product of oxidative phosphorylation), NADPH oxidases, cytochrome P450, xanthine oxidase, lipoxygenase, myeloperoxidase, and uncoupled eNOS (**Figure 3**). While mitochondria act as the major source of ROS in most cardiovascular cells including cardiomyocytes, NADPH oxidases are the major source of intracellular ROS in vascular endothelium. EC derives most of its energy (ATP) from non-mitochondrial glycolysis, rendering it (EC) less likely to have excess ROS from mitochondrial source in physiological condition (**Figure 3**).

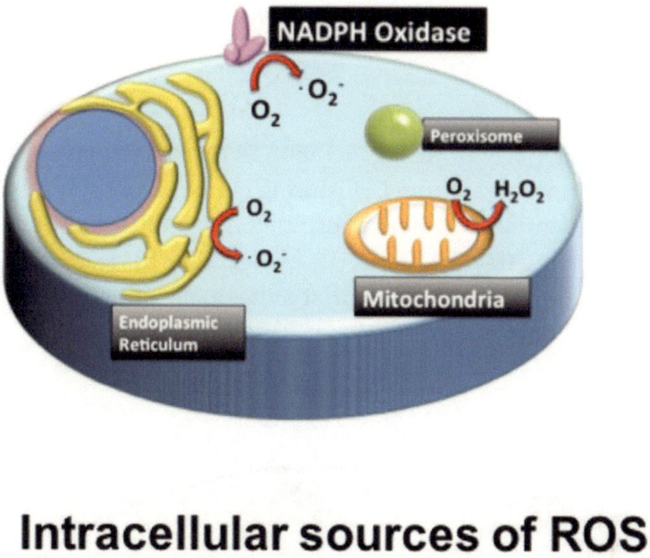

Figure 3. Subcellular sources of ROS include NADPH oxidase, mitochondria, peroxisome, lysosome, endoplasmic reticulum (ER), and cytochrome P450. NAPDH oxidases (Nox) are usually present in the cell membrane and perinuclear and ER membranes. Major species of ROS produced by NADPH oxidase is superoxide (O_2^-). Mitochondria produce ROS as a by-product of respiration/oxidative phosphorylation; electrons leaked from the electron transport chain (ETC), especially from Complexes I and III, produce superoxide in the mitochondrial matrix. Mitochondrial superoxide dismutase (MnSOD) converts superoxide to H_2O_2, which can then cross mitochondrial membrane to enter the cytosol. Nox is also found on the ER.

3.2.1. NADPH oxidase

NADPH oxidase is a multisubunit, membrane-bound protein complex that catalyzes oxidation of NADPH to $NADP^+$ and H^+, and in the process releases an electron. Molecular oxygen accepts this released electron and becomes $O_2^{\bullet -}$. There are several isoforms of NADPH oxidases, such as Rac-1-dependent NADPH oxidase (it contains Nox2/gp91^{phox}, **Figure 2**), Nox1, Nox3, Nox4, and Nox5. All isoforms have been reported to be found in the cardiovascular system except Nox3. With the exception of Nox4 (which is believed to release H_2O_2), all NADPH oxidases produce superoxide. NADPH oxidase is a major source of ROS in vascular endothelium and thus plays important roles in signal transduction in cardiovascular system in health and disease. It has been shown that ECs possess two distinct major signaling pathways, redox-sensitive and redox-independent [24]. While PI3K-Akt-eNOS and Akt-FOXO signaling pathways were shown to be NADPH oxidase-derived ROS-dependent, PLCγ-MAPK-ERK signaling pathways were redox-independent in human coronary vascular ECs (**Figure 4**) [24]. Reduction in Nox-derived ROS resulted in inhibition of EC proliferation and migration [21, 25, 26]. Interestingly, recent findings further demonstrated that above-physiological levels (i.e. twofold increase compared to basal levels) of EC-specific Nox-derived ROS activated AMPK-eNOS signaling pathway in transgenic animals resulting in EC-dependent coronary vasorelaxation [22]. Together, these findings suggest that NADPH oxidase-derived ROS, both at the physiological and above-physiological levels, exert positive effects on EC health, growth, and function (**Figure 4**).

3.2.2. Mitochondria

Mitochondria play a major role in ROS generation in cardiovascular cells with one notable exception in ECs. Electrons leaked from ETC during oxidative phosphorylation in mitochondria produce $O_2^{\bullet-}$. Efficient mitochondrial respiration produces less ROS, however, inefficient oxidative phosphorylation gives rise to excess ROS by leaking electrons from the complexes I and III of the ETC. Mitochondrial antioxidant MnSOD (SOD2) plays a major

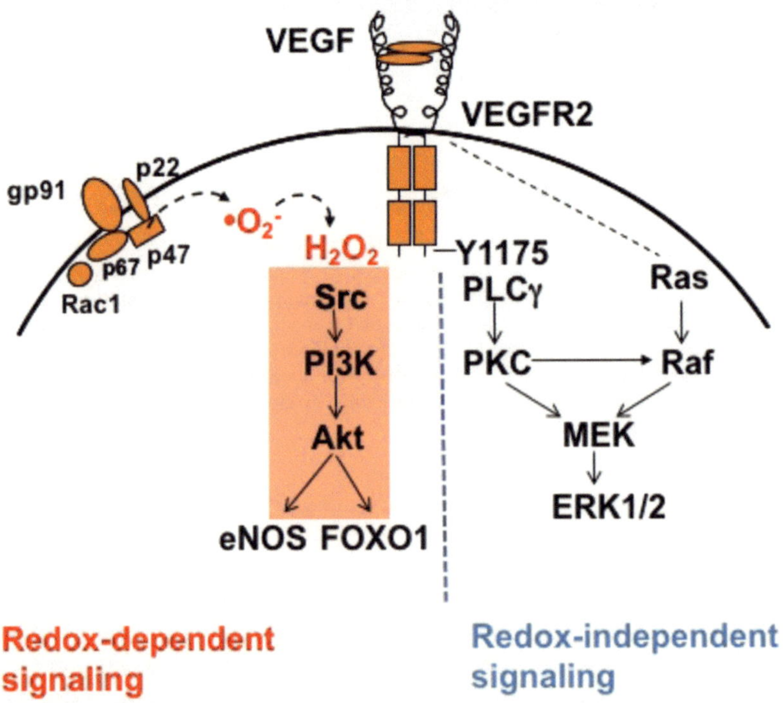

Figure 4. Coronary endothelium possesses two distinct signaling pathways: redox-sensitive PI3K-Akt-eNOS and PI3K-Akt-forkhead (FOXO) signaling (left panel) and redox-independent PLCγ-PKC-MEK-ERK1/2 signaling pathway (right panel).

http://dx.doi.org/10.5772/64570

role in reducing mitochondrial ROS by catalyzing superoxide to H_2O_2; Gpx further catalyzes H_2O_2 to molecular oxygen and water. Mitochondrial ROS may also increase due to increase in NO, which has been reported to inhibit Complex-I and in turn increase superoxide formation by leaking electrons into the matrix of the mitochondria.

3.2.3. Xanthine oxidase

Sulfhydryl oxidation of xanthine dehydrogenase results in xanthine oxidase formation. XO generates superoxide as a byproduct of the reaction where XO catalyzes the conversion of hypoxanthine to xanthine and xanthine to uric acid. XO is believed to produce ROS, especially H_2O_2, in ischemic conditions where oxygen tension is low. However, in ischemia-reperfusion injury, XO has been reported to be generating superoxide [27].

3.2.4. Lipoxygenase

Lipoxygenase plays an important role in hyperlipidemic state. It has been implicated in the oxidation of polyunsaturated fatty acids and in the pathology of atherosclerotic plaque formation and aortic aneurysm development.

3.2.5. Endothelial nitric oxide synthase

As aforementioned, eNOS generates NO. However, it can also produce ROS when uncoupled due to reduced availability of substrates L-arginine and/or co-factor BH4. Peroxynitrite may oxidize BH4, which in turn uncouple eNOS to form superoxide. Increased ROS is, thus, believed to activate a feed forward loop for ROS generation by uncoupling of eNOS.

3.3. Antioxidant enzymes

ROS balance is extremely critical for signal transduction and optimal functions of the cells. "Antioxidant enzymes" play an important role in redox balance. There are many cellular and extracellular enzymes that participate in oxidant metabolism, several of these are evolutionarily conserved. The term "antioxidant" is a misnomer for some of the proteins such as superoxide dismutase (SOD), which on one hand reduces the level of superoxide by converting superoxide to H_2O_2, but on the other hand increases H_2O_2, and thus results in overall increase in ROS levels. Thus, although it is called as antioxidant, SOD may well act like a pro-oxidation enzyme by converting a transient and localized ROS (O_2^-) to stable H_2O_2, which can cross membranes and thus can act farther away from its site of origin (paracrine effect).

3.3.1. Superoxide dismutases (SODs)

The very first step in regulating superoxide levels is catalyzed by this group of enzymes. Superoxide is converted to H_2O_2 by SOD. Most cells in the body including ECs have three isoforms of SOD, such as cytosolic SOD1 (Cu-Zn SOD), which catalyzes cytosolic superoxide to H_2O_2. SOD1 knockout mice have been shown to have impaired EC-dependent vasodilation [28]. In contrast, mitochondrial SOD2 (MnSOD) deletion was found to be embryonic lethal. SOD2 is a nuclear gene which upon protein translation translocated to mitochondrial matrix.

Heterozygous SOD2 mice demonstrated to have hypertension [29]. Excess ROS (e.g. ONOO) may inactivate SOD2; nitrosylation of MnSOD by ONOO has been reported to inhibit the antioxidant activity of the enzyme. Thus, increase in ONOO due to elevated ROS may result in increased mitochondrial ROS by inhibiting MnSOD activity. The "extracellular" SOD3 (Cu/ZnSOD) is a secreted protein which is localized in the outer part of the cell membrane. Deletion of SOD3 is not lethal; however, defective neovascularization has been reported in SOD3 null animals [30].

3.3.2. Glutathione peroxidase (Gpx)

Gpx catalyzes the conversion of H_2O_2 to water. Gpx is more abundantly expressed in cardiovascular cells including EC than catalase. It is also a major antioxidant protein in the mitochondria and is believed to have more critical role than catalase in regulating endothelial ROS. Gpx null animals have endothelial dysfunction [31]. It has also been reported to have severe ischemic-reperfusion injury [32] and defective angiogenesis compared to wild-type control [33].

3.3.3. Catalase

Functionally, catalase is similar to Gpx as it converts H_2O_2 to molecular oxygen and water. Structurally, catalase is a 4-heme containing enzyme. Knockout of catalase is not lethal.

3.3.4. Peroxidoredoxin (Prx)

Prx is a group of enzymes abundantly expressed in cardiovascular system. Functionally, they are similar to Gpx. Probably the most important role of Prx is to protect hemoglobin (Hb) in red blood cells (erythrocytes) where a lack of Prx has been shown to be associated with oxidation of Hb resulting in anemia.

3.3.5. Thioredoxin (Trx)

There are two isoforms of Trx present in the cardiovascular tissues, Trx-1 being present in the cytosol and Trx-2 in the mitochondria. They catalyze thiol-disulfide exchange on the cysteine residues present in the protein and thus convert the oxidized thiols of the proteins to their reduced (SH) forms. This protective action by reducing oxidized pools of proteins in the cells is crucial for redox balance. Overexpression of Trx has been shown to have protective effects against oxidative stress on cardiovascular function [34].

4. Understanding subcellular ROS is critical in CVD

It is obvious from the aforementioned discussion that endogenous ROS levels in specific subcellular compartments regulate certain signaling pathways, survival, proliferation, and pathophysiology in cardiovascular tissues. Precise understanding of the *spatial* (i.e. at different subcellular locations such as in the cytosol, mitochondria) and *temporal role of redox* (i.e. changes in the role of ROS with time) to selectively activate downstream signaling pathways, maintain an intact and continuous EC layer throughout the cardiovascular system, maintain vasodilation in resistance arterioles, and induce a proangiogenic environment in ischemic myocardium is critical for the development of future therapeutic modalities for microvascular disease. In case of redox regulation, failure of the "all or none" approach (e.g. using global antioxidants as in the HOPE trial) also points to the end of an era that has treated any increase in cellular ROS levels as "deleterious." Instead, it is high time to consider ROS as signaling molecules, increase of which may also have "beneficial" effects during a cellular or cardiovascular crisis such as inflammation, ischemia-reperfusion, myocardial infarction, or other cardiovascular injuries including stroke. For example, an initial increase in endothelial ROS by Rac1-dependent NADPH oxidase (Nox) may have positive effects on EC survival during a time of crisis; increase in EC-specific Nox-ROS has been shown to activate a survival pathway (e.g. activation of pro-survival kinase AMPK) and improve endothelial function (coronary vasodilation) by inducing AMPK-eNOS-NO [22]. Thus, it is of utmost importance to understand the roles of modulation (increase or decrease) of subcellular (cytosolic vs. mitochondrial vs. peroxisomal/lysosomal) ROS levels in health and disease.

Sources of funding

This work was supported by an Institutional Development Award (IDeA) from the National Institute of General Medical Sciences of the National Institutes of Health under grant number P20GM103652 (Project-3, to MRA), American Heart Association Grant-inAid 14GRNT20460291 (to MRA), and by NHLBI grant HL46716 (to FWS).

Author details

M. Ruhul Abid* and Frank W. Sellke

*Address all correspondence to: Ruhul_Abid@brown.edu

Cardiothoracic Surgery Division, Department of Surgery, Rhode Island Hospital, Brown University Warren Alpert Medical School, Providence, RI, USA

References

[1] Lassegue B and Griendling KK. NADPH oxidases: functions and pathologies in the vasculature. Arterioscler Thromb Vasc Biol. 2010;30:653-661.

[2] Datla SR and Griendling KK. Reactive oxygen species, NADPH oxidases, and hypertension. Hypertension. 2010;56:325-330.

[3] Luo Z, Teerlink T, Griendling K, Aslam S, Welch WJ and Wilcox CS. Angiotensin II and NADPH oxidase increase ADMA in vascular smooth muscle cells. Hypertension. 2010;56:498-504.

[4] Fukai T and Ushio-Fukai M. Superoxide dismutases: role in redox signaling, vascular function, and diseases. Antioxid Redox Signal. 2011;15:1583-1606.

[5] Frey RS, Ushio-Fukai M and Malik AB. NADPH oxidase-dependent signaling in endothelial cells: role in physiology and pathophysiology. Antioxid Redox Signal. 2009;11:791-810.

[6] Bjelakovic G, Nikolova D, Gluud LL, Simonetti RG and Gluud C. Mortality in randomized trials of antioxidant supplements for primary and secondary prevention: systematic review and meta-analysis. JAMA. 2007;297:842-857.

[7] Willcox BJ, Curb JD and Rodriguez BL. Antioxidants in cardiovascular health and disease: key lessons from epidemiologic studies. Am J Cardiol. 2008;101:75D-86D.

[8] Kris-Etherton PM, Lichtenstein AH, Howard BV, Steinberg D and Witztum JL. Antioxidant vitamin supplements and cardiovascular disease. Circulation. 2004;110:637-641.

[9] Frei B. Cardiovascular disease and nutrient antioxidants: role of low-density lipoprotein oxidation. Crit Rev Food Sci Nutr. 1995;35:83-98.

[10] Bagi Z, Feher A and Beleznai T. Preserved coronary arteriolar dilatation in patients with type 2 diabetes mellitus: implications for reactive oxygen species. Pharmacol Rep. 2009;61:99-104.

[11] Ye Y, Li J and Yuan Z. Effect of antioxidant vitamin supplementation on cardiovascular outcomes: a meta-analysis of randomized controlled trials. PLoS One. 2013;8:e56803.

[12] Feng J, Damrauer SM, Lee M, Sellke FW, Ferran C and Abid MR. Endothelium-dependent coronary vasodilatation requires NADPH oxidase-derived reactive oxygen species. Arterioscler Thromb Vasc Biol. 30:1703-1710.

[13] Zhang Q, Malik P, Pandey D, Gupta S, Jagnandan D, Belin de Chantemele E, Banfi B, Marrero MB, Rudic RD, Stepp DW and Fulton DJ. Paradoxical activation of endothelial nitric oxide synthase by NADPH oxidase. Arterioscler Thromb Vasc Biol. 2008;28:1627-1633.

[14] Sawada N, Salomone S, Kim HH, Kwiatkowski DJ and Liao JK. Regulation of endothelial nitric oxide synthase and postnatal angiogenesis by Rac1. Circ Res. 2008;103:360-368.

[15] Mozaffarian D, Benjamin EJ, Go AS, Arnett DK, Blaha MJ, Cushman M, Das SR, de Ferranti S, Despres JP, Fullerton HJ, Howard VJ, Huffman MD, Isasi CR, Jimenez MC, Judd SE, Kissela BM, Lichtman JH, Lisabeth LD, Liu S, Mackey RH, Magid DJ, McGuire DK, Mohler ER 3rd, Moy CS, Muntner P, Mussolino ME, Nasir K, Neumar RW, Nichol G, Palaniappan L, Pandey DK, Reeves MJ, Rodriguez CJ, Rosamond W, Sorlie PD, Stein

J, Towfighi A, Turan TN, Virani SS, Woo D, Yeh RW and Turner MB. Heart disease and stroke statistics-2016 update: a report from the American Heart Association. Circulation. 2015. Jan 27;131(4):e29–322. doi: 10.1161/CIR.0000000000000152.]

[16] Chilian WM, Penn MS, Pung YF, Dong F, Mayorga M, Ohanyan V, Logan S and Yin L. Coronary collateral growth-back to the future. J Mol Cell Cardiol. 2012 Apr;52(4):905–11. doi: 10.1016/j.yjmcc.2011.12.006.]

[17] Deussen A, Ohanyan V, Jannasch A, Yin L and Chilian W. Mechanisms of metabolic coronary flow regulation. J Mol Cell Cardiol. 2012 Apr;52(4):794–801. doi: 10.1016/j.yjmcc.2011.10.001.]

[18] Schaper W. Collateral circulation: past and present. Basic Res Cardiol. 2009;104:5-21.

[19] Sabe AA, Elmadhun NY, Sadek AA, Chu LM, Bianchi C and Sellke FW. Differential effects of atorvastatin on autophagy in ischemic and nonischemic myocardium in Ossabaw swine with metabolic syndrome. J Thorac Cardiovasc Surg. 2014;148:3172-3178.

[20] Elmadhun NY, Sabe AA, Lassaletta AD, Chu LM, Kondra K, Sturek M and Sellke FW. Metabolic syndrome impairs notch signaling and promotes apoptosis in chronically ischemic myocardium. Journal Thorac Cardiovasc Surg. 2014;148:1048-1055; discussion 1055.

[21] Abid MR, Kachra Z, Spokes KC and Aird WC. NADPH oxidase activity is required for endothelial cell proliferation and migration. FEBS Lett. 2000;486:252-256.

[22] Shafique E, Choy WC, Liu Y, Feng J, Cordeiro B, Lyra A, Arafah M, Yassin-Kassab A, Zanetti AV, Clements RT, Bianchi C, Benjamin LE, Sellke FW and Abid MR. Oxidative stress improves coronary endothelial function through activation of the pro-survival kinase AMPK. Aging (Albany NY). 2013;5:515-530.

[23] Anilkumar N, Weber R, Zhang M, Brewer A and Shah AM. Nox4 and Nox2 NADPH oxidases mediate distinct cellular redox signaling responses to agonist stimulation. Arterioscler Thromb Vasc Biol. 2008;28(7):1347-1354.

[24] Abid MR, Spokes KC, Shih SC and Aird WC. NADPH oxidase activity selectively modulates vascular endothelial growth factor signaling pathways. J Biol Chem. 2007;282:35373-35385.

[25] Abid MR, Tsai JC, Spokes KC, Deshpande SS, Irani K and Aird WC. Vascular endothelial growth factor induces manganese-superoxide dismutase expression in endothelial cells by a Rac1-regulated NADPH oxidase-dependent mechanism. FASEB J. 2001;15:2548-2550.

[26] Ushio-Fukai M, Tang Y, Fukai T, Dikalov SI, Ma Y, Fujimoto M, Quinn MT, Pagano PJ, Johnson C and Alexander RW. Novel role of gp91(phox)-containing NAD(P)H oxidase in vascular endothelial growth factor-induced signaling and angiogenesis. Circ Res. 2002;91:1160-1167.

[27] Brown DI and Griendling KK. Regulation of signal transduction by reactive oxygen species in the cardiovascular system. Circ Res. 2015;116(3):531-549.

[28] Didion SP. Increased superoxide and vascular dysfunction in CuZnSOD-deficient mice. Circ Res. 2002;91(10):938-944.

[29] Rodriguez-Iturbe B, Sepassi L, Quiroz Y, Ni Z and Vaziri ND. Association of mitochondrial SOD deficiency with salt-sensitive hypertension and accelerated renal senescence. J Appl Physiol. 2006;102(1):255-260.

[30] Kim HW, Lin A, Guldberg RE, Ushio-Fukai M and Fukai T. Essential role of extracellular SOD in reparative neovascularization induced by hindlimb ischemia. Circ Res. 2007;101(4)409-419.

[31] Forgione, MA, Weiss N, Heydrick S, Cap A, Klings ES, Bierl C, Eberhardt RT, Farber HW and Loscalzo J. Cellular glutathione peroxidase deficiency and endothelial dysfunction. Am J Physiol Heart Circ Physiol. 2001;282(4):207-12.

[32] Maulik N, Yoshida T and Das DK. Regulation of cardiomyocyte apoptosis in ischemic reperfused mouse heart by glutathione peroxidase. Stress Adaptation, Prophylaxis and Treatment. Kluwer Academic Publishers, Dordrecht, the Netherlands [Das, DK, Ed]. 1999; pp. 13–21.

[33] Galasso, G., et al. Impaired angiogenesis in glutathione Peroxidase-1-Deficient mice is associated with endothelial progenitor cell dysfunction. Circ Res. 2006;98(2):254-261.

[34] Shioji K, Nakamura H, Masutani H and Yodoi J. Redox regulation by thioredoxin in cardiovascular diseases. Antioxid Redox Signal. 2003;5(6):795-802.

Chapter 15

Free Radicals and Neuronal Recovery from an Ischaemic Penumbra: A Review

Cleva Villanueva, Robert D. Kross and
Luis Pérez-Astudillo

Additional information is available at the end of the chapter

http://dx.doi.org/10.5772/63366

Abstract

Stroke remains the second leading cause of death worldwide. The major problem is that the therapeutic window is short and no accepted treatment is completely efficient. Even though there is evidence of free radical participation in the pathophysiology of stroke, no beneficial effects of antioxidants have been demonstrated in clinical assays. Moreover, some reports paradoxically indicate that antioxidants could be harmful and that oxidative stress preconditioning could reduce the long-term effects of stroke. There are two major areas within the ischaemic zone: (1) the core, where neuronal necrosis develops in minutes, and (2) the penumbra surrounding the core, where some neurons could eventually be recovered over an extended time. The present review specifically focuses on the role of free radicals in the life or death of brain cells (mainly neurons) within the ischaemic penumbra. It also analyses the effects of oxidative stress on blood-brain barrier disruption. In conclusion, we postulate a cascade of events that follow cerebral ischaemia and what type of therapeutic approach could eventually change the effect of free radicals on neuronal recovery from an ischaemic penumbra.

Keywords: free radicals, ischaemic penumbra, oxidative stress, antioxidants, stroke

1. Introduction

According to the Global Burden of Disease Study (GBD 2010), stroke was the leading cause of mortality and the third leading cause of disability-adjusted life-years (DALYs) worldwide [1]. The highest incidence rates of ischaemic stroke are in Eastern Europe, Central Asia, East Asia and North Africa/Middle East [2]. Using the GBD 2013 methods it was determined that from

1990 to 2013 there was a significant increase of prevalent cases, total deaths and DALYs due to haemorrhagic and ischaemic stroke in younger adults (20–64 years), mainly in developing countries [3].

Intravenous thrombolysis remains the standard therapy for ischaemic stroke, but the window for therapy is narrow (3–4.5 hours after a stroke) and not completely effective, primarily in patients with large vessel thromboses. Some clinical trials suggest that intra-arterial thrombolysis plus a stent application could be the best therapy in large artery thrombosis. However, such treatment requires a thorough examination of the patient (24 hour computed tomography angiogram service), trained radiologists and quick location of the clot, as well as a rapid triaging of the patients to the stroke intervention centre [4]. The main limitations of thrombolysis are [5] (1) the long delay from the onset of stroke to treatment, (2) the irreversible cell damage caused by ischaemia over time, (3) that ischaemia can result in haemorrhaging caused by thrombolytics and (4) collateral effects of thrombolytics. Time and an understanding of the pathophysiology of neuronal and brain cell death in stroke are critical.

The role of oxidative stress in stroke has been intensively explored. References in the PubMed database alone ("oxidative stress" AND stroke, abstract/title) reveal a total of 1,852 papers (from two in 1991 to 234 in 2015). Even though several studies show beneficial effects of antioxidant supplements for stroke, no meta-analyses (clinical studies) thus far have strongly validated the protective effects of any post-stroke antioxidant supplement. Moreover, there is no meta-analysis supporting the beneficial effects of antioxidant preventive supplementation [6–8]. Indeed, antioxidant supplements actually could be dangerous [9]. A meta-analysis including 4,875 subjects with a follow-up period of 7–15 years demonstrated that the daily intake of more than 300 mg of vitamin C was associated with an increased risk of cardiovascular diseases, coronary artery disease and stroke in diabetic patients [7]. However, there are controversies regarding the effects of dietary antioxidants on stroke. A meta-analysis including 116,117 participants and 1,989 cases demonstrated that circulating lycopene, not simply dietary lycopene, was associated with a significantly decreased stroke risk [10], whereas high flavonol intake, compared to low intake, was associated with a higher stroke risk [11].

Exercise can increase the endogenous antioxidant defence for changing stroke risk. Hooker et al. published an interesting prospective study performed in a total of 46,406 men and 15,282 women who had no cardiovascular disease at the beginning of the study and who carried out a treadmill test to evaluate their cardiorespiratory fitness. The subjects were followed from 1970 to 2001. There was an inverse relationship between cardiorespiratory fitness and the incidence of fatal or non-fatal stroke [12]. An interesting study performed with 31,696 Swedish women who were followed for 10.5 years concluded that a low-risk lifestyle was related to a low stroke risk. A low-risk lifestyle was defined as a healthy diet (to 50% of Recommended Food Score), moderate alcohol consumption (5–15 g/day), not smoking, physical activity (walking/bicycling ≥ 40 min/day and exercising ≥ 1 hour/week) and a body mass index < 25 kg/m^2 [13].

Stroke has been significantly associated with environmental pollution in different countries. Short-term exposure to air pollution has been related to stroke in Denmark [14] and in Sweden [15]. Recent studies in Israel and Germany concluded that long-term exposure to fine-particle dust was associated with a higher risk of stroke [16, 17]. It is relevant that the study in Israel found a relationship of pollution to stroke in young adults [17]. A large epidemiologic study performed with 114,537 women (Nurses' Health Study) in the USA found that the association between long-term pollution exposure and stroke was stronger in diabetic women [18]. Experimentally (though not fully demonstrated in people naturally exposed to pollution), the effects of pollution do seem to be related to oxidative stress. Oxidative stress could simply be defined as the condition where the balance between antioxidants and free radicals tilts in favour of free radicals [9].

2. The ischaemic penumbra

Depending on the location and diameter of the obstructed vessel, the interruption of blood flow and the consequent hypoxia and lack of nutrients produces an ischaemic core where Adenosine triphosphate (ATP) levels reach around 15% of the basal values within minutes. This results in neuronal death from which is impossible to recover [19]. The area that surrounds the ischaemic core is termed the penumbra (from the Latin *paene*, almost; *umbra*, shadow). ATP levels in the penumbra are around 50–70% of the basal values [19], indicating that neuronal death is delayed, and this is where therapeutic strategies should be directed to ensure that neurons survive and recover. Mechanisms leading to neuronal death in the penumbra seem to be triggered by hypoxia and the fall of glucose. Actually the ischaemic penumbra is highly dynamic with a rapid evolution that leads to cell death.

Dirnagl et al. [20] published an interesting paper in 1999 based on experimental and clinical (autopsy histopathological) studies of patients who died from stroke. The paper showed a time-course of damaging events in focal ischaemia. The author updated that time-course in 2012 [21]. Everything starts with blood interruption, and within minutes there is a high wave of excitotoxicity and peri-infarct depolarisation with an accumulation of glutamate, calcium and reactive oxygen species (ROS); in the following hours the mediators that were liberated and induced in the first stages trigger inflammation through the activation of cyclooxygenase-2, caspases, metalloproteinases (MMPs) and the liberation of inflammatory interleukins. After several days apoptosis takes place and the penumbra area becomes part of the death core, although repairing processes are also activated; and there are scar formation, neurogenesis and vasculogenesis [20, 21].

It has been experimentally demonstrated that there are two flow thresholds during stroke evolution, the first being a functional threshold that leads to reversible functional changes and the second producing irreversible membrane failure and morphological damage. The penumbra is between these thresholds [22].

Returning to the time-course concept, when the decrease of blood flow reaches about 20% of preocclusion values, there are a tremendous ionic disequilibrium, osmotic swelling and, finally, within minutes, terminal depolarisation at the core occurs. The blood flow around the core reaches 20 to 50% of preocclusion values within 6 hours, and by that time irreversible damage expands around the core. It is calculated that infarct volume increases more than 20% (from core to penumbra) within the first 3 hours after occlusion [22]. Blood flow-dependent damage explains the short therapeutic window and the lack of thrombolytic therapeutic efficacy. It has been demonstrated experimentally that the biggest effect of thrombolytics occurs within 90 min because acute arterial occlusion and the reduction of blood flow can be tolerated only 1–2 hours before irreversible damage occurs [23]. Optimal treatment time is supposed to be around 3 hours, and between three and 4.5 hours, they only provide small effects [4, 23].

3. Role of oxidative stress in death and survival of brain cells in an ischaemic penumbra

The penumbra area includes neurons and other brain cells and structures such as astrocytes, endothelial cells, pericytes, smooth muscle cells, microglia, basement membrane, as well as extracellular matrix, all of which become activated by the lack of blood flow and thereafter interact to produce free radicals, inflammation and a cascade of events leading to cell death but also regenerative processes that could eventually limit the core progression [5]. It is important to recognise that the cascade of events triggered by stroke goes beyond the core and penumbra and includes the contralateral hemisphere and the whole organism. Cells of the neurovascular unit (see above), cells that migrate to the insult area (neutrophils, monocytes, T cells, B cells) and stem cells from the brain and blood participate in the damage and recovery associated with cerebral ischaemia [21].

Free radicals are produced soon after ischaemia and contribute to both the expansion of neuronal death and neuronal recovery from the ischaemic penumbra. The primary and rapidly produced free radical is probably superoxide, generated by mitochondrial dysfunction induced by hypoxia. Some time thereafter superoxide is produced from other sources at the penumbra, such as the nicotinamide adenine dinucleotide phosphate oxidase (NADPHox) complex, xanthine oxidase, lipoxygenase, cyclooxygenase (COX), cytochrome p450 and, probably (though not yet demonstrated), uncoupled endothelial nitric oxide synthase (eNOS) [24, 25]. Superoxide dismutase (SOD) catalyses the dismutation of superoxide into hydrogen peroxide that is then decomposed into water and oxygen by catalase or glutathione peroxidase (GPx) [9]. Hydrogen peroxide could eventually produce hydroxyl radical (more toxic than superoxide) if it reacts with iron (Fenton reaction). It is well known that hydrogen peroxide stimulates nuclear factor kappa B (NF-kB), which in turn induces the transcription of SOD genes [26]. Even though the redox stimulation of NF-kB has been long known, it is not clear if the stimulation is provided by hydrogen peroxide and/or superoxide itself.

The stimulation of SOD synthesis by ROS does not guarantee antioxidant protection. The continuous production of superoxide in cerebral ischaemia (first stimulated by hypoxia and later by other sources) could eventually turn SOD toxic. If superoxide production exceeds catalase activity and/or glutathione sources are exhausted, SOD could lead to the accumulation of the hydroxyl radical. This is precisely one of the handicaps of experimental models of cerebral ischaemia. The latter are usually produced in normal animals that have been subjected to occlusion of cerebral arteries. This is far from the clinical setting, where cerebral ischaemia usually develops in patients with comorbidities or environmental conditions that constitute a risk for stroke (e.g., diabetes, hypertension, obesity, atherosclerosis, smoke, air pollution). In such conditions there is already an elevated basal oxidative stress with probably poor endogenous antioxidant defence. Moreover, strategies to protect from cerebral ischaemia are far from realistic (e.g., antioxidant supplements are often given before stroke occurs). There are other circumstances that could interfere in the attempted extrapolation of experimental results to a clinical therapeutic design. Usually the experiments on cerebral ischaemia involve a combination of ischaemia/reperfusion, with the rationale being the aggravation of oxidative stress during reperfusion [21]. It would be exceptional to believe that an occluded vessel becomes permeable within a short time, i.e., reperfusion to an ischaemic territory is usually given by neoformation of vessels (angiogenesis). Another drawback of experimental assays is that measures to prevent bias are not common: e.g., randomisation of the animals, appropriate inclusion/exclusion criteria, a low number of cases and thus a low positive predictive value [21]. Even with those disadvantages mentioned, there is experimental evidence which helps to understand the events that lead penumbra cells to either die or survive.

Responses to superoxide production in the penumbra are fast. It has been shown that copper zinc superoxide dismutase (CuZnSOD), the cytosolic form, is increased in the penumbra 1 hour after middle cerebral artery occlusion (MCAO)/reperfusion (MCAOR), whereas manganese SOD (MnSOD, mitochondrial) increases in the penumbra and core 3 hours after MCAOR [27]. Nitric oxide (NO) is another free radical liberated in the ischaemic penumbra. The source of the earlier production of NO in the penumbra seems to be the neuronal nitric oxide synthase (nNOS). This enzyme has been shown to increase in the penumbra 1 hour after MCAO in the rat [28]. Later on, when the inflammatory reaction is present, the inducible NOS (iNOS) is responsible for the high concentrations of NO in the ischaemic penumbra [29]. The coincidence of large quantities of superoxide and NO in the proximity of the core (where the pH is low) facilitates the interaction of those free radicals to form peroxynitrite. Indeed nitrotyrosine (a marker of peroxynitrite production) has been detected in the penumbra 4 hours after MCAOR in the rat [29]. Tyrosine nitration by peroxynitrite can actually inactivate SOD [30].

Besides SOD, other antioxidant defence mechanisms are activated after cerebral ischaemia although they take a longer time. Nuclear factor (erythroid-derived 2)-like 2 (Nrf2), which is an important brain defence against oxidative stress, is upregulated in neurons [31, 32], microglia [31] and astrocytes [31, 32] of the ischaemic penumbra (not in the core), 24 hours after MCAOR in the rats and mice. Activated Nrf2 induces what is termed "phase II defence enzymes and antioxidant stress proteins" through its interaction with the antioxidant response element in the promoter region of target genes [33]. As a result Nfr2 activation during cerebral ischaemia provides protection through the modulation of microglia dynamics, the protection of astrocytes and neurons and regulation of the expression of antioxidant enzymes and anti-inflammatory mediators [33].

Free radicals produced during cerebral ischaemia contribute to a breakdown of the blood-brain barrier (BBB), an event that has been related to cerebral oedema, and has an important role in the pathophysiology of cerebral ischaemia by allowing the arrival of migrating cells that contribute not only to inflammation but also to eventual angiogenesis, neurogenesis and partial regeneration. The BBB is a complex structure integrated by particular endothelial cells: (a) that do not have fenestrations, (b) that have limited pinocytic activity and (c) that have a high content of mitochondria; tight-junction proteins such as occludin, claudin 5 and zonula occludens 1; and pericytes, astrocytes, extracellular matrix and transporter systems, such as the receptor for advanced glycation end products (RAGEs) [34–37]. Protein leakage (evidence of BBB breakdown) has been demonstrated as early as 30 min after MCAOR [25, 38]. In some studies (but not all), such leakage is prevented by an antioxidant treatment [25]. An important source of free radicals during cerebral ischaemia is the vascular endothelium [25, 39]. Apparently the main contributor to superoxide production in the vessels of the penumbra is NADPHox [39]. Superoxide and other ROS activate MMPs, mainly MMP9 and MMP2, that degrade extracellular matrix and basal lamina around vessels, contributing to BBB disruption during ischaemia [38, 40]. It has been demonstrated that MMP9 is upregulated in the penumbra from 24 to 72 hours after ischaemia [41].

Delayed production of free radicals contributes to blood vessel disintegration in an ischaemic penumbra. The subacute phase of cerebral ischaemia (from 24 to 72 hours after blood flow interruption) is characterised (as mentioned above) by an explosion of free radicals produced by the inflammatory reaction induced during the events that occur in the acute phase. It has been estimated that this second wave of free radical generation coincides with a second opening of the BBB [42]. The main source of inflammatory mediators and free radicals in this phase is the microglia (resident macrophages of the brain and spinal cord). Microglia accumulate in the penumbra several hours after cerebral ischaemia [43], but apparently its active role in ischaemia begins earlier. Jolivel et al. published an interesting paper in 2015 [41] showing data on the time-course of microglia activation in the penumbra during ischaemia: (1) soon after reperfusion microglia become activated in the penumbra; (2) an association of activated microglia with endothelial cells of the penumbra begins as soon as 4 hours after reperfusion; (3) at 24 hours after reperfusion CX3CL1 (a chemokine involved in migration of microglia) significantly co-localises with microglia in the penumbra; (4) at the same time the microglia are associated with claudin 5 in the penumbra, which indirectly indicates the disruption of the BBB; (5) MMP9 is activated 3 hours after reperfusion and it peaks at 24 hours (another indirect evidence of BBB disruption) in the penumbra; and (6) at 24 hours after ischaemia neutrophils invade the penumbra (direct evidence of BBB disruption). Microglia activity seems to last only a few days, from 72 hours after ischaemia the microglia decline and the monocytes migrate to the penumbra; apparently those monocytes also have an inflammatory phenotype and serve to clean up the area [44].

Astrocytes play also an important role in the second wave of free radical production; it seems that they are activated by free radicals to protect and rescue neurons at the ischaemic penumbra. Astrocytes are abundant in the brain and have an important role in potassium homeostasis, synapse formation and BBB regulation [45]. Activated astrocytes give protection in ischaemia through glutathione regulation [33, 45]: (1) liberating glutathione, which has a free radical scavenger function; (2) facilitating the enzyme γ glutamyltranspeptidase (present on the surface of astrocytes) to hydrolyse extracellular glutathione, producing glycine and cysteine, that are then captured by neurons to synthesise their own glutathione; and (3) liberating glutamine that is also captured by neurons to synthesise glutathione. Astrocytes also provide protection by removing excess glutamate, producing neurotrophic factors and transforming dehydroascorbate to ascorbate, which is liberated to neurons and works as an antioxidant [33, 46]. **Figure 1** shows an illustration of a hypothetical thrombosis of the middle cerebral artery (superior division) in humans with high-risk factors. **Figure 1** represents a cascade based on the data described above.

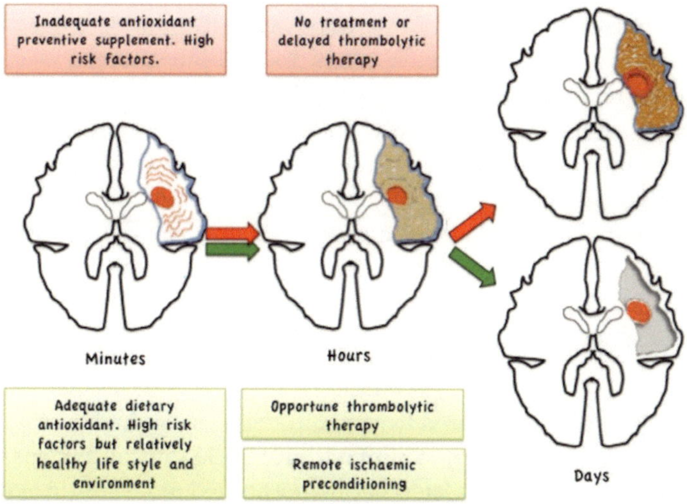

Figure 1. An illustration of a hypothetical thrombosis of the middle cerebral artery (superior division) in humans with high-risk factors. If the patient had received inadequate treatment with antioxidant supplements before cerebral ischaemia and/or the thrombolytic treatment is delayed, the ischaemic penumbra will be part of the core. If the patient has a relatively healthy lifestyle (see Ref. [13]) in a beneficial environment and receives opportune thrombolytic therapy and possibly remote ischaemic preconditioning, the consequences of the cerebral ischaemia will be smaller as compared with the conditions mentioned previously.

4. Preconditioning and survival in the ischaemic penumbra

Preconditioning can be defined as a biphasic response to a noxious stimulus, with a low dose (often accumulated low doses) providing protection when a higher dose is applied [47]. Preconditioning beneficial effects are usually explained by adaptive mechanisms such as changes in homeostasis thresholds or an increase of the endogenous defence. Oxidative preconditioning explains the protective effects of exercise [48]. Preconditioning has been used to increase neuronal survival at the ischaemic penumbra [49].

Several varieties of preconditioning have been used in cerebral ischaemia, such as hyperbaric oxygen (HBO), normobaric hyperoxia (NBH), hypoxia, ischaemic preconditioning and limb remote ischaemic preconditioning (RIsP). In the rat model of MCAOR HBO has been demonstrated to reduce oxidative stress as well as apoptosis in the penumbra, and it increases survival time [50, 51]. Several mechanisms have been related to the beneficial effects of HBO preconditioning. HBO (2.5 ATA, 100% oxygen, 1 hour, every 12 hours, four times before MCAOR) increases SOD and catalase (not GPx) in the penumbra [50]. Longer HBO preconditioning (5 days before MCAOR) increases SirT1 (a class III histone deacetylase whose activity promotes lifespan in lower organisms) in the penumbra [52]. Interestingly, the protective effects of physical activity on cardiovascular ageing have been precisely associated with the increase of SOD and SirT1 [48].

NBH (100% oxygen, 1.0 ATA) has been also used for preconditioning to ameliorate cerebral ischaemia. NBH applied 30 min after ischaemia (MCAOR in a rat model, with 90 min of ischaemia) significantly reduced oxidative stress and apoptosis in the penumbra (with the greatest effect after 8 hours of NBH) [53]. It is important to mention that there are indications of potential harmful effects of HBO and NBH on cerebral ischaemia. Rink et al. [54] published an interesting paper in 2010 showing that HBO and NBH applied just during ischaemia in rats and mice submitted to MCAOR (90 min of ischaemia and 90 min of reperfusion) significantly decreased the infarct volume and also decreased oxidative stress, but increased pO_2 in the penumbra. However, when those therapies were administered during reperfusion the effect was the opposite. The findings are important because in the clinical setting it is difficult to establish the time-course of cerebral ischaemia and that administering HBO or NBH could be dangerous.

Hypoxic preconditioning has been used to promote angiogenesis in the ischaemic penumbra. In an interesting study, Li et al. [55] submitted mice to 30 min of hypoxia before cerebral ischaemia. Twenty-four and 72 hours later they demonstrated protection (a reduction of infarct volume and the neurophysiological index) and a significant increase of vascular endothelial growth factor (VEGF) as well as platelet endothelial cell adhesion molecule 1 (CD31, an index of angiogenesis) in both neurons and the vascular cells of the ischaemic penumbra.

Brain ischaemia preconditioning (BIP) has been extensively studied. Classically the model consists of submitting animals to a short period of transient MCAO, and then 1 day later, the animals are subjected to permanent MCAO or MCAOR [56]. Different mechanisms have been associated with BIP such as adaptation to glutamate activation of the N-methyl-D-aspartic acid (NMDA) receptor and the signal transduction pathways stimulated by this receptor including phosphorylation of cyclic AMP-responsive element binding protein (CREB) in the penumbra, persistent activation of protein kinase B (Akt) and decreased apoptosis in the penumbra [49]. Recently, Liu et al. [57] showed that rats submitted to BIP (one and 4 days before MCAOR) showed smaller infarct volumes and increased brain immunoreactivity to VEGF 7 days after MCAOR, which indicates similarities to the hypoxia preconditioning mechanisms.

Preconditioning, as described above, has been used in a number of experimental studies. In the last few years, a therapeutic strategy based on preconditioning principia has been applied not only in experimental but in clinical studies as well. RIsP simply consists of producing transient ischaemia in the upper or lower members, by inflation or deflation of a blood pressure cuff [58]. RIsP has been used in humans in a variety of applications such as in sports [59], for subarachnoid haemorrhages [60], and in cardiovascular surgery [61, 62]. There are experimental validations of the utility of RIsP in recovering the penumbra following cerebral

http://dx.doi.org/10.5772/63366

ischaemia. Rats were subjected to MCAOR (90 min of ischaemia), immediately after ischaemia RIsP was applied in three cycles of occlusion and release, lasting 10 min each. After 48 hours it was demonstrated that the treatment (1) diminished the infarct volume, (2) improved the neurologic deficit and (3) decreased BBB breakdown (demonstrated by preventing an occludin protein decrease, Evans blue extravasation and MMP9 activation) [40]. Different mechanisms have been suggested for the protective effects of RIsP. Interestingly, in a clinical study of acute mountain sickness prevention by RIsP [59], it was clearly demonstrated (by electron paramagnetic resonance) that protection was not associated with the reduction of systemic oxidative stress. It seems that RIsP effects are associated with the liberation of the hypoxia-inducible factor α [58] and stimulation of eNOS [63]. **Figure 2** shows the modified **Figure 1**, adding molecular mechanisms and RIsP.

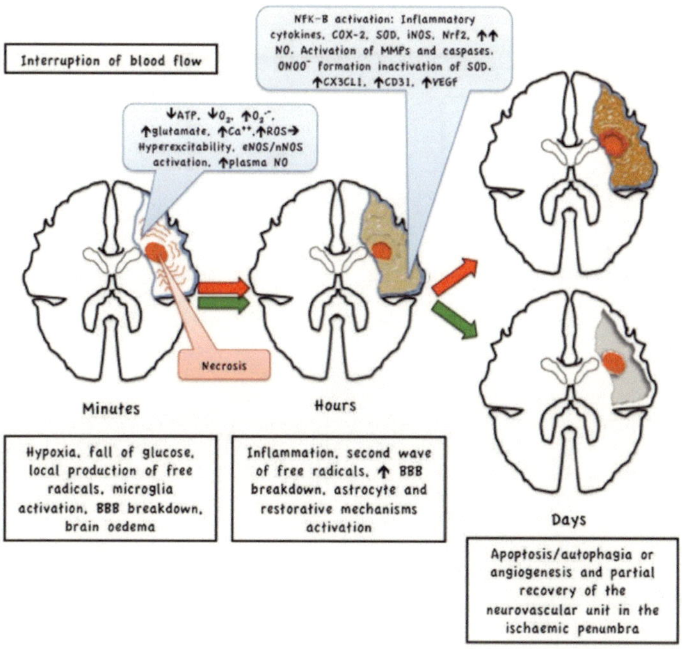

Figure 2. A hypothetical cascade of events leading to cell death or survival in the ischaemic penumbra. The cascade begins with an interruption of the blood supply that leads to hypoxia and the fall of glucose and consequently ATP. Within minutes there is necrosis in the core, and the subsequent ischaemic penumbra is characterised by an increase of superoxide ($O_2^{\bullet-}$), glutamate, calcium (Ca^{2+}) and other ROS, leading to hyperexcitability. eNOS and nNOS are activated (possibly not exclusively in the ischaemic penumbra) and nitric oxide (NO) levels increase in the plasma. Those phenomena produce a blood-brain barrier (BBB) breakdown and consequently brain oedema. From 1 to 7 days after blood interruption, there are a tremendous inflammatory reaction and a second wave of free radical production, activation of the NF-kB stimulating the synthesis of cyclooxygenase 2 (COX-2), superoxide dismutase (SOD), inducible NOS (iNOS) and the (erythroid-derived 2)-like 2 factor (Nrf2). NO increases additionally and interacts with $O_2^{\bullet-}$, producing peroxynitrite ($ONOO^-$), which in turn inactivates SOD through tyrosine nitration. Caspases and metalloproteinases (MMPs) are activated. The CX3CL1 and the endothelial cell adhesion molecule (CD31) increase. The restorative mechanisms begin with astrocyte activation. Part of the restorative mechanism is the induction of the vascular endothelial growth factor (VEGF) and CD31. If therapy is not effective or appropriate, the cells in the ischaemic penumbra will die from apoptosis or autophagy, which extends the core area. Otherwise the ischaemic penumbra is partially recovered.

The organism not only adapts to noxious stimuli but also to protective treatments, which is precisely one of the pitfalls of "preventive" antioxidant supplements. In an ongoing study (not yet published), our group found that daily doses (10 mg/kg per day for 7 days) of (−)-epicatechin ((−)-Epi) (one of the flavonols contained in chocolate) significantly increased the infarct volume 18 hours after permanent MCAO was produced in rats (**Figure 3**). It is important to note that cerebral ischaemia was produced in healthy (10-week-old) male Wistar rats, which could explain the results. We think that the treatment decreased the endogenous antioxidants and, when the ischaemia was produced, there was insufficient defence. We also think that the results would have been different if the treatment had been administered to animals that previously had high oxidative stress.

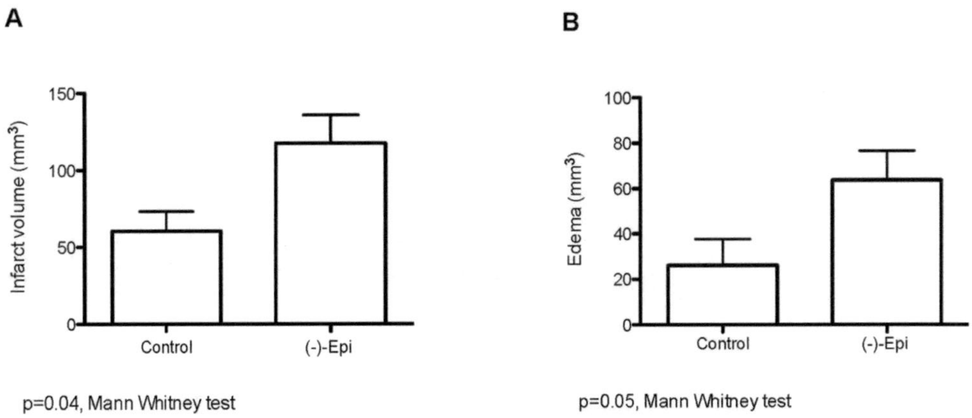

Figure 3. The significant increment of infarct volume (A) in rats treated with (−)-epicatechin ((−)-Epi) that were submitted to permanent occlusion of the middle cerebral artery (MCAO). And even though there was no significant difference in cerebral oedema (B), there was a tendency for the group treated with (−)-Epi to be higher.

5. Conclusions

Cerebral ischaemia remains a challenge in medical therapeutics because of the narrow window of time during which treatment can be applied, as well as its low efficacy. Brain cells in the ischaemic core cannot be recovered; they die within minutes from necrosis, whereas the death of those in the ischaemic penumbra is briefly delayed; and the mechanism of death is apoptosis and autophagy. Therapeutic strategies should be precisely directed to optimise all possible processes for recovering cells from the ischaemic penumbra. The neurovascular unit in the ischaemic penumbra is dynamically changing, switching off and on the pathways that could lead to cell death or survival. Free radicals are an important part of those pathways and can play a role in either cell loss or recovery. Even though results of preclinical studies are optimistic, the effects of antioxidant supplements have not been clinically validated in cerebral ischaemia. Moreover, there are increasing data showing warning signs. "Preventive" antioxidant supplements could decrease the endogenous antioxidant defence that is needed at the precise moment of cerebral ischaemia. Antioxidant treatment (dietary or supplemental) should be carefully managed, depending on the basal conditions and the endogenous antioxidant defence of every person. There is some hope for applying RIsP in cerebral ischaemia, since it seems to have beneficial effects on the clinical physiological and pathological conditions associated with oxidative stress. Preclinical studies, even with their disadvantages, help to elucidate the pathophysiology of cerebral ischaemia and thereby the design of future treatments.

Acknowledgements

This work was supported by Consejo Nacional de Ciencia y Tecnología, Mexico (Grant CONACTY 202483), Instituto Politécnico Nacional, Mexico (Grant SIP 20150654), and Kross Link Laboratories (NY, USA).

Author details

Cleva Villanueva[1*], Robert D. Kross[2] and Luis Pérez-Astudillo[3]

*Address all correspondence to: villanuevacleva3@gmail.com

1 Instituto Politecnico Nacional, Escuela Superior de Medicina, Mexico City, Mexico

2 Kross-Link Laboratories, Bellmore, NY, USA

3 Biotest S.C. Cd Sahagun, Hidalgo, Mexico

References

[1] Appel LJ. Reducing sodium intake to prevent stroke: time for action, not hesitation. Stroke. 2014;45: 909–911. DOI: 10.1161/STROKEAHA.113.002870.

[2] Bennett DA, Krishnamurthi RV, Barker-Collo S, Forouzanfar MH, Naghavi M, Connor M, *et al.* The global burden of ischemic stroke: findings of the GBD 2010 study. Global Heart. 2014;9: 107–112. DOI: 10.1016/j.gheart.2014.01.001.

[3] Krishnamurthi RV, Moran AE, Feigin VL, Barker-Collo S, Norrving B, Mensah GA, *et al.* Stroke prevalence, mortality and disability-adjusted life years in adults aged 20–64 years in 1990–2013: data from the Global Burden of Disease 2013 Study. Neuroepidemiology. 2015;45: 190–202. DOI: 10.1159/000441098.

[4] Sekhar A. Intra-arterial treatment in acute ischaemic stroke: what we learn from the MR CLEAN trial. J R Coll Physicians Edinb. 2015;45: 43–44. DOI: 10.4997/JRCPE.2015.110.

[5] Liu R, Yuan H, Yuan F, Yang SH. Neuroprotection targeting ischemic penumbra and beyond for the treatment of ischemic stroke. Neurological Res. 2012;34: 331–337. DOI: 10.1179/1743132812Y.0000000020.

[6] Bin Q, Hu X, Cao Y, Gao F. The role of vitamin E (tocopherol) supplementation in the prevention of stroke. A meta-analysis of 13 randomised controlled trials. Thrombosis Haemost. 2011;105: 579–585. DOI: 10.1160/TH10-11-0729.

[7] Sarmento RA, Silva FM, Sbruzzi G, Schaan BD, Almeida JC. Antioxidant micronutrients and cardiovascular risk in patients with diabetes: a systematic review. Arq Bras Cardiol. 2013;101: 240–248. DOI: 10.5935/abc.20130146.

[8] Ye Y, Li J, Yuan Z. Effect of antioxidant vitamin supplementation on cardiovascular outcomes: a meta-analysis of randomized controlled trials. PLoS One. 2013;8: e56803. DOI: 10.1371/journal.pone.0056803.

[9] Villanueva C, Kross RD. Antioxidant-induced stress. Int J Mol Sci. 2012;13: 2091–2109. DOI: 10.3390/ijms13022091.

[10] Li X, Xu J. Dietary and circulating lycopene and stroke risk: a meta-analysis of prospective studies. Sci Rep. 2014;4: 1–8. DOI: 10.1038/srep05031.

[11] Hollman PCH, Geelen A, Kromhout D. Dietary flavonol intake may lower stroke risk in men and women. J Nutr. 2010;140: 600–604. DOI: 10.3945/jn.109.116632.

[12] Hooker SP, Sui X, Colabianchi N, Vena J, Laditka J, LaMonte MJ, *et al*. Cardiorespiratory fitness as a predictor of fatal and nonfatal stroke in asymptomatic women and men. Stroke. 2008;39: 2950–2957. DOI: 10.1161/STROKEAHA.107.495275.

[13] Larsson SC, Akesson A, Wolk A. Healthy diet and lifestyle and risk of stroke in a prospective cohort of women. Neurology. 2014;83: 1699–1704. DOI: 10.1212/WNL.0000000000000954.

[14] Andersen ZJ, Olsen TS, Andersen KK, Loft S, Ketzel M, Raaschou-Nielsen O. Association between short-term exposure to ultrafine particles and hospital admissions for stroke in Copenhagen, Denmark, Eur Heart J. 2010;31: 2034–2040. DOI: 10.1093/eurheartj/ehq188.

[15] Oudin A, Stromberg U, Jakobsson K, Stroh E, Bjork J. Estimation of short-term effects of air pollution on stroke hospital admissions in southern Sweden. Neuroepidemiology. 2010;34: 131–142. DOI: 10.1159/000274807.

[16] Hoffmann B, Weinmayr G, Hennig F, Fuks K, Moebus S, Weimar C, *et al*. Air quality, stroke, and coronary events: results of the Heinz Nixdorf Recall Study from the Ruhr Region. Dtsch Arztebl Int. 2015;112: 195–201. DOI: 10.3238/arztebl.2015.0195.

[17] Yitshak Sade M, Novack V, Ifergane G, Horev A, Kloog I. Air pollution and ischemic stroke among young adults. Stroke. 2015;46: 3348–3353. DOI: 10.1161/STROKEAHA. 115.010992.

[18] Hart JE, Puett RC, Rexrode KM, Albert CM, Laden F. Effect modification of long-term air pollution exposures and the risk of incident cardiovascular disease in US women. J Am Heart Assoc. 2015;4: e002301. DOI: 10.1161/JAHA.115.002301.

[19] Li V, Bi X, Szelemej P, Kong J. Delayed neuronal death in ischemic stroke. In: Balestrino M, editor. Molecular Pathways and Advances in the Preclinical Study of Ischemic Stroke. Rijeka: InTech; 2012. p. 117–144.

[20] Dirnagl U, Iadecola C, Moskowitz MA. Pathobiology of ischaemic stroke: an integrated view. Trends Neurosci. 1999;22: 391–397. DOI: 10.1016/SO166-2236(99)1401-0.

[21] Dirnagl U. Pathobiology of injury after stroke: the neurovascular unit and beyond. Ann N Y Acad Sci. 2012;1268: 21–25. DOI: 10.1111/j.1749-6632.2012.06691.x.

[22] Heiss WD. The ischemic penumbra: how does tissue injury evolve? Ann N Y Acad Sci. 2012;1268: 26–34. DOI: 10.1111/J.1749-6632.2012.06668.x.

[23] Grotta J. Timing of thrombolysis for acute ischemic stroke: "timing is everything" or "everyone is different". Ann N Y Acad Sci. 2012;1268: 141–144. DOI: 10.1111/J. 1749-6632.2012.06690.x.

[24] Pamenter ME, Ali SS, Tang Q, Finley JC, Gu XQ, Dugan LL, *et al*. An in vitro ischemic penumbral mimic perfusate increases NADPH oxidase-mediated superoxide production in cultured hippocampal neurons. Brain Res. 2012;1452: 165–172. DOI: 10.1016/ j.brainres.2012.03.004.

[25] Fraser PA. The role of free radical generation in increasing cerebrovascular permeability. Free Radic Biol Med. 2011;51: 967–977. DOI. 10.1016/j.freeradbiomed.2011.06.003.

[26] Schmidt KN, Amstad P, Cerutti P, Baeuerle PA. The roles of hydrogen peroxide and superoxide as messengers in the activation of transcription factor NF-kappa B. Chem Biol. 1995;2: 13–22. DOI: 10.1016/1074-5521(95)90076-4.

[27] Bonova P, Danielisova V, Nemethova M, Matiasova M, Bona M, Gottlieb M. Scheme of ischaemia-triggered agents during brain infarct evolution in a rat model of permanent focal ischaemia. J Mol Neurosci. 2015;57: 73–82. DOI: 10.1007/sl2031-015-0578-6.

[28] Shen J, Ma S, Chan P, Lee W, Fung PC, Cheung RT, *et al*. Nitric oxide down-regulates caveolin-1 expression in rat brains during focal cerebral ischemia and reperfusion injury. J Neurochem. 2006;96: 1078–1089. DOI: 10.1111/j.1471-4159.2005.03589.x.

[29] Suzuki M, Tabuchi M, Ikeda M, Tomita T. Concurrent formation of peroxynitrite with the expression of inducible nitric oxide synthase in the brain during middle cerebral artery occlusion and reperfusion in rats. Brain Res. 2002;951: 113–120. DOI: 10.1016/ S0006-8993(02)03145.1.

[30] Yamakura F, Taka H, Fujimura T, Murayama K. Inactivation of human manganese-superoxide dismutase by peroxynitrite is caused by exclusive nitration of tyrosine 34 to 3-nitrotyrosine. J Biol Chem. 1998;273: 14085–14089. DOI: 10.1074/jbc.273.23.14085.

[31] Dang J, Brandenburg LO, Rosen C, Fragoulis A, Kipp M, Pufe T, *et al.* Nrf2 expression by neurons, astroglia, and microglia in the cerebral cortical penumbra of ischemic rats. J Mol Neurosci. 2012;46: 578–584. DOI: 10.1007/SL2031-011-9465.9.

[32] Takagi T, Kitashoji A, Iwawaki T, Tsuruma K, Shimazawa M, Yoshimura S, *et al.* Temporal activation of Nrf2 in the penumbra and Nrf2 activator-mediated neuroprotection in ischemia-reperfusion injury. Free Radic Biol Med. 2014;72: 124–133. DOI: 10-1016/j.freeradbiomed.2014.04.009.

[33] Alfieri A, Srivastava S, Siow RC, Modo M, Fraser PA, Mann GE. Targeting the Nrf2-Keap1 antioxidant defence pathway for neurovascular protection in stroke. J Physiol. 2011;589: 4125–4136. DOI: 10.1113/jphysiol.2011.210294.

[34] Yang Y, Thompson JF, Taheri S, Salayandia VM, McAvoy TA, Hill JW, *et al.* Early inhibition of MMP activity in ischemic rat brain promotes expression of tight junction proteins and angiogenesis during recovery. J Cereb Blood Flow Metab. 2013;33: 1104–1114. DOI: 10.1038/jcbfm.2013.56.

[35] Ronaldson PT, Davis TP. Targeting transporters: promoting blood–brain barrier repair in response to oxidative stress injury. Brain Res. 2015;1623: 39–52. DOI: 10.1016/j.brainres.2015.03.018.

[36] Kook SY, Hong HS, Moon M, Ha CM, Chang S, Mook-Jung I. Abeta(1)(-)(4)(2)-RAGE interaction disrupts tight junctions of the blood–brain barrier via Ca(2)(+)-calcineurin signaling. J Neurosci. 2012;32: 8845–8854. DOI: 10.1532/JNEUROSCI.6102-11.2012.

[37] Khatri R, McKinney AM, Swenson B, Janardhan V. Blood–brain barrier, reperfusion injury, and hemorrhagic transformation in acute ischemic stroke. Neurology. 2012;79: S52–S57. DOI: 10.1212/WNL.0b013e3182697e70.

[38] Chen H, Yoshioka H, Kim GS, Jung JE, Okami N, Sakata H, *et al.* Oxidative stress in ischemic brain damage: mechanisms of cell death and potential molecular targets for neuroprotection. Antioxid Redox Signal. 2011;14: 1505–1517. DOI: 10.1089/ars.2010.3576.

[39] Zehendner CM, Librizzi L, Hedrich J, Bauer NM, Angamo EA, de Curtis M, *et al.* Moderate hypoxia followed by reoxygenation results in blood–brain barrier breakdown via oxidative stress-dependent tight-junction protein disruption. PLoS One. 2013;8: e82823. DOI: 10.1371/journal.pone.0082823.

[40] Ren C, Li N, Wang B, Yang Y, Gao J, Li S, *et al.* Limb ischemic preconditioning attenuates blood–brain barrier disruption by inhibiting activity of MMP-9 and

occludin degradation after focal cerebral ischemia. Aging Dis. 2015;6: 406–417. DOI: 10.14336/AD.2015.0812.

[41] Jolivel V, Bicker F, Biname F, Ploen R, Keller S, Gollan R, *et al*. Perivascular microglia promote blood vessel disintegration in the ischemic penumbra. Acta Neuropathol. 2015;129: 279–295. DOI: 10.1007/s00401-014-1372-1.

[42] Yang Y, Rosenberg GA. Blood–brain barrier breakdown in acute and chronic cerebrovascular disease. Stroke. 2011;42: 3323–3328. DOI: 10.1161/STROKEAHA.110.68257.

[43] Zendedel A, Habib P, Dang J, Lammerding L, Hoffmann S, Beyer C, *et al*. Omega-3 polyunsaturated fatty acids ameliorate neuroinflammation and mitigate ischemic stroke damage through interactions with astrocytes and microglia. J Neuroimmunol. 2015;278: 200–211. DOI: 10.1016/j.jneuroim.2014.11.007.

[44] Ritzel RM, Patel AR, Grenier JM, Crapser J, Verma R, Jellison ER, *et al*. Functional differences between microglia and monocytes after ischemic stroke. J Neuroinflammation. 2015;12: 106–117. DOI: 10.1186/s12974-015-0329-1.

[45] Ouyang YB, Xu L, Yue S, Liu S, Giffard RG. Neuroprotection by astrocytes in brain ischemia: importance of microRNAs. Neurosci Lett. 2014;565: 53–58. DOI: 10.1016/j.neulet.2013.11.015.

[46] Li Y, Liu Z, Xin H, Chopp M. The role of astrocytes in mediating exogenous cell-based restorative therapy for stroke. Glia. 2014;62: 1–16. DOI: 10.1002/glia.22585.

[47] Mattson MP. Hormesis defined. Ageing Res Rev. 2008;7: 1–7. DOI: 10.1016/j.arr.2007.08.007.

[48] Corbi G, Conti V, Russomanno G, Rengo G, Vitulli P, Ciccarelli AL, Filipelli A, Ferrara N. Is physical activity able to modify oxidative damage in cardiovascular aging? Oxid Med Cell Longev. 2012;2012: 1–6. DOI: 10.1155/2012/728547.

[49] Liu XQ, Sheng R, Qin ZH. The neuroprotective mechanism of brain ischemic preconditioning. Acta Pharm Sin. 2009;30: 1071–1080. DOI: 10.1038/aps.2009.105.

[50] Li J, Liu W, Ding S, Xu W, Guan Y, Zhang JH, *et al*. Hyperbaric oxygen preconditioning induces tolerance against brain ischemia–reperfusion injury by upregulation of antioxidant enzymes in rats. Brain Res. 2008;1210: 223–229. DOI: 10.1016/j.brainres.2008.03.007.

[51] Li JS, Zhang W, Kang ZM, Ding SJ, Liu WW, Zhang JH, *et al*. Hyperbaric oxygen preconditioning reduces ischemia–reperfusion injury by inhibition of apoptosis via mitochondrial pathway in rat brain. Neuroscience 2009;159: 1309–1315. DOI: 10.1016/j.neuroscience.2009.01.011.

[52] Yan W, Fang Z, Yang Q, Dong H, Lu Y, Lei C, *et al*. SirT1 mediates hyperbaric oxygen preconditioning-induced ischemic tolerance in rat brain. J Cereb Blood Flow Metab. 2013;33 :396–406. DOI: 10.1038/jcbfm.2012.179.

[53] Yuan Z, Pan R, Liu W, Liu KJ. Extended normobaric hyperoxia therapy yields greater neuroprotection for focal transient ischemia–reperfusion in rats. Med Gas Res. 2014;4: 14–22. DOI: 10.1186/2045-912-4-14.

[54] Rink C, Roy S, Khan M, Ananth P, Kuppusamy P, Sen CK, *et al*. Oxygen-sensitive outcomes and gene expression in acute ischemic stroke. J Cereb Blood Flow Metab. 2010;30: 1275–1287. DOI: 10.1038/jcbfm.2010.7.

[55] Li S, Zhang Y, Shao G, Yang M, Niu J, Lv G, *et al*. Hypoxic preconditioning stimulates angiogenesis in ischemic penumbra after acute cerebral infarction. Neural Regen Res. 2013;8: 2895–2903. DOI: 10.3969/j.issn.1673-5374.2013.31.002.

[56] Masada T, Hua Y, Xi G, Ennis SR, Keep RF. Attenuation of ischemic brain edema and cerebrovascular injury after ischemic preconditioning in the rat. J Cereb Blood Flow Metab. 2001;21: 22–33. DOI: 10.1097/00004647-200101000-00004.

[57] Liu Y, Zhu S, Wang Y, Hu J, Xu L, Ding L, *et al*. Neuroprotective effect of ischemic preconditioning in focal cerebral infarction: relationship with upregulation of vascular endothelial growth factor. Neural Regen Res. 2014;9: 1117–1121. DOI: 10.4103/1673-5374.135313.

[58] Weber NC, Riedemann I, Smit KF, Zitta K, van de Vondervoort D, Zuurbier CJ, *et al*. Plasma from human volunteers subjected to remote ischemic preconditioning protects human endothelial cells from hypoxia-induced cell damage. Basic Res Cardiol. 2015;110: 17–28. DOI: 10.1007/S00394-015-0474-9.

[59] Berger MM, Kohne H, Hotz L, Hammer M, Schommer K, Bartsch P, *et al*. Remote ischemic preconditioning delays the onset of acute mountain sickness in normobaric hypoxia. Physiol Rep. 2015;3: e12325–e12334. DOI: 10.14814/phy2.12325.

[60] Koch S, Katsnelson M, Dong C, Perez-Pinzon M. Remote ischemic limb preconditioning after subarachnoid hemorrhage: a phase Ib study of safety and feasibility. Stroke. 2011;42: 1387–1391. DOI: 10.1161/STROKEAHA.110.605840.

[61] Wu Q, Gui P, Wu J, Ding D, Purusram G, Dong N, *et al*. Effect of limb ischemic preconditioning on myocardial injury in patients undergoing mitral valve replacement surgery. A randomized controlled trial. Circ J. 2011;75: 1885–1889. DOI: 10.1253/circj.CJ-10-1130.

[62] Davies WR, Brown AJ, Watson W, McCormick LM, West NE, Dutka DP, *et al*. Remote ischemic preconditioning improves outcome at 6 years after elective percutaneous coronary intervention: the CRISP stent trial long-term follow-up. Circ Cardiovasc Interv. 2013;6: 246–251. DOI: 10.1161/CIRCINTERVENTIONS.112.000184.

[63] Corti P, Gladwin MT. Is nitrite the circulating endocrine effector of remote ischemic preconditioning? Circ Res. 2014;114: 1554–1557. DOI: 10.1161/CIRCRESAHA.114.303960.

Chapter 16

Role of Oxygen Free Radicals in Cancer Development and Treatment

Jalal Pourahmad, Ahmad Salimi and
Enaytollah Seydi

Additional information is available at the end of the chapter

http://dx.doi.org/10.5772/64787

Abstract

It is well known that species derived from oxygen are cytotoxic and are involved in the etiology of cancer. Several carcinogens during metabolism exert their effect by producing reactive oxygen species (ROS). One of the consequences of oxidative damage to cellular DNA is mutated. It plays a vital role in the process of carcinogenesis (especially in the initiation and progression). The alters, including rearrangement of DNA sequence, base modification, DNA miscoding lesions, gene amplification, and the activation of oncogenes, could be implicated in the initiation stage of several cancers. Mitochondrial changes in the cancer cells are well known and as a result are respiratory injured. Mitochondrial dysfunction could lead to a low coupling efficiency of the mitochondrial electron transport chain (mETC), raising electron leakage and increased ROS formation. It has been documented that by reducing and inactivation of antioxidant system, the oxidative stress (OS) in cancer cells is higher. Cancer cells exhibit a higher oxidative stress level compared to normal cells, rendering tumor cells more vulnerable to raise ROS levels. Therefore, increasing ROS levels through redox modulation can be a strategy to selectively kill cancer cells but not normal cells. A promising anti-cancer method named "oxidation therapy" has been developed by causing cytotoxic oxidative stress for cancer therapy. In this chapter, we described the role of ROS as a double-edged sword in cancer development and treatment.

Keywords: cancer, reactive oxygen species, oxidation therapy, mitochondria

1. Introduction

Oxygen, while peremptory required for life, can also take part in the demolition of tissue and/ or damage its ability to normal function. Reactive oxygen species (ROS), or low generally oxygen-free radicals (OFR), are produced by cellular metabolism in living cells. It has been appraised that the medium person has around 15,000 free radicals aggressive each cell per day. In an athlete, this number can be raised by almost 50%. In many instances, ROS are generated specifically to answer necessary biological functions, whereas in other cases, they indicate byproducts of metabolic processes. The production of ROS is an outcome of aerobic life. ROS represent a permanent source of attacks to our genetic material that can be either reduced or enhanced by environmental influences, hormonal and nutritional. Notwithstanding the antioxidant defense system of cell to neutralize oxidative injury from ROS, radical-linked damage of proteins and DNA has been suggested to play a major role in the development of diseases such as neurodegenerative disorders, arthritis, arteriosclerosis, cancer, and others diseases. All ROS have the potential to interact with cellular ingredients containing the deoxyribosyl backbone of DNA or DNA bases to generate strand breaks or damaged bases. ROS can also oxidize proteins or lipids afterward producing mediators that react with DNA by forming adducts. Many oxidative DNA damages are oxidative damage, and promutagenic is suggested to play an important role in the development of some cancers. Now, researchers do not know the correct role that injury by ROS plays a vital role in cancer development and its contributory role with other forms of genetic occurrences accelerating malignant progression and cell transformation. However, it is known that oxidative free radicals and oxidative stress (OS) could take part in the beginning of proliferation of cancerous cells. The result of OS at a given phase of carcinogenesis is immediately linked to the reactivity and the type of the radical species complicated. Nonenzymatic antioxidants accompanied by antioxidant enzymes are involved in ROS transformation. But antioxidant conservation versus ROS damages should be carried out with precaution inasmuch as the function of the antioxidant might indeed motivate the progression of cancer through the raised permanence of tumor cells. In inhibition of ROS-related cancer, the major duty looks to be decrease of exogenous and endogenous origins of ROS and the omission of carcinogens in environment. There is as well as the probability that cancer therapy could make utilization of the findings of ROS researches. Intracellular formation of ROS such as O_2^-, OH•, and H_2O_2 is associated with the suppression of cell proliferation. Similarly, production of oxidative stress in reply to several external motivations has been implicated in the activation of transcription factors and to the triggering of cell death. In this chapter, we run over how radical species induce DNA sequence changes, deletions, mutations, gene rearrangements, and alterations. These changes may lead to the beginning of apoptosis signaling leading to cell death, or to the inactivation of some tumor suppressor genes and/or the activation of several proto-oncogenes. The adjustment of gene expression by means of antioxidants, the redox state, and oxidants stays as a promising therapeutic procedure. Some anticarcinogenic agents have been demonstrated to inhibit ROS formation and oxidative DNA injury, inhibiting tumor development. As well as, new compounds vectors expressing radical-scavenging enzymes reduce apoptosis. Oxidative stress has been implicated in both the pathogenesis and apoptosis of cancer providing designed support for two concepts: free radical species may be raised in tumor cells and oxidant scavenging systems may be effective in cancer remedy. In addition, the production of ROS can be used therapeutically for cancer therapy. In this chapter, we described the role of ROS in cancer development and treatments.

2. Role of ROS in development of cancer

2.1. Mechanisms of free radical-induced DNA base modification and mutagenesis

It has been appraised that in one human cell is exposed to nearly 10^5 oxidative hits such as hydroxyl radical and other such species in a day. Constant change of genetic material resulting from these oxidative damage incidents demonstrates the initial step of carcinogenesis involved in aging and mutagenesis. The mechanisms such as specific and nonspecific repair play an important role in the removal of DNA changes by free radicals. It has been documented that base-excision is one method of repair DNA base damage. The alterations, including base deletion and substitution, play a role of in the DNA damage (misrepairing) and carcinogenesis. Mutagenic potential is directly equal to the number of oxidative DNA changes that flee repair. It is known that repair mechanisms decline with age and so DNA damages accumulate with age. The subsequence specificity of DNA lesion locates modifies the mutation frequency. The particular mechanism by OS which helps to the expansion of carcinogenesis is mainly unknown. However, two distinct mechanisms are supposed to act an important role in the expansion of oxidative and carcinogenesis. The modulation of gene expression by oxidative damage, can affect carcinogenesis. The epigenetic effects on gene expression could lead to the stimulation of proliferation and growth signals. Chromosomal rearrangements are speculated to result from loss of heterozygosity, alterations in gene expression, contributing to genetic amplifications and strand breakage misrepair, which in turn may advance neoplastic progression. Active oxygen species have been shown to motive poly(ADP ribosylation) and protein kinase pathways, thus affecting signal transduction pathways. This can lead to modulation of the expression of necessary genes for tumor promotion and proliferation. One previous study shows that RAS signal transduction pathways play a role in the mediating free radical signaling. Second, free radicals cause genetic changes, including chromosomal rearrangements and mutations, play a vital role in the beginning of carcinogenesis process. The oxidative DNA damage leads to a wide range of chromosomal abnormalities, inducing a wide cytotoxicity and stoppage of DNA duplication. Mutations can happen a failure to arrest in G1, diminishing their capacity to repair damaged DNA. This enhancement in replication errors can begin tumor suppressor gene inactivation and additional oncogene activation, eventually contributing to malignancy. Free radical-induced cytotoxicity may also help the beginning of carcinogenesis by promoting the clonal expansion of more resistant-initiated cells depleting the normal cell population, then increasing the possibility of mutation through incorrect replication or due to misrepair, while chromosomal rearrangements can end strand breakage misrepair. The initiation potential of oxidants might help to induce carcinogenesis as a result of their ability to cause DNA base alterations in tumor suppressor genes and certain oncogenes. Researches have shown that the radicals (especially hydroxyl radicals) are able to activate some oncogenes, including C-Raf-1 and K-ras. On the one hand, the activation launches through N-terminal deletions in these genes and the induction of DNA point mutations in GC base pairs. On the other hand, the base point mutations in CpG dinucleotides are also mostly found in specific tumor suppressor genes, including retinoblastoma and p53, which leading to their inactivation. It is shown that cells containing mutant or absent p53 are attacked by hydroxyl radical, which leading to a failure to arrest in G1 stage, diminishing their ability to repair damaged DNA. This enhancement in replication errors can initiate tumor suppressor gene inactivation and additional oncogene activation, eventually contributing to malignancy. Free radical-induced cytotoxicity may also contribute to the initiation of carcinogenesis by promoting the clonal expansion of more resistant-initiated cells, depleting the normal cell population, then increasing the likelihood of mutation [1].

2.2. Role of ROS in genotoxicity and DNA damage

ROS-caused DNA lesion may be characterized both structurally and chemically and displays a typical schema of modifications. The free radicals-induced DNA lesion was detected in the various cancer tissues. Most of these alterations can be modified in the in vitro situation.

The figures of DNA lesion induced through ROS experimentally include production of base-free sites, modification of all bases, frame shifts, deletions, DNA-protein cross-links, strand breaks, and chromosomal rearrangements. The Fenton chemistry mechanism is one of the reactions involved in DNA damage through the generation of hydroxyl radical form. It is well known that hydroxyl radical responds with all ingredients of the DNA molecule: the pyrimidine bases and purine. Regarding oxidative DNA lesion, main concern has centralized on repair to bases of DNA, with over 20 yields known, but only a few have been investigated with more details. Also, hydroxyl radical is capable to aggravate to twofold bonds of DNA bases at second-order rate constants of $3–10 \times 10^9 M^{-1} s^{-1}$ that grabs an H-atom from the methyl group of thymine and each of the five carbon atoms of 2′ deoxyribose with rate constants of $2 \times 10^9 M^{-1} s^{-1}$. Provided OH-adduct radicals of DNA bases are produced through additional reactions, the carbon-centered sugar radicals and allyl radical of thymine are formed from abstraction reactions. Peroxyl radicals are generated in environments full of oxygen through oxygen addition to OH-adduct radicals and also to carbon-centered radicals at diffusion controlled rates. Further reactions of base and sugar radicals generate a variety of sites, modified bases and sugars, protein of DNA, strand breaks, and cross-links.

Hydroxyl radical attacks to pyrimidines: to the C5 and C6 site of cytosine and thymine, generating C5-OH- and C6-OH-adduct radicals. Oxidative reactions of the C5-OH-adduct radicals of thymine and cytosine followed by release of proton (deprotonation) and addition of OH or water lead to the generation of glycols of cytosine and thymine. Oxygen adds to C5-OH-adduct radicals to produce 5-hydroxy-6-peroxyl radicals that may remove superoxide followed by reaction with water, giving rise to cytosine glycol and thymine glycol. Oxidation of the allyl radical of thymine generates 5-(hydroxymethyl) uracil (5-OHMeUra) and 5-formyluracil. In the lack of O_2, 6-hydroxy-5-hydropyrimidines and 5-hydroxy-6-hydroare generated by reduction of 6-OH- and 5-OH-adduct radicals of pyrimidines, respectively. Hydroxyl radical is as well as capable to attacks to purines giving rise to C4-OH-, C5-OH-, and C8-OH-adducts. One electron oxidation and one electron reduction of C8-OH-adduct radicals yield formamidopyrimidines and 8-hydroxypurines (7,8-dihydro-8-oxopurines). The most studied of these oxidized DNA products is 8-oxo-deoxyguanosine (8-oxo-dG), mainly because it is the most detectable. This base ornamentation falls out in nearly one in 10^5 guanidine residues in a healthy human cell. 8-Hydroxyguanine and 8-hydroxy-29-deoxyguanosine undergo keto-enol tautomerism, which favors the 6, 8-diketo form. Therefore, 8-OH-G is mostly named 8-oxoG or 8-oxy-7-hydroguanine. The nucleoside is thereupon named 8-oxo-7-hydro-29-deoxyguanosine or 8-oxo-dG so, 8-OH-dG and 8-oxo-dG are the identical compounds. Several methods for evaluating oxidative DNA damage exist; a favorite method engages enzymatic digestion of DNA, which releases 8-hydroxypurines for analysis by HPLC usually with electrochemical detector. Another method uses acidic hydrolysis of DNA, which releases the free base, because the glycosidic bond is cleaved by acid. Measurement is through HPLC or, transformation to volatile compounds, through GC-MS. The 8-oxoG damage is main due to it is relatively simply generated and is mutagenic, thus is a main indicator for the detection of carcinogenesis. The studies suggested mutagenic potential of 8-oxo-dG is supported by insertion of adenine opposite the lesions, or a loss of base pairing specificity, misreading of adjacent pyrimidines. Mutations that may arise due to the production of 8-oxo-dG involve GC→TA transversions. Former studies have shown that the mispairing of 8-oxo-dG with adenine appears to be feasible due to the energetically favored syn glycosidic conformation, while coupling with dG assumes the antiform. Studies demonstrated that factors such as day/night shift work, low meat intake, low BMI (<21.8), smoking, and hard physical labor significantly increased the 8-oxo-dG level, whereas medium physical exercise, such as sports, reduced its level. These data propose that the way of life might remarkably affect the level of oxidative lesion. The generation of 2-oxy-dA in the nucleotide unite is another mechanism of mutations. Studies have shown that the incorporation of 2 oxy-dA opposite G caused GC→TA transversions in the chromosomal lac I gene [2].

2.3. Lipid peroxidation and DNA damage

While major consideration has centralized on direct DNA lesion by oxygen free radicals because of the genetic outcomes of such lesion, reactive radical species may also induce damage to other cellular members. Phospholipids in the cell membrane are extremely susceptible to oxidative process and have been discovered to be repeated targets of radical-caused injury that supply them to be involved in free radical chain reactions. Several of the fatty acids are polyunsaturated, have a methylene group between two double bonds that predisposes the fatty acid more susceptible to oxidation. In addition, it is reported that polyunsaturated fatty acids (at high concentration) in phospholipids predisposes play a role of in the free radical chain reactions. Linoleic acid is the most common fatty acid in cell membranes. A set of arachidonic acid oxidation products termed isoprostanes is the best biomarker of lipid peroxidation that generally detected through GC-MS. The first products of unsaturated fatty acid oxidation are short-lived lipid hydroperoxides. When they react with metals, they produce some of products for example epoxides and aldehydes, which are themselves reactive. Malondialdehyde (MDA) is one of the important aldehyde products through lipid peroxidation. This product of lipid peroxidation is mutagenic and carcinogenic in mammalian cells and animals, respectively. MDA can react with DNA bases dA, dC, and dG, to form adducts, M_1A, M_1C, and M_1G. M_1G has been indicated in the several tissues (such as pancreas, liver, and breast). The M_1G content corresponds nearly to 6500 adducts in cell. Many researches have shown that M_1G is an electrophile in the genome. N_2-Oxo-propenyl-dG, as a yield of quantitative and rapid ring-opening of M_1G, is as well as electrophilic, but aims regions of DNA distinct from M_1G. Therefore, the conversion of M_1G and N_2-oxo-propenyl-dG may unfold varying reactive groups of DNA that could take part in the production of DNA-DNA inter-strand cross-links or DNA-protein cross-links. It has been shown that hydroxypropanodeox-oguanosines (OH-PdGs) are exist in rodent and human liver DNA. It has been proposed that these propano adducts are interceded by the reaction of DNA with crotonaldehyde and acrolein, which in turn are products of lipid peroxidation. Crotonaldehyde and acrolein are mutagenic in mammalian cells and bacteria.

There is a few information associated with the repair of OH-PdGs. Studies show that PdG is a main substrate for the nucleotide cut repair complex of mammalian cells and *E. coli* and is identified and repaired through the mismatch repair system. Various exocyclic etheno DNA adducts increasing from lipid peroxidation have been found in DNA from healthy human volunteers. The most important involves etheno-dG, etheno-dC, and etheno-dA. Etheno-dC and etheno-dA are found to be strongly genotoxic but weakly mutagenic [3].

3. Role of ROS in treatment of cancer

3.1. Functions of ROS in the cancer cells

The findings from both *in vitro* and *in vivo* studies have shown that endogenous oxidative stress in cancer cells is higher than normal cells. ROS might function as a double-edged sword and as varied ROS levels could cause various biological responses. A low to moderate raise of ROS may help with the proliferation and survival of cells. But, at a high level, ROS may suppress the antioxidant capacity of the cell and start cell death (**Figure 1**). On the other hand, at the accumulation of ROS, these cells may be more sensitive than normal cells. The normal cells at under physiological status play an important role in maintaining redox homeostasis with a low level of basal ROS by controlling the balance between pro-oxidants and antioxidant capacity. The physiological conditions are affected by ROS inducers (such as hypoxia, metabolic defects, ER stress, and oncogenes) and ROS elimination (such as NRF2, glutathione,

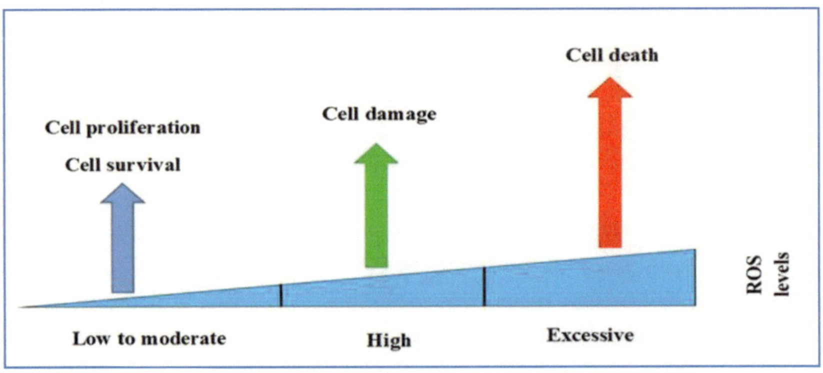

Figure 1. The interaction between different ROS levels in cancer cells. In cancer cells, ROS at low to moderate levels induces cell proliferation and cell survival, at high level induce cell damage and at an excessive level induce cell death.

NADPH, tumor suppressors, and dietary antioxidant agents) [4, 5]. The increase of ROS level of intracellular by activating signaling pathways in cancer cells represents that these cells very more vulnerable than normal cells to ROS-caused cell death. As a result, these cells in comparison to normal cells very more dependent on the capacity of the antioxidant system and more vulnerable to major oxidative stress induced through exogenous ROS-generating agents or compounds that inhibit the antioxidant system. This might constitute a biochemical basis to plan therapeutic strategies to selectively death cancer cells using ROS-moderated mechanisms [4–6].

As described above, the increase of ROS in cancer cells was induced several biological responses. These biological responses (including adaptation, increase in cellular proliferation, cell damage, and cell death) are likely to be dependent on the cellular genetic background, the types of the specific ROS involved, and the levels of ROS at the duration of the oxidative stress [7].

3.2. Antioxidant and oxidation pathways regulate ROS generation

Oxidative stress plays an important role in cell signaling as a sensor and regulator. It was reported that a lot of regulator agents have a considerable effect on up-expression and down-expression of antioxidant genes. In the following, we explain some of the major factors that act directly in the expression of antioxidant genes (**Figure 2**). On the other hand, good understanding of the particular pathways that are affected by these regulators is important before designing therapeutic approaches to the adjustment of ROS levels [4].

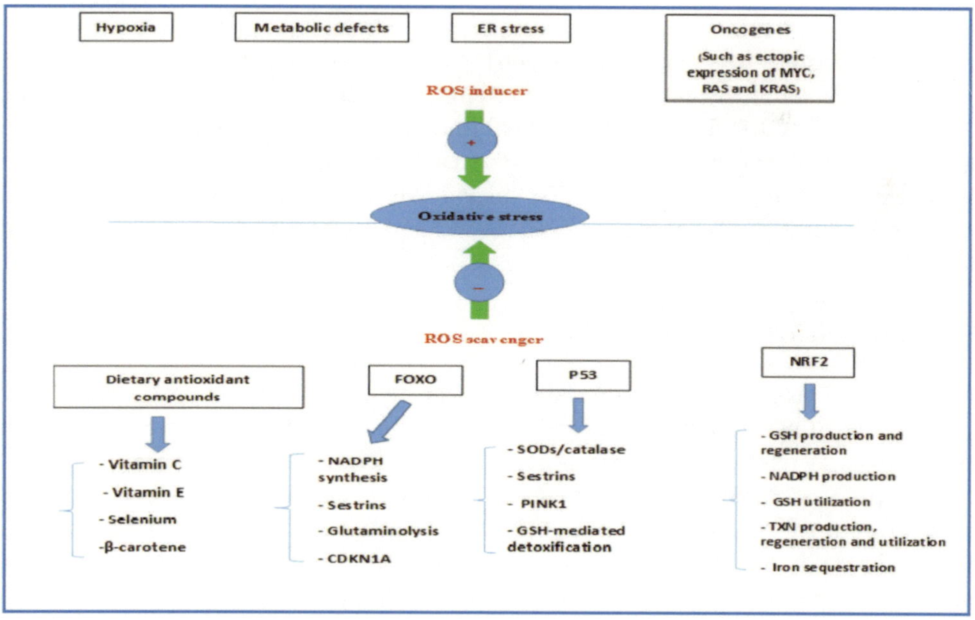

Figure 2. The regulation of ROS level by ROS inducers and ROS scavengers. The oxidative stress/ROS generation increase by agents such as, oncogenes, mitochondrial mutations, hypoxia, ER stress and decrease expression levels of antioxidant proteins that prevent increasing ROS level.

3.3. NRF2 (nuclear factor, erythroid-derived 2, like 2)

NRF2 is an important regulator of the antioxidant system and cellular stress responses in the several cancers. From the support on the function of Nrf2 target genes, one can easily conclude that activation of Nrf2 may protect cells from several stresses imposed through toxic exposure. Actually, it is recognized that NRF2 regulate various anti-oxidative stress responses and for detoxification reactions, its expression in the tissues increases [8, 9].

NRF2 adjust the common various different antioxidant pathways such as GSH production and regeneration, GSH utilization, NADPH production, thioredoxin (TXN) production, regeneration and utilization, Quinone detoxification and Iron sequestration (**Figure 2**). It is directly (through GSH metabolism) and indirectly (controlling free Fe(II) homeostasis) involved in ROS detoxification. NRF2 decreases the generation of harmful hydroxyl radicals from ROS by increasing the release of Fe(II) from haem molecules [4].

It was suggested that phytochemical compounds such as dietary and medicinal plants through the effect on NRF2 pathway played a key role in cancer therapy [8, 9].

3.4. FOXO (Forkhead box O) and p53

FOXO, as a transcription factors, are involved in different signaling pathways and play key roles in some physiological and pathological processes such as cancer. It could play and act as a self-regulatory mechanism, which protects cells from an oxidative damages, via keep in good condition a balance of ROS and antioxidant productions.

FOXO and p53 (as a tumor suppressor) have a key role in inhibiting oxidative stress process through inducing antioxidant gene expression [4]. It was reported that an increase of ROS level leads to up-regulation of anti-oxidative proteins, such as MnSOD and catalase through FOXO3a- and FOXO1 [10]. The p53, as a final transcription factor, has an important role in regulating antioxidant gene expression is p53 and a double-edged (as a pro- and antioxidant) role in ROS controlling. The p53 and FOXO play a role of the regulate antioxidant pathways such as SODs/catalase, PTEN-induced putative kinase 1 (PINK1), NADPH synthesis, and sestrins [4].

3.5. Hypoxia and hypoglycemia

Hypoxic conditions caused by the imbalance between intake and oxygen consumption [4]. The production of ROS through the mitochondrial complex I and III, xanthine oxidase, and NADPH oxidase related to hypoxia is recognized as one of the most harmful causes of oxidative process. Some studies have shown that hypoxia condition-caused superoxide generation occurs through the activation of NADPH oxidase placed in the cell membrane and under moderate condition, NO is generated in mitochondria. Studies suggested that hypoxia-induced loss in mitochondria membrane potential and this and this event is related to raising ROS [11].

Studies have shown that the mitochondria complex III (at the Qo site) at during the transfer of electrons from ubisemiquinone to molecular oxygen is the main source for ROS generation under hypoxia. In addition, it has shown that activation the transcription factor hypoxia-inducible factor (HIF) dependent on ROS level. HIFs regulate physiological responses to hypoxia, such as pathophysiological processes (especially in cancer) [4].

It was reported that, there is a relation between an increase in the level of H_2O_2 generation of mitochondria and an increase in susceptible cancer cells to apoptosis. This susceptibility caused cytotoxicity and also to oxidative stress-induced apoptosis when compared to normal cells [12].

3.6. Oncogenes

The oncogenes such as RAS, c-MYC, and Bcr/Abl, as a ROS-generators, are common agents that induce increase ROS levels in cancer cells by alteration in balance between pro-oxidant and anti-oxidant systems [11]. In the cancer cells, oxidative stress (due to increase ROS level and decrease antioxidant level) is higher than normal cells. At a time when equivalent levels of oxidative stress are added by the administration of exogenous ROS-inducing agents, oxidative stress levels in cancer cells but not normal cells can readily over the threshold of cell death. Hence, cancer cells in compared normal cells are expected to be more vulnerable to cell damage caused by ROS-inducing agents and this vulnerability can be exploited to selectively kill these cells [11].

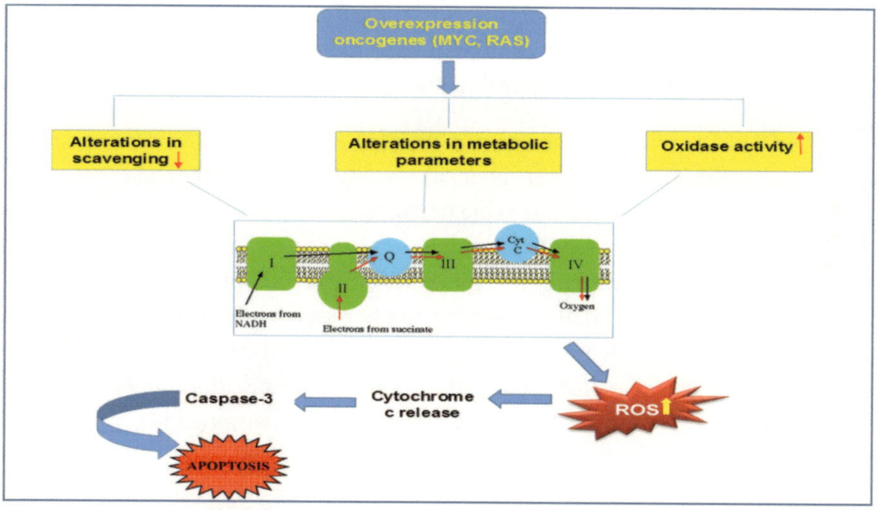

Figure 3. A model for increase ROS and apoptosis signaling by oncogenes such as c-MYC.

The activation of MYC in cancer cells leads to an elevating in intracellular ROS through mechanisms such as changes in scavenging process, metabolic rate, and eventual activation of intracellular oxidases (**Figure 3**). The previous investigations show that the increased expression of c-MYC and E2F1 induces accumulation of ROS and increases ROS by c-MYC and E2F1 sensitizes host cells to apoptosis.

Hypoxia, on the one hand, as a ROS inducer, can also directly induce the raised expression of oncogenes such as MYC and RAS through HIF-2α. On the other hand, MYC increases mitochondrial biogenesis, which adds to the raised ROS generation under hypoxic conditions and the raised mitochondrial ROS generation elevate the oxidative stress process [12].

It has been suggested that RAS, p53, and c-MYC through the mitochondria to regulate ROS generation, thereby affecting apoptosis. RAS in K-Ras-transformed fibroblast cell under the condition that glucose deprivation induces apoptosis through changes in mitochondrial complex gene expression. It has also been reported that RAS in p66SHC overexpression condition in the transformed cells increase ROS generation through mitochondria and p53, MPTP opening and mitochondrial swelling could induce apoptosis (**Figure 3**) [12].

3.7. Mitochondria

In recent decades, several studies have shown that mitochondria organelle plays an important role in human health and disease. These studies led to the emergence of a new field of study named "mitochondrial medicine." In the mitochondria, the molecules that are located on or inside have been considered as an initial pharmacological target and a wide range of efforts are in progress to use these targets to develop targeted treatments for cancer.

It has been confirmed that these organelles are the principal intracellular source of ROS production in most tissues. The under physiological status approximately 2% the O_2 consumed is changed to ROS molecules. In the mitochondria, ROS generation (such as O_2^-) often occurs by complexes I and III respiratory chain. Studies have shown that under physiological condition, complex II respiratory chain could also be a main regulator of ROS generation from mitochondria [13].

In eukaryotic cells, the mitochondrion is an important organelle that plays a main role in several critical processes. The important role of mitochondria is mentioned in the physiology of cancer, such as in energy metabolism and cell cycle regulation. There is powerful documentary evidence to support the rationale for the expansion of anticancer strategies based on mitochondrial targets. This organelle is recognizing to play an important role in the apoptosis mechanism and initiate cell death through various mechanisms that comprise disrupting electron transport and energy metabolism in the respiratory chain, releasing agents or proteins (such as cytochrome c) that mediate apoptosis signaling, and changing the cellular redox status by ROS generation.

The therapeutic targeting of cancer cells based on mitochondria have often depended on the intrinsic various differences between mitochondria in normal and cancer cells, which allow for better options, manipulation different pathways, and destruction of these cancer cells. These differences are including bioenergetics change, disturbance of the mitochondrial DNA (mtDNA), and morphological and physiological changes in the cancer cell (**Table 1**). The mtDNA is one main target of ROS and the lack of sufficient protective histones surrounding the mtDNA in cancer cells makes the mtDNA more easily tending to ROS-caused DNA damage. In addition, various researches have shown that the mitochondria were different in cancer cells than in normal cells, such as grow faster, fewer and smaller, and also had the morphological transformed [13].

	Cancer cells	Normal cell
Bioenergetics process	Aerobic glycolysis condition "Warburg Effect"	Aerobic condition
Mitochondrial DNA (mtDNA)	mtDNA is mutated	mtDNA is normal
Morphological and physiological differences (shape and count)	Size and shape: smaller	Size and shape: larger
MMP level	Higher (~60 mV)	Lower
ROS level	Higher	Lower
Intracellular pH	Acidic	No acidic
Metabolic rates	Higher	Lower

Table 1. Some differences between cancer and normal cells such as bioenergetics process, MMP and ROS level, and morphological and physiological differences.

Today, several mitochondria targeted strategies for cancer therapy have been focused on the development of agents that manage increased the ROS generation in mitochondria from the cancer cells without effect on the normal cells. It has been shown that ROS generation in the mitochondria is evaluated through the rates of both mitochondria ROS (mtROS) disposal and production, and ROS levels in mitochondria are regulated by several agents, including mitochondria O_2 levels, mitochondrial membrane potential (MMP or $\Delta\psi m$), the metabolic condition of mitochondria, and other factors (**Figure 4**). A number of recent researches reveal the fact that mtROS at low to high levels act as several functions. That is it at low levels, involved in the hypoxia adaptation process, at moderate levels, involved in controlling inflammatory response, and at high level involved in regulating apoptosis signaling.

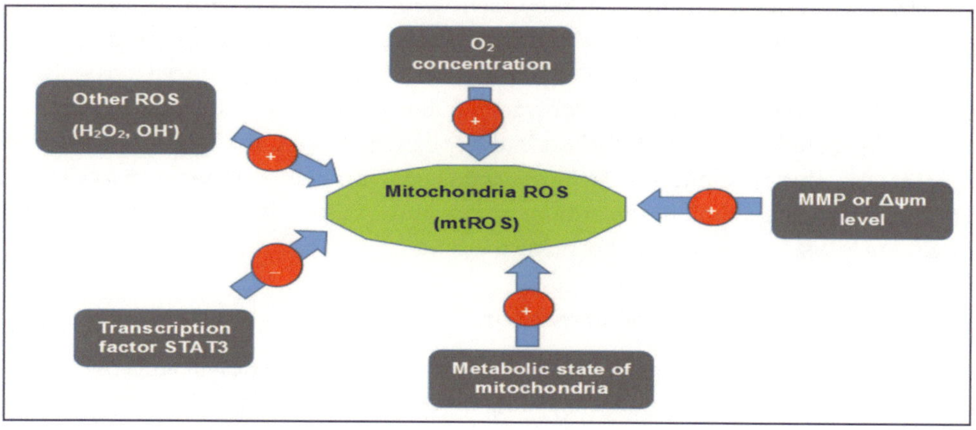

Figure 4. Adjustment of mitochondria ROS (mtROS) generation. Several agents such as MMP, the metabolic state of mitochondrial, O_2 level and STAT3 adjust the generation of mtROS.

As mentioned in the previous section, the increase of ROS level of intracellular by sever agents through activating signaling pathways in cancer cells represents that these cells are more vulnerable than normal cells to ROS-caused cell death. The results of the studies suggest that ROS (such as H_2O_2) could affect the extrinsic apoptosis pathway through changing the intracellular space. The up-regulation of receptor shows in various systems with increase ROS by exogenous ROS and ROS causing agents. It has also been found to sensitize cancer cells, but not normal cells to TRAIL-caused apoptosis.

Adenine nucleotide translocator (ANT), as an inner mitochondrial protein, is also a target of ROS regulation by integrity of its redox-sensitive cysteines, supplying an extra mechanism by which drug-caused ROS generation may activate mitochondrial apoptosis signaling. In addition, it has shown that $O_2{\bullet}^-$ plays a key role, on the one hand, to regulate the function of voltage-dependent anion channel (VDAC) to promote cytochrome c explosion. On the other hand, ROS also could regulate protein complexes inner place the mitochondrial electron transport chain (mETC), activate caspases-3 and initiate apoptosis signaling.

Today, agents that are used in the treatment of cancer through the mechanism of ROS generation are known as an important drug class. Some studies have shown that several mitochondria-targeted drugs have potency useful in selective cancer cell killing and no effect on normal cells in pre-clinical and clinical testing, such as ROS regulators. It has been shown that cancer cells in comparison with normal cells are more vulnerable to irreversible damage induced by stress oxidative and subsequent apoptosis. Researchers in previous studies have been used of the differences between the mitochondria between cancer and normal cells as a means to kill cancer cells by anti-cancer drugs. The phrase "mitocan" has been suggested to categorize mitochondria-targeted anticancer drugs, particularly those that caused increase ROS generation in mitochondria.

A promising anti-cancer strategy named "oxidation therapy" has been expanded by inducing cytotoxic oxidative stress in cancer cells and no effect on normal cells through several mechanisms for cancer treatment. Developing cancer therapies based on increasing further the high ROS level in cancer cells to a toxic level by the several mechanisms such as triggering ROS accumulation directly and inhibiting the antioxidant systems display powerful phenomenon of selectively killing cancer cells [6]. A number of drugs class have been recognized as increasing ROS production. It is well documented that some of chemotherapeutic agents can induce ROS generation through mitochondrial respiratory chain complexes in patients during cancer therapy. These compounds can be separated into various categories such as alkylating agents, anthracycline antibiotics, platinum compounds, mitotic inhibitors, antimetabolites, biological response modifiers, and hormone therapies.

3.8. Targeting mitochondrial respiratory chain

Arsenic trioxide (ATO) is used in the treatment of acute promyelocytic leukemia (APL). It was reported that ATO induces apoptosis signaling in several cancer cells such as lung, leukemia, and myeloma cancer through the induction of ROS. The mechanism by which ATO cause increased ROS generation is not completely well known. The most recent investigations indicated that ATO can impair the function of respiratory chain in the mitochondria, leading to increased generation of superoxide, likely by causing leakage of electrons from the mitochondrial respiratory chain complexes (**Figure 5**). On the other hand, ATO could be used in mixture with several anticancer drugs, which play a role through increasing ROS production.

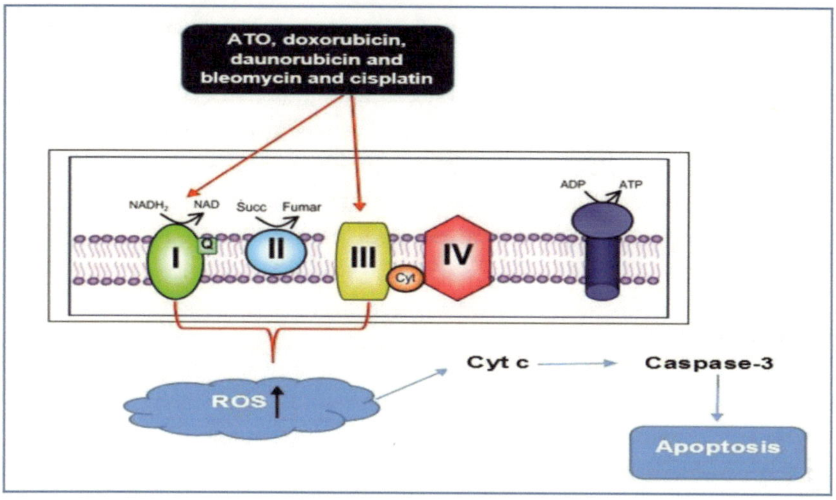

Figure 5. Mechanism of ROS generation and apoptosis induction by the ATO, doxorubicin, daunorubicin and bleomycin (anthracycline antibiotics) and cisplatin. These drugs, leading to increased generation of ROS, likely by causing leakage of electrons from the mitochondrial respiratory chain complexes.

The doxorubicin, daunorubicin, and bleomycin are an anthracycline antibiotics, cisplatin is a platinum compound, and amitriptyline as a tricyclic antidepressant are used in the treatment of several types of cancer. The mechanism of doxorubicin bleomycin, cisplatin, and amitriptyline in the ROS production is the same of ATO. These drugs with impair the function of respiratory chain in the mitochondria, leading to increase generation of superoxide. These compounds due to this mechanism (ROS generation) are used for the treatment of several types of cancers (**Figure 5**).

Studies have shown that other drugs such as dequalinium chloride (preclinical) and metformin (preclinical and clinical, Phase I) through inhibition of mitochondrial complex 1 have the ability to produce ROS.

3.9. Targeting VDACs

VDACs, also known as mitochondrial porins, show high similarity between some animals (especially mice) and humans. VDAC play an important role in the cell, such as regulating mitochondrial shape and structural changes, regulating apoptosis signaling, regulating ATP and calcium transport. Several studies have demonstrated the role of VDAC in the regulation of apoptosis signaling and VDAC is being studied as a cancer-specific target.

Erastin (Phase I/II) and Lanperasone (FDA-approved), as a modified form of tolperisone, down-regulate mitochondrial VDACs and alter the mitochondrial membrane permeability induce increase ROS generation. As has been mentioned, these drugs promote ROS production through the disturbance of VDAC and cause non-apoptotic form of cell death in KRAS.

3.10. Targeting NOX

Several studies have shown that some drugs and agents including, paclitaxel (taxol), ionizing radiation, niclosamide, AGX-891, AG-221 with effect on NOX induces ROS generation. Taxol is a mitotic inhibitory drug and it has been shown that induced ROS production/accumulation in the cell. The recent results from both *in vitro* and *in vivo* studies have shown that this drug causes the translocation of Rac1, which favorably regulates the activity of NOX, thereby furthering ROS (H_2O_2) production. It was reported that taxol can raise the levels of ROS in the extracellular and subsequently induced cancer cell death resulting in the release of cytochrome *c* from the mitochondria.

3.11. Targeting p53

P53 act as a transcription factor to regulate the expression of many pro-oxidant genes. The 5-fluorouracil (5-FU) is an antimetabolites and pyrimidine analog. It is used for therapies for several types of cancers, such as gastrointestinal, colon, rectal, and head and neck cancer, through inducing intracellular increase in superoxide. The mechanism by which 5-FU cause increased ROS generation from mitochondria is through a p53-dependent pathway [4]. The level of ROS production is different among these compounds and thus that anthracyclines (such as, doxorubicin), alkylating agents (such as, cyclophosphamide), platinum complexes are considered as the highest generation of ROS and taxanes, vinca alkaloids, and nucleotide/nucleoside analogs such as 5-FU as the lowest generation of ROS.

3.12. Targeting antioxidant system

It has been confirmed that GSH, catalase, and thioredoxin (TXN), as an antioxidant system, play a main role in equivalent pro-oxidant/antioxidant system through the scavenging various types of ROS. The two pathways GSH through enzymes such as GPX and GST and catalase can act directly on scavenging ROS in cells. For that reason, oxidative stress can be promoted with methods based on the loss of the reduced GSH storage and other antioxidant sources. A number of drugs class have been recognized as increasing oxidative stress process and ROS generation through targeting antioxidant system [4, 5].

These drugs are, including buthionine sulfoximine (BSO), imexon, phenylethyl isothiocyanate, mangafodipir, 2-methoxyestradiol, tetrathiomolybdate (ATN-224), and auranofin, used in the treatment of various types of cancer. For example, BSO through inhibition of the antioxidant system (especially GSH) in cancer cells (such as ovarian and breast cancers) can induce an accumulation of ROS due to the high basal ROS output in ovarian and breast cancers, and initiate cell death [4, 5]. Other studies have shown that imexon through decrease GSH pool and subsequently increase the production of ROS and decrease mitochondria function was induced apoptosis. Other studies have shown that some other drugs, including ascorbic acid and diethylmaleate are able effects on GSH (GSH depletion). One the other hand, mercaptosuccinic acid, aminotriazol, and 2-Methoxyoestradiol were able to inhibit of GPx, catalase, and SOD, respectively, and thereby increase ROS production [7].

4. Conclusion

Cancer is a multistage disease including initiation, promotion, and progression. The increased ROS causes DNA damage, which may lead to DNA damage or gene mutation, resulting in the progression of cancer. Increased generation of ROS and an altered redox status have observed in cancer cells, and investigations suggest that this biochemical property of cancer cells can be exploited for cancer therapy. For treatment of cancer, since high levels of ROS can induce cell death, treatment of radiation, chemotherapy, and molecule compounds all can increase the level of intracellular ROS to induce cancer cell death and apoptosis. The increased intracellular ROS levels could make cancer cells more vulnerable than normal cells to oxidative stress-induced cell death.

Author details

Jalal Pourahmad[1*], Ahmad Salimi[2] and Enaytollah Seydi[3]

*Address all correspondence to: j.pourahmadjaktaji@utoronto.ca

1 Department of Pharmacology and Toxicology, School of Pharmacy, Shahid Beheshti University of Medical Sciences, Tehran, Iran

2 Department of Pharmacology and Toxicology, School of Pharmacy, Ardabil University of Medical Science, Ardabil, Iran

3 Department of Occupational Health Engineering, Research Center for Health, Safety and Environment (RCHSE), Alborz University of Medical Sciences, Karaj, Iran

References

[1] Dizdaroglu M, Jaruga P, Birincioglu M, Rodriguez H. Free radical-induced damage to DNA: mechanisms and measurement 1, 2. Free Radical Biology and Medicine. 2002;32(11):1102-15.

[2] Waris G, Ahsan H. Reactive oxygen species: role in the development of cancer and various chronic conditions. Journal of Carcinogenesis. 2006;5(1):14.

[3] Marnett LJ. Oxy radicals, lipid peroxidation and DNA damage. Toxicology. 2002;181:219-222.

[4] Gorrini C, Harris IS, Mak TW. Modulation of oxidative stress as an anticancer strategy. Nature Reviews Drug Discovery. 2013;12(12):931-947.

[5] Trachootham D, Alexandre J, Huang P. Targeting cancer cells by ROS-mediated mechanisms: a radical therapeutic approach? Nature Reviews Drug Discovery. 2009;8(7):579-591.

[6] Nogueira V, Hay N. Molecular pathways: reactive oxygen species homeostasis in cancer cells and implications for cancer therapy. Clinical Cancer Research. 2013;19(16): 4309-4314.

[7] Pelicano H, Carney D, Huang P. ROS stress in cancer cells and therapeutic implications. Drug Resistance Updates. 2004;7(2):97-110.

[8] Alexander C-M. The involvement of NRF2 in lung cancer. Oxidative Medicine and Cellular Longevity. 2013;2013.

[9] Lau A, Villeneuve NF, Sun Z, Wong PK, Zhang DD. Dual roles of Nrf2 in cancer. Pharmacological Research. 2008;58(5):262-270.

[10] Weidinger C, Krause K, Klagge A, Karger S, Fuhrer D. Forkhead box-O transcription factor: critical conductors of cancer's fate. Endocrine-related Cancer. 2008;15(4):917-929.

[11] Suzuki-Karasaki Y, Suzuki-Karasaki M, Uchida M, Ochiai T. Depolarization controls TRAIL-sensitization and tumor-selective killing of cancer cells: crosstalk with ROS. Frontiers in Oncology. 2014;1–4.

[12] Ralph SJ, Rodríguez-Enríquez S, Neuzil J, Saavedra E, Moreno-Sánchez R. The causes of cancer revisited: "mitochondrial malignancy" and ROS-induced oncogenic transformation–why mitochondria are targets for cancer therapy. Molecular Aspects of Medicine. 2010;31(2):145-170.

[13] Modica-Napolitano JS, Weissig V. Treatment strategies that enhance the efficacy and selectivity of mitochondria-targeted anticancer agents. International Journal of Molecular Sciences. 2015;16(8):17394-17421.

Chapter 17

Role of Dietary Antioxidant Agents in Chronic Kidney Disease

Dianelena Eugenio-Pérez,
Liliana Yazmín Medina-Fernández,
Jennyfer Andrea Saldivar-Anaya,
Eduardo Molina-Jijón and José Pedraza-Chaverri

Additional information is available at the end of the chapter

http://dx.doi.org/10.5772/63669

Abstract

Chronic kidney disease (CKD) is defined as the atrophy of the kidney or progressive decline of renal function mainly caused by chronic diseases such as diabetes mellitus and hypertension. CKD affects more than 10% of the world's population. Moreover, there is no single treatment to improve kidney function in CKD patients. Consequently, this condition is considered a worldwide public health problem. The development of novel CKD therapies is highly needed because current treatment methods are ineffective. Since oxidative stress plays a critical role in CKD, the study of the effect of antioxidants in this pathology is highly important. Dietary antioxidant agents have shown protective effects in CKD. Hence, they may be key for the development of feasible therapies. The aim of this chapter is to provide recent information about the therapeutic role of dietary antioxidants in experimental models of CKD and clinical trials, as well as to describe the mechanisms through which antioxidants exert nephroprotection. The dietary antioxidants revised in this chapter are curcumin, sulforaphane, resveratrol, quercetin, proanthocyanidins, flavan-3-ols, soy protein, red propolis, and Mediterranean diet.

Keywords: natural compounds, chronic kidney disease, diabetic nephropathy, oxidative stress, inflammation

1. Introduction

1.1. Function of the kidney

The aim of this overview on kidney function is to introduce readers unfamiliar with renal physiology to basic principles that are required for a better understanding of chronic kidney disease (CKD). A detailed and state-of-the-art description of the morphology and function of the kidneys and the structure of the nephrons can be found in standard handbooks of renal physiology [1, 2].

Human kidney contains around 1–3 millions of functioning units called nephrons. Each nephron consists of a glomerulus and a tubular system. The glomerulus filters the blood free of cells and large proteins (filtration), and produces an ultrafiltrate composed of small circulating elements. The ultrafiltrate enters the tubule, which is highly specialized at various segments, to produce the final urine by removing substances from the tubular fluid

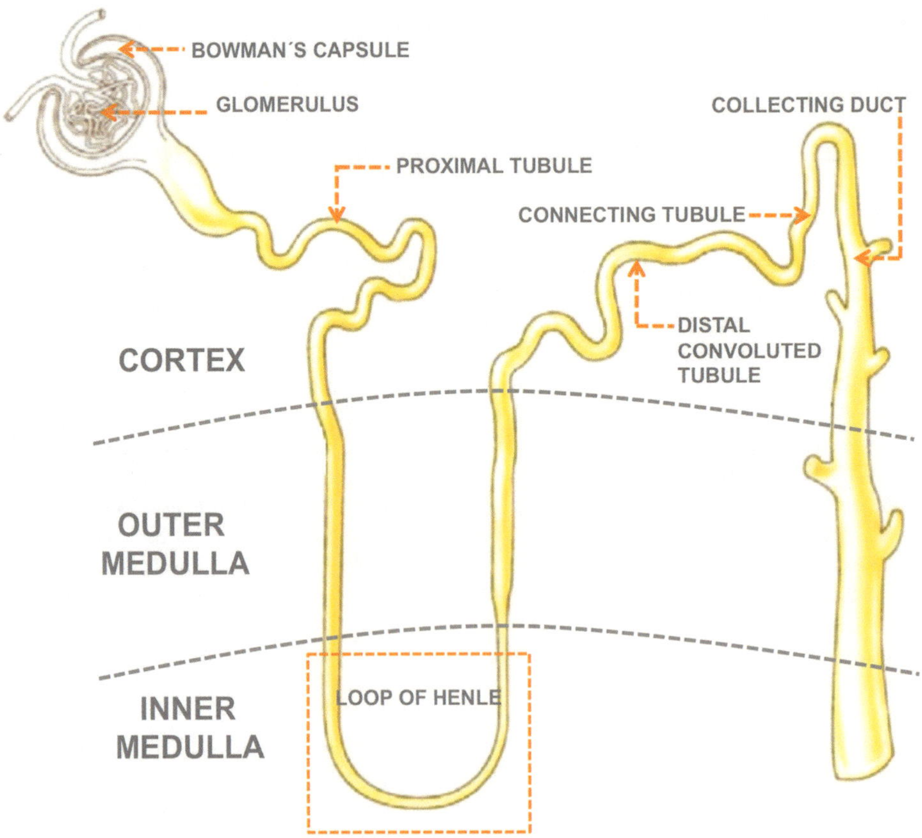

Figure 1. Structure of the nephron. Nephrons are constituted by glomeruli and the tubular system which encompasses the proximal tubule, the loop of Henle, the distal convoluted and connecting tubules and the collecting duct. Macroscopically nephrons can be divided into cortex, outer and inner medulla.

(reabsorption) or adding substances to the tubular fluid (secretion). Filtration, reabsorption, and secretion keep the organism in balance in terms of water, minerals, electrolytes, and hydrogen ion concentration and eliminate the toxic substances produced by the body.

Plasma is constantly equilibrated with the interstitial fluid of the extracellular space and with the intracellular space. Organs such as kidneys, lungs, and intestine maintain the physiological composition of the body fluids of mammals. The kidney carries out this process through the excretion of xenobiotics, solutes, water, and metabolic wastes by producing the urine. In the kidney, blood is filtered through the glomerulus, which is a capillary network composed of endothelial and mesangial cells and podocytes; this process is called ultrafiltration, whose driving force depends on blood pressure and filtration pressure in the glomerular capillaries. Filtered water and solutes still of use for the body are efficiently recycled to the circulation by obligatory and regulated reabsorptive processes in the tubular sections of the nephrons.

Primary ultrafiltrate contains essential nutrients and electrolytes that need to be actively reabsorbed to avoid critical losses and ensuing deficiencies. On the contrary, the kidney actively secretes some metabolic wastes since their rate of production exceeds their rate of glomerular filtration. All these selective processes are carried out by the nephrons, epithelial tubular structures that consist of several interconnected segments with specific morphological and functional characteristics, the proximal tubule (PT) with its convoluted segments S1 and S2 (proximal convoluted tubule, PCT) and straight segment S3, the loop of Henle (LOH), the distal tubule (DT) with its convoluted segment (distal convoluted tubule, DCT) and connecting tubule, and finally the collecting duct (CD) (**Figure 1**).

By these means, about 180 L of primary filtrate is generated every day to produce about 1–3 L of final urine. This indicates that about 99% of the primary urine is reabsorbed along the more than two million nephrons.

1.2. Chronic kidney disease

CKD is defined as the atrophy of the kidney or progressive decline of renal function [3]. CKD affects more than 10% of the world population [4]. Furthermore, treatment methods such as dialysis or transplantation are expensive or ineffective; therefore, this condition is considered a public health problem [5]. Renal dysfunction can be identified when the glomerular filtration rate (GFR) is below 60 mL/min/1.73 m^2 for more than 3 months and when albuminuria, defined as an albumin-to-creatinine ratio above 30 mg/g per day, is present [5].

Among different factors that induce CKD, diabetes mellitus and hypertension are the most important causes of this pathology [6]. Diabetic nephropathy (DN) is the main microvascular complication of diabetes often leading to CKD. As a matter of fact, DN is the main cause of dialysis admissions (34% of admissions) [7]. DN occurs when high blood glucose concentrations impair the function of renal blood vessels and glomerular and epithelial tubular cells [8]. Hypertension is the second leading cause of CKD [9]. Hypertensive nephropathy patients are advised to maintain their blood pressure to 130/80 mm Hg to prevent CKD development [10]. Several mechanisms are involved in CKD pathogenesis; some of them include inflammation, glomerulosclerosis, tubulointerstitial fibrosis, and mainly oxidative stress [11]. Oxidative stress is a common phenomenon in CKD lesions, and it is considered to play a critical role in both the progression of CKD and related complications [12–15]. There is no single treatment to improve kidney function in CKD. Approaches to retard the progression of this disease are limited to normalization of blood pressure, blood glucose, and insulin. In this context, several antioxidants have been tested in CKD studies.

1.3. Oxidative stress

An imbalance between reactive oxygen (ROS) and nitrogen (RNS) species and cellular antioxidants, in favor of oxidant species, is termed oxidative stress [16, 17].

Oxidant formation is physiologically important in the process of tissue repair as a result of inflammation and in the self-defense mechanism against microorganisms and other foreign antigens. However, when this process occurs in chronic pathological conditions, such as CKD, it has a detrimental effect and contributes to cell and tissue damage.

ROS are produced when oxygen is partially reduced. Some ROS are free radicals as they have an unpaired electron in their outer orbit. Free radicals include superoxide ($O_2^{\bullet -}$) and hydroxyl ($^{\bullet}OH$) radicals while non-radicals include hydrogen peroxide (H_2O_2), and singlet oxygen ($^1\Delta_g$ O_2). Sources of ROS include the mitochondrial electron transport chain, endothelial cells (xanthine oxidase reaction), inflammatory cells (myeloperoxidase and nicotinamide adenine dinucleotide phosphate (NADPH) oxidase), catecholamine oxidation, and metabolism of arachidonic acid. The physiological formation of ROS is detoxified by endogenous antioxidants, which are classified into two types: enzymatic and non-enzymatic. Enzymatic antioxidants include superoxide dismutase (SOD), catalase (CAT), glutathione peroxidase (GPx), glutathione reductase (GR), and glutathione S-transferase (GST). Glutathione (GSH) is the most abundant nonenzymatic antioxidant in the cell. Also, exogenous antioxidants obtained from daily food intake are classified as nonenzymatic antioxidants, which can be hydrophilic (ascorbic acid/vitamin C and flavonoids) or lipophilic (α-tocopherol/vitamin E and carotenoids).

Oxidative stress plays a critical role in CKD progression, directly by inducing glomerular and tubular damage or indirectly associated with inflammation, hypertension, and/or endothelial dysfunction [17]. Factors that cause oxidative stress are activation of NADPH oxidases, uncoupled endothelial nitric oxide synthase and mitochondrial dysfunction together with decreased antioxidant defenses such as decreased expression and activity of antioxidant enzymes and intracellular GSH content. In this context, ROS oxidize a wide variety of cellular components such as lipids, proteins, carbohydrates, and nucleic acids. Hence, the products of oxidant damage can be used as markers of oxidative stress. In fact, in patients with CKD, increased products of low-density lipoprotein (LDL) oxidation (ox-LDL) and levels of thiobarbituric acid-reactive substances (TBARS), which are markers of lipid peroxidation, have been found [18]. Antioxidants are widely used as a therapy to reduce oxidative stress. Therefore, the aim of this chapter is to provide recent information about the therapeutic role of dietary antioxidants in experimental models of CKD and clinical trials, as well as to describe the mechanisms through which antioxidants exert nephroprotection.

2. Dietary antioxidants

Dietary antioxidants encompass a wide range of molecules. The structures of some of the antioxidants reviewed in this chapter are shown in **Figure 2**. In addition, a scheme summarizing the mechanism of action of dietary compounds and their antioxidant properties in CKD is shown in **Figure 3**.

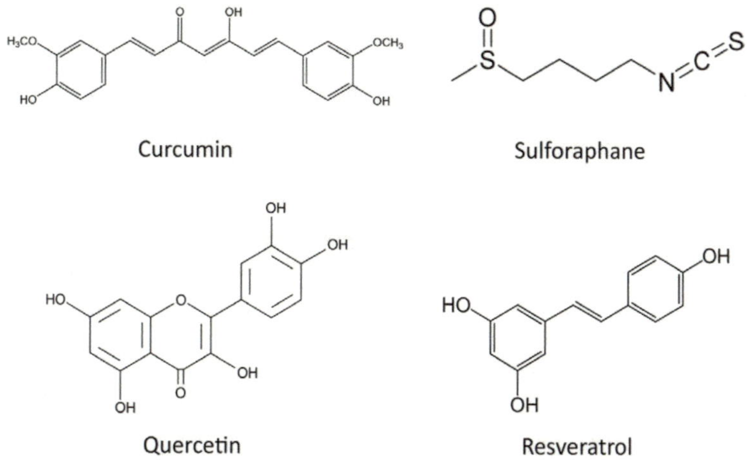

Figure 2. Molecular structure of the dietary antioxidants curcumin, sulforaphane, quercetin, and resveratrol.

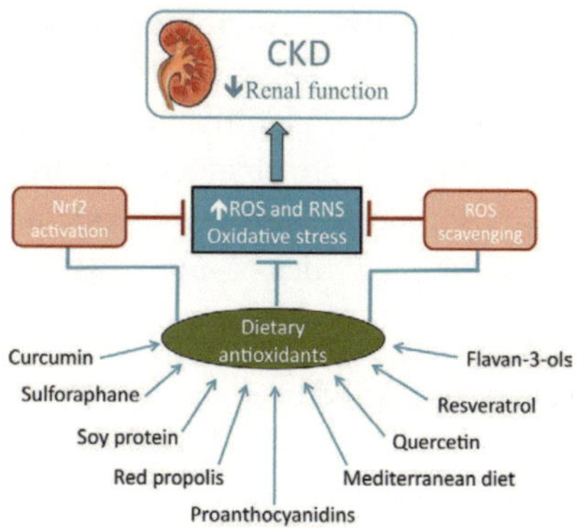

Figure 3. Beneficial properties of dietary antioxidants and its role in chronic kidney disease (CKD). Dietary compounds decrease renal dysfunction in CKD by inducing Nrf2 nuclear localization and scavenging reactive oxygen species (ROS) decreasing oxidative stress. Nrf2, nuclear factor E2-related factor 2; RNS, reactive nitrogen species.

2.1. Curcumin

Curcumin is the main curcuminoid found in turmeric (*Curcuma longa*), which is used as a spice or food colorant in curry, mustard, cheese, yogurt, soups, and cereals [19]. Curcumin is classified as a bifunctional antioxidant agent due to its ability to scavenge ROS and to modulate cellular localization of nuclear factor E2-related factor 2 (Nrf2). Curcumin is able to scavenge superoxide anion ($O_2^{\cdot-}$) [20–22], hydroxyl radicals (·OH) [22, 23], H_2O_2 [20, 22, 23], singlet oxygen [22, 24], nitric oxide [25, 26], peroxynitrite [22, 27], and peroxyl radicals (ROO·) [22, 23].

Curcumin also exhibits anti-inflammatory properties [28, 29]. One of the main targets of curcumin are the pro-inflammatory transcriptional factors, such as nuclear factor (NF)-κB and activator protein (AP)-1, which have an important role in mediating inflammatory responses by modulating the production of pro-inflammatory cytokines [30].

Curcumin has been reported to reverse 5/6 nephrectomy (5/6 Nx)-induced damage in rats. Curcumin administration (120 mg/kg) 30 days after 5/6 Nx from day 31 to 60 was reported to reverse glomerular hypertension and hyperfiltration, induce cell proliferation and nuclear localization of Nrf2, and ameliorate 5/6 Nx-induced oxidative stress and decrease in antioxidant enzymes [31]. Moreover, curcumin administration (75 mg/kg) 7 days after 5/6 Nx for 9 weeks was reported to decrease blood urea nitrogen (BUN) and plasma creatinine levels, and attenuate proteinuria, segmental sclerosis, and tubular dilatation [32]. Furthermore, curcumin administration (60 mg/kg) for 7 days before and 30 days after 5/6 Nx was reported to attenuate proteinuria, systemic and glomerular hypertension, hyperfiltration, glomerular sclerosis, interstitial fibrosis, interstitial inflammation, and increased plasma creatinine and BUN. These effects were associated with Nrf2 nuclear translocation [33]. In addition, curcumin (75 mg/kg) administration 2 weeks after surgery for 11 weeks was also reported to decrease BUN and plasma creatinine levels, as well as ameliorate proteinuria [34].

Curcumin has also been reported to exert nephroprotection in DN models [29]. Sharma et al. [35] evaluated the effect of curcumin on renal function and oxidative stress in streptozotocin (STZ)-induced diabetic rats. Rats were given curcumin (15 or 30 mg/kg) 4 weeks after STZ administration for 2 weeks. STZ-induced diabetic rats showed polyuria, increased blood glucose, and decreased body weight compared with age-matched control rats. After 6 weeks, diabetic rats also exhibited renal dysfunction, as evidenced by reduced creatinine and urea clearance and increased proteinuria, along with a marked increase in oxidative stress, as determined by lipid peroxidation and activities of antioxidant enzymes. Curcumin was able to ameliorate both renal dysfunction and oxidative stress in diabetic rats [35].

Moreover, clinical trials have been conducted to evaluate the effect of turmeric on DN [36, 37]. In a randomized, double-blind and placebo-controlled study, patients with DN received turmeric (22.1 mg of curcumin, three times a day) for 2 months. Serum levels of transforming growth factor-β (TGF-β) and interleukin-8 (IL-8), and urinary levels of IL-8 were significantly decreased after turmeric supplementation. Moreover, proteinuria in DN patients was effectively improved by turmeric without adverse effects [36].

In another randomized, double-blind, and placebo-controlled study, patients under hemodialysis were randomly divided into control and trial groups [37]. Trial group received turmeric (22.1 mg of curcumin, three times a day) for 8 weeks, whereas control group received starch. Patients in both groups also received Nephrovit tablet as a previous regimen at least for 3 months. Plasma malondialdehyde (MDA) level decreased in both groups, the ratio of decrease was significantly higher in the trial group. Activities of GPx, GR and CAT in red blood cells increased in both groups, the ratio of CAT increment was significantly higher in the trial group. Furthermore, a significant increment in albumin plasma level in the trial group was observed [37]. Therefore, turmeric attenuates oxidative stress and renal damage in hemodialysis patients.

2.2. Sulforaphane

Sulforaphane (SFN) is a naturally occurring isothiocyanate synthesized by the enzymatic action of myrosinase on glucoraphanin, a glucosinolate found in cruciferous vegetables of the genus Brassica as broccoli, brussel sprouts, mustard, cabbage, and cress [34]. SFN is classified as an indirect antioxidant agent due to its ability to increase Nrf2 nuclear localization. It has been proposed that Nrf2 activation may occur by disruption of interactions between Nrf2 and Kelch-like ECH-associated protein (Keap)-1 or by mitogen-activated protein kinases (MAPK) pathways activation [38–40].

The renoprotective effect of SFN has been evidenced in several *in vivo* studies [41–44]. In a STZ-induced diabetic mouse model, SFN treatment (started 2 weeks after STZ injection) was reported to improve metabolic dysfunction associated with diabetes, albuminuria, and glomerular sclerosis. This study further revealed that SFN attenuates high glucose-induced mesangial cell hypertrophy by Nrf2-mediated TGF-β signaling repression [41]. In addition, SFN administration (0.5 mg/kg) for 3 months was reported to prevent STZ-induced renal fibrosis and increment in albumin-to-creatinine ratio [42]. Moreover, SFN has shown beneficial effects in the unilateral ureteral obstruction (UUO) model. In rats, SFN was reported to preserve Nrf2 levels and attenuate mitochondrial-induced oxidative damage and renal fibrosis [43]. An additional study of UUO in rats showed that structural renal damage was improved by SFN treatment [44].

2.3. Quercetin

Quercetin is the main flavonol in human nutrition [45]. Quercetin is present in nuts, red onions, grapes, berries, citrus fruits, tea, pepper, coriander, fennel, radish, broccoli, tomatoes, apples, and red wine [46, 47]. Quercetin is a potent natural antioxidant and scavenger of ROS and RNS [48, 49].

The effect of quercetin in the STZ-induced diabetic rat model was evaluated. Four weeks after STZ injection, quercetin (10 mg/kg) was given orally for 4 weeks. At the end of the experiment, quercetin treatment reduced proteinuria, serum creatinine, and BUN [50]. Gomes et al. [51] evaluated whether quercetin could also have beneficial effects in concurrent STZ-induced DN and spontaneous atherosclerosis, using apolipoprotein E-deficient mice (apoE (−/−)). Six weeks after STZ or vehicle injection, mice were randomly divided into control mice, diabetic apoE (−/−) mice, and diabetic apoE (−/−) + quercetin (10 mg/kg) mice. Quercetin treatment diminished polyuria and glycemia, and normalized hypertriglyceridemia. Moreover, quercetin decreased serum creatinine and proteinuria. Furthermore, protective effects on renal structural changes, as normalization of the index of glomerulosclerosis and kidney weight/body weight, were observed. Thus, quercetin could be a therapeutic option for DN, including diabetes-associated dyslipidemia [51].

2.4. Resveratrol

Resveratrol (RSV) is a polyphenolic compound found in berries, nuts, peanuts, grapes, red wine, coffee, legumes, and chocolate [52]. RSV is classified as a bifunctional antioxidant agent; it is able to scavenge $^{\bullet}OH$, $O_2^{\bullet -}$ and metal-induced radicals [53] as well as induce gene expression of antioxidant enzymes, such as SOD and GPx [54].

Sharma et al. [55] evaluated RSV effect on renal function and oxidative stress in STZ-induced diabetic rats. Rats were divided into four groups: control, diabetes, and diabetes + RSV (5 or 10 mg/kg) groups. Four weeks after STZ injection, RSV was administered from week 4 to 6. STZ-induced diabetic rats showed polyuria, an increase in blood glucose and a decrease in body weight. After 6 weeks, diabetic rats also exhibited renal dysfunction, as evidenced by reduced creatinine and urea clearance and increased proteinuria along with enhanced oxidative stress, as evidenced by increased MDA and decreased GSH level and SOD and CAT activities. RSV treatment significantly attenuated renal dysfunction and oxidative stress [55].

RSV effect on renal fibrosis induced by UUO was evaluated in mice by Liang et al. [56]. Mice were divided into three groups: control, UUO, and UUO + RSV (20 mg/kg) groups. RSV treatment attenuated renal injury including extracellular matrix deposition and tubulointerstitial damage. Renal cortical mRNA levels of intercellular adhesion molecule (ICAM)-1, tumor necrosis factor (TNF)-α, and TGF-β, protein expression of fibronectin, and mothers against decapentaplegic homolog 3 (Smad3) acetylation were significantly upregulated in the UUO group. RSV treatment decreased the expression of these proteins. Furthermore, RSV increased SOD activity and decreased MDA and 8-hydroxy-2′-deoxyguanosine (8-OHdG) levels [56].

There is no clinical evidence showing RSV effects on CKD; however, several studies suggest it may exert beneficial effects on CKD patients. RSV supplementation in type 2 diabetic patients reduced insulin resistance and urinary excretion of ortho-tyrosine, a marker of oxidative stress [57]. Moreover, dietary supplementation with red grape juice exerted antioxidative and anti-inflammatory effects in hemodialysis patients [58, 59]. In 2006, red grape juice supplementation was reported to increase antioxidant capacity of plasma and decrease oxidized LDL and monocyte chemoattractant protein-1, an inflammatory biomarker, concentration in plasma [58]. Furthermore, in 2008, red grape juice supplementation was reported to decrease the neutrophil NADPH oxidase activity [58].

2.5. Proanthocyanidins

Proanthocyanidins are flavonoids found in cinnamon, sorghum, red wine, chocolate, berries, plums, apples, nuts, and grapes [52]. Anti-inflammatory and antioxidant properties have been attributed to proanthocyanidins [60].

The associations between habitual proanthocyanidin intake, renal function, and the risk of clinical renal outcomes in elderly women were studied by Ivey et al. [61]. Women aged over

75 years old, free of prevalent renal disease at baseline, were selected for this study. Proanthocyanidin intake was determined using a food frequency questionnaire and the US Department of Agriculture proanthocyanidin food content database. Fasting serum cystatin C and creatinine were assessed at baseline. Renal failure hospitalizations and deaths were assessed over 5 years of follow-up. Participants in the highest tertile of proanthocyanidin intake had a 9% lower cystatin C concentration than participants with lower proanthocyanidin consumption. High proanthocyanidin consumers were at 50% lower risk of moderate chronic kidney insufficiency, and 65% lower risk of experiencing a 5-year renal disease event. Therefore, a high proanthocyanidin intake is associated with renal health preservation [61].

Recently, the effect of grape seed proanthocyanidin extract (GSPE) on renal injury in type 2 diabetic rats was evaluated [62]. Rats were divided into control and diabetic groups; this later was induced diabetes by a high-carbohydrate/high-fat diet and a low STZ dose. Diabetic rats were further divided into control and three experimental groups. Experimental groups received 125, 250, or 500 mg/kg bw of GSPE. After 16 weeks, GSPE administration increased body weight and decreased food and water consumption, and urine volume in rats. Diabetic rats treated with GSPE showed decreased fasting blood glucose, serum insulin, glycated hemoglobin (HbA1c), and systolic blood pressure. GSPE significantly improved renal function parameters, reduced the expression of tissue inhibitor of metalloproteinase 1 and also increased the activity of matrix metalloproteinase 9. Furthermore, GSPE increased the activity of antioxidant enzymes and reduced the levels of C reactive protein (CRP) in the serum and the expression of TNFα, monocyte chemoattractant protein 1, and ICAM1 in the kidney. Hence, the GSPE protective effect on renal injury in type 2 diabetic rats might be associated with decreased renal inflammation and oxidative stress [62].

2.6. Flavan-3-ols

Flavan-3-ols are naturally occurring flavonoids. Epigallocatechin-3-gallate (EGCG) and catechin are flavan-3-ols whose effect has been evaluated in CKD models. EGCG is found in green tea, berries, red grapes, plums, apples, and peaches, whereas catechins are found in tea, cacao, red wine, and fruit [52].

Nakagawa et al. [63] evaluated the effect of EGCG on methylguanidine (MG) production in adenine-induced CKD rats. MG is a strong uremic toxin produced from creatinine. Under CKD conditions, MG synthesis increases. Rats were divided into control and CKD groups; CKD group was fed a 0.75% adenine diet. After 25 days, BUN levels were measured, and rats with CKD were divided into five groups. Control group was divided into two groups. Four CKD groups were given water or EGCG (20, 100, and 500 mg/kg bw) orally 30 min before and after creatinine intraperitoneal injection (100 mg/100 g bw). One group of normal rats also received creatinine injections (100 mg/100 g bw) and water was given orally 30 min before and after creatinine injection. One CKD and one control group received water 30 min before and after physiological saline injection. MG production was significantly increased in rats with adenine-induced CKD. However, EGCG administration inhibited MG production [63].

Furthermore, Yamabe et al. [64] evaluated the effect of oral EGCG (25, 50, or 100 mg/kg) administration in rats with subtotal nephrectomy plus STZ-injection. After a 50-day administration period, rats treated with EGCG showed suppressed hyperglycemia, proteinuria, and lipid peroxidation; however, there were only weak effects on the levels of serum creatinine and glycosylated protein. Further, EGCG reduced the renal accumulation of advanced glycation end-product and its related protein expression in the kidney cortex as well as associated pathological conditions [64].

Varatharajan et al. [65] evaluated the antioxidant and pro-oxidant effects of catechins-rich oil palm leaves extract (OPLE) on DN. Rats were divided into control, diabetes, and diabetes + OPLE groups. Diabetes and diabetes + OPLE groups were administered an intraperitoneal STZ injection. Seventy-two hours later, OPLE group received 1000 mg/kg of OPLE for 4 or 12 weeks. OPLE administration for 4 weeks attenuated renal dysfunction (hyperfiltration and proteinuria) and the development of glomerulosclerosis and tubulointerstitial fibrosis. Suppression of increased oxidative stress markers (8-OHdG and lipid peroxides) and the fibrotic cytokine, TGF-β1, was observed. OPLE also reduced renal expression of NADPH oxidase subunits $p22^{phox}$and $p67^{phox}$. Surprisingly, identical dose of OPLE when administered to diabetic animals for 12 weeks caused worsening of renal dysfunction and elevation of lipid peroxides and TGF-β1. These unfavorable effects were accompanied by increased expression of $p22^{phox}$. Therefore, OPLE exerts both antioxidant and pro-oxidant effects in DN depending on the duration of the treatment [65].

2.7. Soy protein

Soy has a high biologic value due to its essential amino acids, biologic active peptides, and nonprotein compounds, such as isoflavones, content.

Azadbakht and Esmaillzadeh [66] evaluated the effect of soy protein consumption on DN patients. A crossover clinical trial was conducted among 14 patients. One diet included 0.8 g/kg of protein of which 70% was animal protein and 30% vegetable protein. The other diet included the same protein amount of which 35% was animal protein, 35% soy protein, and 30% other vegetables protein. Both diets were prescribed in each phase of the trial for 7 weeks. There was a 4-week washout between the two phases of the study. As showed by the results, soy protein consumption was able to reduce proteinuria in DN patients [66].

Yeh et al. [67] investigated the effect of soybean β-conglycinin on DN. Forty rats were induced diabetes by STZ intravenous injection. Then, rats were divided into five groups: control group fed with standard diet and four groups fed with NaCl. DN rats were divided into control group, DN + soy protein 7% group, DN + soybean β-conglycinin 1.75 % group, and DN + soybean β-conglycinin 3.5% group. Results shown that soy protein and β-conglycinin were able to retard the progression of DN by increasing insulin sensitivity, regulating lipid metabolism, improving renal function, and inhibiting angiotensin-converting enzyme activity [67].

2.8. Red propolis

Propolis is a natural polyphenol-rich resinous substance collected by honeybees from a variety of plant sources [68]. Propolis is thought to improve human health and prevent disease [69].

Health-promoting properties are attributed to its polyphenolic composition. Red propolis (RP) has been classified as a separate type of propolis based on its unique chemical composition, particularly rich in isoflavonoids [70]. Anti-inflammatory and antioxidant properties have been attributed to RP [71, 72].

Teles et al. [73] evaluated the effect of RP in the 5/6 nephrectomy model. Rats underwent nephrectomy and, 30 days after surgery, they were divided into untreated nephrectomy and RP-treated nephrectomy groups. Animals were observed for 90 days after surgery; RP-treated group showed significant reduction of hypertension, proteinuria, serum creatinine, glomerulosclerosis, renal macrophage infiltration, and oxidative stress when compared to untreated rats.

RP treatment attenuated hypertension and structural renal damage in 5/6 nephrectomy model. Reduction of renal inflammation and oxidative stress could be involved in this protective effect.

2.9. Mediterranean diet

Nutritionists elaborated Mediterranean diet (MD) model from observations of the Northern Mediterranean countries food habits. These included consumption of whole grain cereals, vegetables and fruit, legumes, nuts, herbs, spices, fresh cheese from sheep and goat milk, fish, seafood, olive oil, and wine [74].

MD provides a high and varied intake of antioxidant compounds. For instance, virgin olive oil contains carotenes and phenolics [75]; white wine contains simple phenols; and whole grain cereals, nuts, fish, and seafood contain omega-3 fatty acids.

Migliori et al. [76] evaluated the effect of white wine and extra-virgin olive oil on inflammatory markers in 10 patients with CKD and 10 healthy volunteers. Two weeks before the study patients were not allowed to drink alcoholic beverages, then, they were randomized to a cross-over design A–B or B–A of a 2-week treatment with white wine (4 ml/kg) and extra-virgin olive oil (treatment A) or extra-virgin olive oil alone (treatment B). The two study periods were separated by 2 weeks in which patients were not allowed again to drink any alcoholic beverage. Plasma levels of inflammatory markers CRP, interleukin-6 (IL-6), TNF-α, and IL-8 were determined. During treatment A, plasma levels of CRP and IL-6 decreased in CKD patients and healthy volunteers. No significant variation versus baseline was observed during treatment B. Plasma markers of chronic inflammation were significantly reduced in CKD patients during the combined consumption of white wine and olive oil. Thus, this nutritional intervention could be effective as a therapy in CKD. The protective effect of omega-3 fatty acids in CKD has also been evaluated.

Gopinath et al. [77] evaluated the association between polyunsatured fatty acids (PUFA; n-3, n-6, and α-linolenic acid) and fish consumption and the prevalence of CKD. Two-thousand six-hundred Blue Mountains Eye Study (1997–1999) participants aged ≥50 years were evaluated. Dietary data were collected using a semiquantitative food frequency questionnaire, and PUFA and fish intakes were calculated. Baseline biochemistry including serum creatinine was measured. Moderate CKD was defined as an estimated GFR of <60 ml/min per 1.73 m^2.

Participants in the highest quartile of long-chain n-3 PUFA consumption had a significantly reduced possibility of having CKD compared with those in the lowest quartile. α-linolenic acid intake was positively associated with CKD. Total n-3 PUFA or total n-6 PUFA were not significantly associated with CKD. The highest compared with the lowest quartile of fish intake was associated with a reduced possibility of having CKD. Hence, an increased dietary intake of long-chain n-3 PUFA and fish reduces the prevalence of CKD [77].

3. Conclusions and future directions

CKD is considered a public health problem because its incidence is about 10% of world population and treatment methods are ineffective or expensive. Consequently, the development of novel therapies is highly needed. This chapter summarizes information about dietary antioxidant agents, which have shown nephroprotection on CKD, showing what has been found and leading to future studies. Future studies might aim to study physical and chemical properties of these compounds as well as the mechanisms involved in nephroprotection. A better understanding of these aspects will be key in the improvement of therapies, which have been studied on clinical trials as well as in the design of clinical trials of those compounds, which have not been studied in humans.

In that way, therapies will be not only effective but also viable because of the easy access to these compounds.

Acknowledgements

This work was supported by CONACYT 220046 and 252008 and PAPIIT IN201316

Author details

Dianelena Eugenio-Pérez[1], Liliana Yazmín Medina-Fernández[1],
Jennyfer Andrea Saldivar-Anaya[1], Eduardo Molina-Jijón[1,2] and José Pedraza-Chaverri[1*]

*Address all correspondence to: pedraza@unam.mx

1 Department of Biology, Faculty of Chemistry, National Autonomous University of Mexico (UNAM), University City, D.F., Mexico

2 Department of Biosciences and Engineering, CIIEMAD-IPN, Mexico City, Mexico

References

[1] Taal M.W., Chertow G.M., Marsden P.A., Skorecki K., Yu A.S.L. and Brenner B.M. Brenner & Rector's The Kidney. 9th ed. Philadelphia: Saunders; 2012.

[2] Alpern J., Caplan M.J. and Moe O.W. Seldin and Giebisch's The Kidney: Physiology & Pathophysiology. 5th ed. London: Academic Press; 2013.

[3] Levey A.S., Eckardt K.U., Tsukamoto Y., Levin A., Coresh J., Rossert J., et al. Definition and classification of chronic kidney disease: A position statement from Kidney Disease: Improving Global Outcomes (KDIGO). Kidney Int. 2005;67(6):2089–2100. DOI: 10.1111/j1523-1755.2005.00365.x.

[4] James M.T., Hemmelgarn B.R., Tonelli M. Early recognition and prevention of chronic kidney disease. Lancet. 2010;375(9722):1296–309. DOI: 10.1016/S0140-6736(09)62004-3.

[5] Levey A.S., Coresh J., Balk E., Kausz A.T., Levin A., Steffes M.W., et al. National Kidney Foundation practice guidelines for chronic kidney disease: Evaluation, classification, and stratification. Ann Intern Med. 2003;139(2):137–47. DOI: 10.7326/0003-4819-139-2-200307150-00013.

[6] Laliberté F., Bookhart B.K., Vekeman F., Corral M., Duh M.S., Bailey R.A., et al. Direct all-cause health care costs associated with chronic kidney disease in patients with diabetes and hypertension: A managed care perspective. J Manag Care Pharm. 2009;15(4):312–22.

[7] Flores J., Alvo M., Borja H., Morales J., Vega J., Zuñiga C., et al. Chronic kidney disease: classification, identification, management, and complications. Rev med Chile. 2009;137(1):137–77. DOI: 10.4067/S0034-98872009000100026.

[8] Roshan B., Stanton R.C. A story of microalbuminuria and diabetic nephropathy. J Nephropathol. 2013;2(4):234–40. DOI: 10.12860/JNP.2013.37.

[9] Hart P.D., Bakris G.L. Hypertensive nephropathy: Prevention and treatment recommendations. Expert Opin Pharmacother. 2010;11(16):2675–86. DOI: 10.1517/14656566.2010.485612.

[10] Kidney Disease Outcomes Quality Initiative (K/DOQI). K/DOQI clinical practice guidelines on hypertension and antihypertensive agents in chronic kidney disease. Am J Kidney Dis. 2004;43(5 Suppl 1):S1–290. DOI: 10.1053/j.ajkd.2004.03.003.

[11] Chokhandre M.K., Mahmoud M.I., Hakami T., Jafer M., Inamdar A.S. Vitamin D & its analogues in type 2 diabetic nephropathy: A systematic review. J Diabetes Metab Disord. 2015;14:58. DOI: 10.1186/s40200-015-0186-6.

[12] Vaziri N.D. Oxidative stress in uremia: Nature, mechanisms, and potential consequences. Semin Nephrol. 2004;24(5):469–73. DOI:10.1016/j.semnephrol.2004.06.026.

[13] Himmelfarb J., Stenvinkel P., Ikizler T.A., Hakim R.M. The elephant in uremia: Oxidant stress as a unifying concept of cardiovascular disease in uremia. Kidney Int. 2002;62(5): 1524–38. DOI: 10.1046/j.1523-1755.2002.00600.x.

[14] Himmelfarb J., Hakim R.M. Oxidative stress in uremia. Curr Opin Nephrol Hypertens. 2003;12(6):593–8. DOI: 10.1097/01.mnh.0000098764.18213.4f.

[15] Ruiz S., Pergola P.E., Zager R.A., Vaziri N.D. Targeting the transcription factor Nrf2 to ameliorate oxidative stress and inflammation in chronic kidney disease. Kidney Int. 2013;83(6):1029–41. DOI: 10.1038/ki.2012.439.

[16] Locatelli F., Canaud B., Eckardt K.U., Stenvinkel P., Wanner C., Zoccali C. Oxidative stress in end-stage renal disease: An emerging threat to patient outcome. Nephrol Dial Transplant . 2003;18(7):1272–80. DOI: 10.1093/ndt/gfg074.

[17] Kuo K., Tarng D. Oxidative stress in chronic kidney disease. Adaptive Med. 2010;2(2): 87–94. DOI: 10.4247/AM.2010.ABA010.

[18] Costa-Hong V., Bortolotto L.A., Jorgetti V., Consolim-Colombo F., Krieger E.M., Lima J.J. Oxidative stress and endothelial dysfunction in chronic kidney disease. Arq Bras Cardiol. 2009;92(5):381–6. DOI: 10.1590/S0066-782X2009000500013.

[19] Trujillo J., Chirino Y.I., Molina-Jijón E., Andérica-Romero A.C., Tapia E., Pedraza-Chaverrí J. Renoprotective effect of the antioxidant curcumin: Recent findings. Redox Biol. 2013;1:448–56. DOI: 10.1016/j.redox.2013.09.003.

[20] Ak T., Gülçin I. Antioxidant and radical scavenging properties of curcumin. Chem Biol Interact. 2008;174(1):27–37. DOI: 10.1016/j.cbi.2008.05.003.

[21] Sreejayan N., Rao M.N. Free radical scavenging activity of curcuminoids. Arzneimittelforschung. 1996;46(2):169–71.

[22] Trujillo J., Molina-Jijón E., Medina-Campos O.N., Rodríguez-Muñoz R., Reyes J.L., Loredo M.L., et al. Curcumin prevents cisplatin-induced decrease in the tight and adherents junctions: Relation to oxidative stress. Food Funct. DOI: 10.1039/C5FO00624D.

[23] Barzegar A., Moosavi-Movahedi A.A. Intracellular ROS protection efficiency and free radical-scavenging activity of curcumin. PLoS One. 2011;6(10):e26012. DOI: 10.1371/journal.pone.0026012.

[24] Das K.C., Das C.K. Curcumin (diferuloylmethane), a singlet oxygen ((1)O(2)) quencher. Biochem Biophys Res Commun. 2002;295(1):62–6. DOI: 10.1016/S0006-291X(02)00633-2.

[25] Sreejayan, Rao M.N. Nitric oxide scavenging by curcuminoids. J Pharm Pharmacol. 1997;49(1):105–7. DOI: 10.1111/j.2042-7158.1997.tb06761.x.

[26] Sumanont Y., Murakami Y., Tohda M., Vajragupta O., Matsumoto K., Watanabe H. Evaluation of the nitric oxide radical scavenging activity of manganese complexes of

curcumin and its derivative. Biol Pharm Bull. 2004;27(2):170–3. DOI: 10.1248/bpb.27.170.

[27] Kim J.E., Kim A.R., Chung H.Y., Han S.Y., Kim B.S., Choi J.S. In vitro peroxynitrite scavenging activity of diarylheptanoids from *Curcuma longa*. Phytother Res . 2003;17(5): 481–4. DOI: 10.1002/ptr.1179.

[28] He Y., Yue Y., Zheng X., Zhang K., Chen S., Du Z. Curcumin, Inflammation, and chronic diseases: How are they linked?. Molecules. 2015;20(5):9183–213. DOI: 10.3390/molecules20059183.

[29] Soetikno V., Suzuki K., Veeraveedu P.T., Arumugam S., Lakshmanan A.P., Sone H., et al. Molecular understanding of curcumin in diabetic nephropathy. Drug Discov Today. 2013;18(15–16):756–63. DOI: 10.1016/j.drudis.2013.04.009.

[30] Gupta S.C., Patchva S., Koh W., Aggarwal B.B. Discovery of curcumin, a component of golden spice, and its miraculous biological activities. Clin Exp Pharmacol Physiol. 2012;39(3):283–99. DOI: 10.1111/j.1440-1681.2011.05648.x.

[31] Tapia E., Zatarain-Barrón Z.L., Hernández-Pando R., Zarco-Márquez G., Molina-Jijón E., Cristóbal-García M., et al. Curcumin reverses glomerular hemodynamic alterations and oxidant stress in 5/6 nephrectomized rats. Phytomedicine. 2013;20(3–4):359–66. DOI: 10.1016/j.phymed.2012.11.014.

[32] Ghosh S.S., Massey H.D., Krieg R., Fazelbhoy Z.A., Ghosh S., Sica D.A., et al. Curcumin ameliorates renal failure in 5/6 nephrectomized rats: role of inflammation. Am J Physiol Renal Physiol. 2009;296(5):F1146–57. DOI: 10.1152/ajprenal.90732.2008.

[33] Tapia E., Soto V., Ortiz-Vega K.M., Zarco-Márquez G., Molina-Jijón E., Cristóbal-García M., et al. Curcumin induces Nrf2 nuclear translocation and prevents glomerular hypertension, hyperfiltration, oxidant stress, and the decrease in antioxidant enzymes in 5/6 nephrectomized rats. Oxid Med Cell Longev. 2012;2012:269039. DOI: 10.1155/2012/269039.

[34] Soetikno V., Sari F.R., Lakshmanan A.P., Arumugam S., Harima M., Suzuki K., et al. Curcumin alleviates oxidative stress, inflammation, and renal fibrosis in remnant kidney through the Nrf2-keap1 pathway. Mol Nutr Food Res. 2013;57(9):1649–59. DOI: 10.1002/mnfr.201200540.

[35] Sharma S., Kulkarni S.K., Chopra K. Curcumin, the active principle of turmeric (*Curcuma longa*), ameliorates diabetic nephropathy in rats. Clin Exp Pharmacol Physiol. 2006;33(10):940–5. DOI: 10.1111/j.1440-1681.2006.04468.x.

[36] Khajehdehi P., Pakfetrat M., Javidnia K., Azad F., Malekmakan L., Nasab M.H., Dehghanzadeh G., et al. Oral supplementation of turmeric attenuates proteinuria, transforming growth factor-β and interleukin-8 levels in patients with overt type 2 diabetic nephropathy: A randomized, double-blind and placebo-controlled study. Scand J Urol Nephrol. 2011;45(5):365–70. DOI: 10.3109/00365599.2011.585622.

[37] Pakfetrat M., Akmali M., Malekmakan L., Dabaghimanesh M., Khorsand M. Role of turmeric in oxidative modulation in end-stage renal disease patients. Hemodial Int. 2015;19(1):124–31. DOI: 10.1111/hdi.12204.

[38] Guerrero-Beltrán C.E., Mukhopadhyay P., Horváth B., Rajesh M., Tapia E., García-Torres I., et al. Sulforaphane, a natural constituent of broccoli, prevents cell death and inflammation in nephropathy. J Nutr Biochem. 2012;23(5):494–500. DOI: 10.1016/j.jnutbio.2011.02.004.

[39] Dinkova-Kostova A.T., Kostov R.V. Glucosinolates and isothiocyanates in health and disease. Trends Mol Med . 2012;18(6):337–47. DOI: 10.1016/j.molmed.2012.04.003.

[40] Vasanthi H.R., Mukherjee S., Das D.K. Potential health benefits of broccoli – a chemico-biological overview. Mini Rev Med Chem. 2009; 9(6):749–59. DOI: 10.2174/138955709788452685.

[41] Zheng H., Whitman S.A., Wu W., Wondrak G.T., Wong P.K., Fang D., et al. Therapeutic potential of Nrf2 activators in streptozotocin-induced diabetic nephropathy. Diabetes. 2011;60(11):3055–66. DOI: 10.2337/db11-0807.

[42] Cui W., Bai Y., Miao X., Luo P., Chen Q., Tan Y., et al. Prevention of diabetic nephropathy by sulforaphane: Possible role of Nrf2 upregulation and activation. Oxid Med Cell Longev. 2012;2012:821936. DOI: 10.1155/2012/821936.

[43] Chung S.D., Lai T.Y., Chien C.T., Yu H.J. Activating Nrf-2 signaling depresses unilateral ureteral obstruction-evoked mitochondrial stress-related autophagy, apoptosis and pyroptosis in kidney. PLoS One. 2012;7(10):e47299. DOI: 10.1371/journal.pone.0047299.

[44] Noorafshan A., Karbalay-Doust S., Poorshahid M. Stereological survey of the ameliorative effects of sulforaphane and quercetin on renal tissue in unilateral ureteral obstruction in rats. Acta Clin Croat. 2012;51(4):555–62.

[45] Hollman P.C., de Vries J.H., van Leeuwen S.D., Mengelers M.J., Katan M.B. Absorption of dietary quercetin glycosides and quercetin in healthy ileostomy volunteers. Am J Clin Nutr. 1995;62(6):1276–82.

[46] Gibellini L., Pinti M., Nasi M., De Biasi S., Roat E., Bertoncelli L., et al. Interfering with ROS metabolism in cancer cells: The potential role of quercetin. Cancers (Basel). 2010;2(2):1288–311. DOI: 10.3390/cancers2021288.

[47] Aras A., Khokhar A.R., Qureshi M.Z., Silva M.F., Sobczak-Kupiec A., Pineda E.A., et al. Targeting cancer with nano-bullets: Curcumin, EGCG, resveratrol and quercetin on flying carpets. Asian Pac J Cancer Prev. 2014;15(9):3865–71. DOI: 10.7314/APJCP.2014.15.9.3865.

[48] Coballase-Urrutia E., Pedraza-Chaverri J., Camacho-Carranza R., Cárdenas-Rodríguez N., Huerta-Gertrudis B., Medina-Campos O.N., et al. Antioxidant activity of Heterotheca inuloides extracts and of some of its metabolites. Toxicology. 2010;276(1):41–8. DOI: 10.1016/j.tox.2010.06.013.

[49] Boots A.W., Haenen G.R., Bast A. Health effects of quercetin: from antioxidant to nutraceutical. Eur J Pharmacol. 2008;585(2–3):325–37. DOI: 10.1016/j.ejphar.2008.

[50] Anjaneyulu M., Chopra K. Quercetin, an anti-oxidant bioflavonoid, attenuates diabetic nephropathy in rats. Clin Exp Pharmacol Physiol. 2004;31(4):244–8. DOI: 10.1111/j.1440-1681.2004.03982.x.

[51] Gomes I.B., Porto M.L., Santos M.C., Campagnaro B.P., Gava A.L., Meyrelles S.S., et al. The protective effects of oral low-dose quercetin on diabetic nephropathy in hypercholesterolemic mice. Front Physiol. 2015;6:247. DOI: 10.3389/fphys.2015.00247.

[52] Álvarez-Parrilla E., de la Rosa L.A., González-Aguilar G.A., Ayala-Zavala J.F. Antioxidants in food and health. 1st ed. México: Clave Editorial; 2012.

[53] Leonard S.S., Xia C., Jiang B.H., Stinefelt B., Klandorf H., Harris G.K., et al . Resveratrol scavenges reactive oxygen species and effects radical-induced cellular responses. Biochem Biophys Res Commun. 2003;309(4):1017–26. DOI: 10.1016/j.bbrc.2003.08.105.

[54] Spanier G., Xu H., Xia N., Tobias S., Deng S., Wojnowski L., et al. Resveratrol reduces endothelial oxidative stress by modulating the gene expression of superoxide dismutase 1 (SOD1), glutathione peroxidase 1 (GPx1) and NADPH oxidase subunit (Nox4). J Physiol Pharmacol. 2009;60 Suppl 4:111–6.

[55] Sharma S., Anjaneyulu M., Kulkarni S.K., Chopra K. Resveratrol, a polyphenolic phytoalexin, attenuates diabetic nephropathy in rats. Pharmacology. 2006;76(2):69. DOI: 10.1159/000089720.

[56] Liang J., Tian S., Han J., Xiong P. Resveratrol as a therapeutic agent for renal fibrosis induced by unilateral ureteral obstruction. Ren Fail. 2014;36(2):285–91. DOI: 10.3109/0886022X.2013.844644.

[57] Brasnyo P., Molnar G.A., Mohas M., Marko L., Laczy B., Cseh J., et al. Resveratrol improves insulin sensitivity, reduces oxidative stress and activates the Akt pathway in type 2 diabetic patients. Br J Nutr. 2011;106(3):383–9. DOI: 10.1017/S0007114511000316.

[58] Castilla P., Davalos A., Teruel J.L., Cerrato F., Fernandez-Lucas M., Merino J.L., et al. Comparative effects of dietary supplementation with red grape juice and vitamin E on production of superoxide by circulating neutrophil NADPH oxidase in hemodialysis patients. Am J Clin Nutr. 2008;87(4):1053–61.

[59] Castilla P., Echarri R., Davalos A., Cerrato F., Ortega H., Teruel J.L., et al. Concentrated red grape juice exerts antioxidant, hypolipidemic, and antiinflammatory effects in both hemodialysis patients and healthy subjects. Am J Clin Nutr. 2006;84(1):252–62.

[60] Fine A.M. Oligomeric proanthocyanidin complexes: history, structure, and phytopharmaceutical applications. Altern Med Rev. 2000;5(2):144–51.

[61] Ivey K.L., Lewis J.R., Lim W.H., Lim E.M., Hodgson J.M., Prince R.L. Associations of proanthocyanidin intake with renal function and clinical outcomes in elderly women. PLoS One. 2013;8(8):e71166. DOI: 10.1371/journal.pone.0071166.

[62] Bao L., Zhang Z., Dai X., Ding Y., Jiang Y., Li Y., et al. Effects of grape seed proanthocyanidin extract on renal injury in type 2 diabetic rats. Mol Med Rep. 2015;11(1):645–52. DOI: 10.3892/mmr.2014.2768.

[63] Nakagawa T., Yokozawa T., Sano M., Takeuchi S., Kim M., Minamoto S. Activity of (-)-epigallocatechin 3-O-gallate against oxidative stress in rats with adenine-induced renal failure. J Agric Food Chem. 2004;52(7):2103–7. DOI: 10.1021/jf030258j.

[64] Yamabe N., Yokozawa T., Oya T., Kim M. Therapeutic potential of (-)-epigallocatechin 3-O-gallate on renal damage in diabetic nephropathy model rats. J Pharmacol Exp Ther. 2006;319(1):228–36. DOI: 10.1124/jpet.106.107029.

[65] Varatharajan R., Sattar M.Z., Chung I., Abdulla M.A., Kassim N.M., Abdullah N.A. Antioxidant and pro-oxidant effects of oil palm (*Elaeis guineensis*) leaves extract in experimental diabetic nephropathy: A duration-dependent outcome. BMC Complement Altern Med. 2013;13:242. DOI: 10.1186/1472-6882-13-242.

[66] Azadbakht L., Esmaillzadeh A. Soy-protein consumption and kidney-related biomarkers among type 2 diabetics: A crossover, randomized clinical trial. J Ren Nutr. 2009;19(6):479–86. DOI: 10.1053/j.jrn.2009.06.002

[67] Yeh W.J., Yang H.Y., Chen J.R. Soy β-conglycinin retards progression of diabetic nephropathy via modulating the insulin sensitivity and angiotensin-converting enzyme activity in rats fed with high salt diet. Food Funct. 2014;5(11):2898–904. DOI: 10.1039/c4fo00379a.

[68] da Costa M.F., Libório A.B., Teles F., Martins Cda S., Soares P.M., Meneses G.C., et al. Red propolis ameliorates ischemic-reperfusion acute kidney injury. Phytomedicine. 2015;22(9):787–95. DOI: 10.1016/j.phymed.2015.03.017.

[69] Daleprane J.B., Abdalla D.S. Emerging roles of propolis: antioxidant, cardioprotective, and antiangiogenic actions. Evid Based Complement Alternat Med. 2013;2013:175135. DOI: 10.1155/2013/175135

[70] Righi A.A., Negri G., Salatino A. Comparative chemistry of propolis from eight brazilian localities. Evid Based Complement Alternat Med. 2013;2013:267878. DOI: 10.1155/2013/267878

[71] Bueno-Silva B., Alencar S.M., Koo H., Ikegaki M., Silva G.V., Napimoga M.H., et al. Anti-inflammatory and antimicrobial evaluation of neovestitol and vestitol isolated from Brazilian red propolis. J Agric Food Chem. 2013;61(19):4546–50. DOI: 10.1021/jf305468f

[72] Enis Yonar M., Yonar S.M., Ural M.S., Silici S., Düsükcan M. Protective role of propolis in chlorpyrifos-induced changes in the haematological parameters and the oxidative/

antioxidative status of Cyprinus carpio carpio. Food Chem Toxicol. 2012;50(8):2703–8. DOI: 10.1016/j.fct.2012.05.032.

[73] Teles F., da Silva T.M., da Cruz Júnior F.P., Honorato V.H., de Oliveira Costa H., Barbosa A.P. Brazilian red propolis attenuates hypertension and renal damage in 5/6 renal ablation model. PLoS One. 2015;10(1):e0116535. DOI: 10.1371/journal.pone.0116535.

[74] Gerber M., Hoffman R. The Mediterranean diet: Health, science and society. Br J Nutr. 2015;113 Suppl 2:S4–10. DOI: 10.1017/S0007114514003912.

[75] Servili M., Montedoro G. Contribution of phenolic compounds to virgin olive oil quality. Eur J Lipid Sci Technol. 2002;104(9–10):602–13. DOI: 10.1002/1438-9312(200210)104:9/10<602::AID-EJLT602>3.0.CO;2-X.

[76] Migliori M., Panichi V., de la Torre R., Fitó M., Covas M., Bertelli A., et al. Anti-inflammatory effect of white wine in CKD patients and healthy volunteers. Blood Purif. 2015;39(1–3):218–23. DOI: 10.1159/000371570.

[77] Gopinath B., Harris D.C., Flood V.M., Burlutsky G., Mitchell P. Consumption of long-chain n-3 PUFA, α-linolenic acid and fish is associated with the prevalence of chronic kidney disease. Br J Nutr. 2011;105(9):1361–8. DOI: 10.1017/S0007114510005040.

Chapter 18

Novel Antioxidant Therapy Against Myocardial Ischemia–Reperfusion Injury During Percutaneous Coronary Angioplasty

Pablo Parra and Ramón Rodrigo

Additional information is available at the end of the chapter

http://dx.doi.org/10.5772/63658

Abstract

Acute myocardial infarction (AMI) is the leading cause of mortality worldwide. Major advances in the treatment have included coronary interventions, such as systemic thrombolysis and percutaneous coronary angioplasty (PCA). These procedures have been aimed to recover the blood flow in the cardiac zones affected by the occlusion of a branch of the coronary artery. However, damage is generated in the heart tissue known as myocardial reperfusion injury, an event associated with increased oxidative stress. Reactive oxygen species (ROS) are able to trigger cell death pathways, and myocardial structural and functional impairment. Studies on animal models of AMI suggest that lethal reperfusion accounts for up to 50% of the final size of a myocardial infarct, a part of the damage likely to be prevented. Although a number of strategies have been aimed to ameliorate lethal reperfusion injury, up to date the beneficial effects in clinical settings remain elusive. The accumulated body of evidence suggests that redox balance is a crucial determinant of ischemia–reperfusion injury, with clear mechanistic insights into pharmacological approaches. This chapter presents the molecular basis for a novel cardioprotection of patients with AMI subjected to PCA, based on a reinforcement of the antioxidant system.

Keywords: acute myocardial infarction, ischemia–reperfusion, oxidative stress, antioxidant therapy, coronary angioplasty

1. Introduction

According to the World Health Organization, a total of 56 million deaths occurred worldwide during 2012 and 17.5 million (31.25%) were due to cardiovascular diseases, still the principal cause of death by noncommunicable diseases. In addition, deaths due to ischemic heart disease (IHD) in 2012 were estimated as 7.4 million (13.2%), remaining as the leading cause of death over the past decade [1, 2], with a considerable social impact due to mortality, morbidity, loss of quality of life and high economic cost. In IHD, severe and prolonged myocardial ischemic events occur through thrombotic complications from atherosclerotic plaques in pericardial coronary arteries, leading to cardiomyocyte death. The latter becomes more significant when ischemia is caused by complete coronary occlusion, generating an acute myocardial infarction (AMI) where the coronary microcirculation is significantly reduced, affecting most of the left ventricular wall thickness together with structural and functional impairments, scarring and adverse remodeling [3, 4]. The most effective therapeutic intervention for reducing the size of a myocardial infarct and improving the clinical outcome is timely and effective restoring of coronary flow using either thrombolytic therapy or percutaneous coronary angioplasty (PCA), but this process can itself induce further viable cardiomyocyte death and increased infarct size, a phenomenon known as myocardial reperfusion injury (MRI), thus reducing the beneficial effects. The MRI causes four types of cardiac dysfunction, the first two being reversible and the others irreversible: (i) reperfusion-induced arrhythmias; (ii) myocardial stunning; (iii) microvascular obstruction or no-reflow phenomenon; and (iv) lethal myocardial reperfusion injury (LMRI). LMRI is the most important because may account for up to 50% of the myocardial infarct (MI) final size as shown in both experimental ischemia–reperfusion (I/R) models and patients with ST-segment elevation MI applying therapeutic interventions solely at the onset of myocardial reperfusion [5, 6]. In addition, several experimental studies have shown the important role of oxidative stress in MRI and it has been postulated as a therapeutic target for cardioprotection [7–13]. However, the clinical trials have shown mixed results with no clear confirmation of the beneficial effects of exogenous antioxidant therapy at the onset of myocardial revascularization, possibly due to differences in the design and methodology [14]. Next, we describe the pathophysiological mechanisms involved in MRI and the molecular basis for a novel cardioprotective treatment of patients with AMI subjected to PCA, based on a reinforcement of the antioxidant system.

2. Oxidative stress and the pathophysiology of myocardial ischemia–reperfusion injury

Occlusion of a coronary artery decreases blood flow to myocardial tissue causing a state of prolonged ischemia. The lack of oxygen and nutrients triggers a series of abrupt metabolic and biochemical changes within the cardiomyocyte that lead to several mechanisms of cell death, which are enhanced in the reperfusion (**Figure 1**).

During acute myocardial ischemia, the absence of oxygen in the mitochondrial electron transport chain (mETC) causes a drop in the production of adenosine triphosphate (ATP), and the glycolytic pathway generates a shift to anaerobic respiration with intracellular accumulation of lactic acid [9, 15]. In addition, the Krebs cycle stops and CO_2 cannot be eliminated from the extracellular space due to blood flow arrest. Therefore, a decrease in the intracellular pH

(<7.0) occurs, which increases the Na^+ influx through the Na^+/H^+ exchanger, while the ATP depletion stops Na^+ efflux through Na^+/K^+-ATPase. This intracellular Na^+ accumulation activates Na^+/Ca^{2+} exchangers in the reverse direction leading to cytosolic Ca^{2+} overload [16], where the sarcoplasmic reticulum is unable of uptaking Ca^{2+} from the cytosol because sarco(endo)plasmic reticulum Ca^{2+}-ATPase (SERCA) transporter needs ATP to function [17]. High levels of intracellular Ca^{2+} induce the conversion, via limited proteolysis and sulfhydryl oxidation, of xanthine dehydrogenase to xanthine oxidase (XO) in endothelial cells mainly, an isoform that produces superoxide anion and hydrogen peroxide (H_2O_2) from oxygen [18]. The acidic conditions exert a strong inhibitory effect on the mitochondrial permeability transition pore (mPTP) [19], despite the presence of inducing factors opening such as Ca^{2+} and inorganic phosphate overload, oxidative stress and ADP. The mPTP is an inner mitochondrial membrane protein channel that, when it is open under certain conditions, mediates non-selective permeability to molecules less than 1.5 kDa, collapsing the mitochondrial membrane potential and uncoupling oxidative phosphorylation, leading to ATP depletion, mitochondrial matrix swelling and cell death through apoptosis and necrosis [20]. In addition, acidosis and low levels of ATP reduces the myocardial contractile activity [21].

The coronary revascularization postmyocardial ischemia rapidly increases the level of tissue oxygenation, which triggers a series of mechanisms producing LMRI. The most important mediators of this process are described below.

2.1. Oxidative stress

During the first minutes of the onset of myocardial reperfusion, a burst of ROS occurs, in accordance with several experiments demonstrating direct measurements of free radicals in isolated hearts and *in vivo* I/R models [8, 10–13]. The potential enzymatic sources of ROS production in cardiac tissue exposed to I/R are xanthine oxidase (XO) in endothelial cells, nicotinamide adenine dinucleotide phosphate (NADPH) oxidase (NOX) in neutrophils, mETC, uncoupled nitric oxide synthase (uncNOS), cytochrome P450, lipoxygenase/cyclooxygenase and monoamine oxidase [22]. XO activation and ATP catabolism to hypoxanthine occur in ischemic period, generating high levels of ROS together with uric acid from oxygen and accumulated hypoxanthine (or xanthine), when blood flow is restored [18]. The important role of NOX family in the MRI has been shown in experimental studies where NOX-isoform-specific knockout mice have significantly reduced infarct sizes compared to wild-type (WT) controls, confirming these results in buffer-perfused Langendorff models [23]. Cardiolipin peroxidation and cytochrome oxidase uncoupling in ischemic period results in the inhibition of electron flux through mETC, ATP depletion and increased superoxide anion generation, a situation that persists in the reperfusion where the Krebs cycle is reactivated and high levels of tissue oxygen can lead to increased ROS production [24]. Tetrahydrobiopterin (BH_4), a NOS cofactor, suffers oxidation to dihydrobiopterin in prolonged ischemia, resulting in loss of NOS enzyme affinity by the substrate L-citrulline together with a shift in the generation of nitric oxide (NO), a potent vasodilator, to superoxide anion during reperfusion [24, 25].

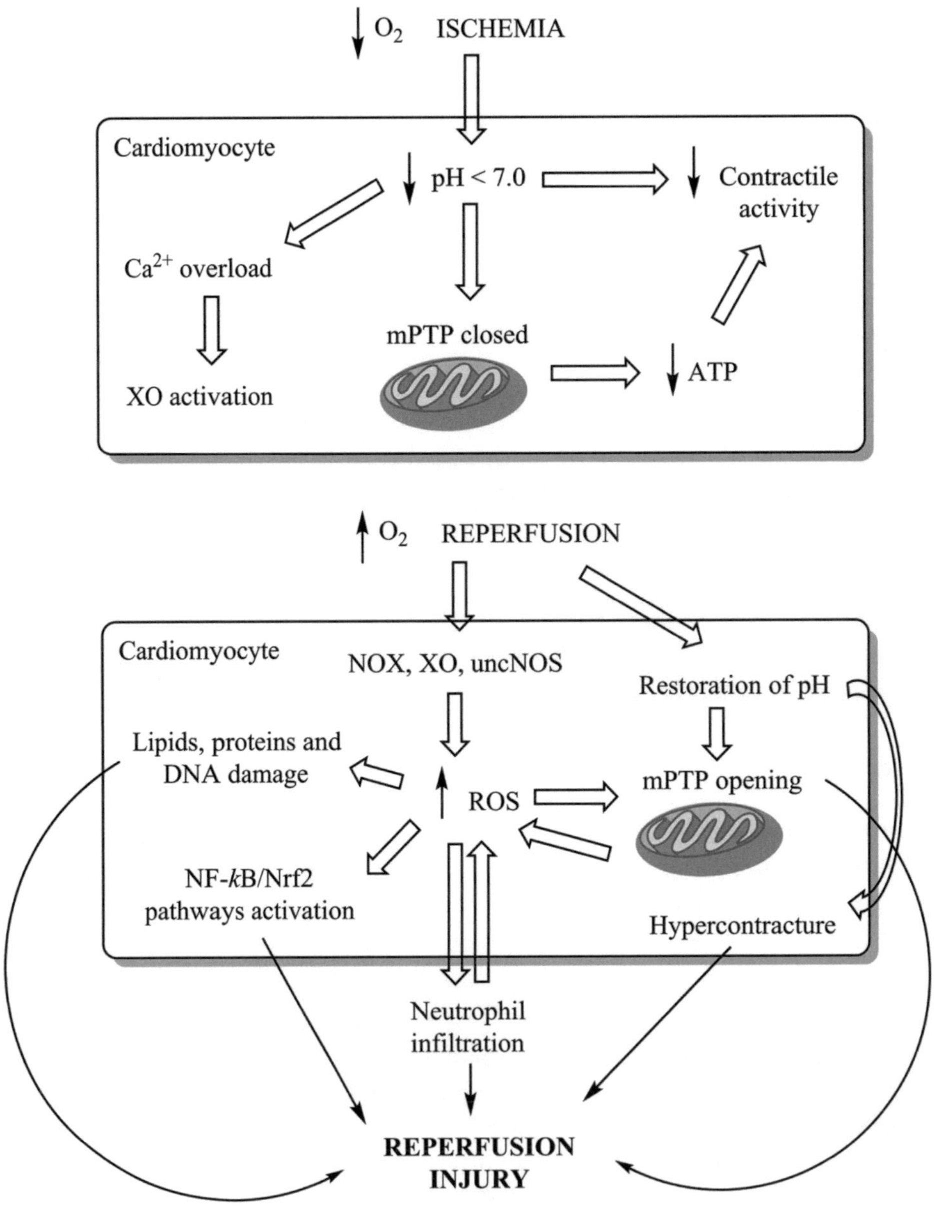

Figure 1. Schematic representation of the pathophysiological mechanism involved in myocardial damage due to I/R. ATP, adenosine triphosphate; mPTP, mitochondrial permeability transition pore; NOX, NADPH oxidase; NF-κB, nuclear factor kappa B; Nrf2, nuclear factor-erythroid 2-related factor 2; ROS, reactive oxygen species; uncNOS, uncoupled nitric oxide synthase; XO, xanthine oxidase; Ca^{2+}, calcium; DNA, deoxyribonucleic acid.

Exacerbation of oxidative stress during postischemia myocardial reperfusion overwhelms the endogenous antioxidant defenses, causing free radical propagation reactions with direct damage to cellular biomolecules as lipid peroxidation, protein oxidation/nitration and DNA damage [24, 26]. The main effecter of ROS-induced damage is the highly reactive hydroxyl radical generated from Fenton/Haber–Weiss reactions and peroxynitrite (reviewed in Section 3) [24], demonstrating its formation in a postischemia reperfused heart [11]. In addition, ROS can induce activation both of nuclear factor kappa B (NF-κB) and nuclear factor-erythroid 2-related factor 2 (Nrf2)-signaling pathways, although the ROS concentration threshold has not been experimentally determined [27]. NF-κB proteins are a family of transcription factors with a central role in regulating the expression of genes related with inflammation, immune response, cell proliferation and apoptosis [28–30], and different levels of ROS can both activate and inhibit NF-κB-signaling, depending on the context, with a high degree of complexity [31]. On the other hand, Nrf2 is a transcription factor that positively regulates the human antioxidant response element (ARE), leading to the gene expression of endogenous antioxidant defence system. Kelch-like ECH-associated protein 1 (Keap1) is a suppressor protein anchored in the cytoplasm that physically binds Nrf2, but oxidative stress facilitates the complex dissociation and Nrf2 nuclear translocation to ARE-containing promoters [32]. A study demonstrated that Nrf2 is indispensable for the regulation of both constitutive and inducible expression of antioxidants and phase-2 enzymes in mouse primary cardiomyocytes [33]. In clinical trials, the antioxidant therapy at the onset of reperfusion, in patients with AMI subjected to PCA, has mainly considered the use, alone or combined, of ROS scavengers, inhibitors of ROS sources, human recombinant antioxidant enzymes and reduced glutathione donor [14].

2.2. Intracellular pH

The intracellular acidic pH generated in ischemia returns to physiological values during myocardial reperfusion [9]. Bond et al. [34] simulated I/R conditions in cultured neonatal rat cardiac myocytes, demonstrating that when intracellular acidic pH increases to 7.4 hypercontracture and cell death occur. In addition, free Ca^{2+} increases during simulated ischemia and in simulated reperfusion. Under conditions of ischemia, it was shown in cultured cardiac myocytes and perfused papillary muscles that inhibition of Na^+/H^+ exchanger delayed the increase of intracellular pH after reperfusion and prevented reperfusion-induced cell killing, but not reduce the increase in intracellular-free Ca^{2+} [35]. By contrast, reperfusion with inhibition of Na^+/Ca^{2+} exchanger decreases intracellular free Ca^{2+} but did not reduce cell killing. These results suggest that acidotic pH is generally protective in I/R, and Na^+/H^+ exchanger contributes to reperfusion washout effect on intracellular acidic pH, leading to a Ca^{2+}-independent lethal reperfusion injury in cardiomyocytes.

2.3. The mPTP opening

Recently, it has been proposed that various potential protein components either to form the molecular structure of the mPTP or to regulate its opening [20, 36]. It was shown that the mPTP opening occurs within the first few minutes postischemia myocardial reperfusion [37], with both burst of oxidative stress and intracellular pH normalization (possibly due to the inhibitory effect of acid pH on mPTP is removed) as the main contributing factors [38, 39]. On the other hand, Ca^{2+} overload seems not to be a causative factor in I/R model. In adult rat myocytes, both cytosolic and mitochondrial Ca^{2+} increased during ischemia but decreases to basal levels in the first minutes of reperfusion. Ca^{2+} overload occurred late in both compartments, event that was prevented by mPTP inhibitors. Besides, intramitochondrial Ca^{2+} chelation did not prevent cell death after reperfusion. Thus, Ca^{2+} overload appears to be the consequence of bioenergetic failure after mPTP opening [38]. Another study showed that, at the onset of reperfusion, there is a transient increase in cytosolic Ca^{2+} levels together with a simultaneous transient sarcoplasmic reticulum Ca^{2+} depletion [40], corroborating the latter. The mPTP is a potential pharmacological target for prevent LMRI, and experimental studies with mPTP inhibitors (such as cyplosporin A), at the onset of myocardial reperfusion, has been reported to reduce MI size by 40–50% [41–44].

2.4. Inflammation

Ischemia is associated with slow infiltration of neutrophils, but recruitment toward the necrotic zone is favored after reperfusion by increased ROS exacerbation that triggers upregulation of adhesion molecules (P-selectin, CD11/CD18, ICAM-1) in cardiomyocytes, with cytokines (TNFα, IL-1, IL-6, IL-8, NAP-1, PAF, MIP-2) and complement, which are released from ischemic-reperfused myocardium. Neutrophils adhesion to coronary vascular endothelium occurs rapidly (within minutes) after onset of reperfusion, with abundant accumulation into the infarct zone during the following 6 hours. Neutrophils release more than 20 different proteolytic enzymes (hydrolases, metalloproteinases, and proteases) and are a major ROS source by generating superoxide anions through NOX, positioning them as important contributors to MRI [45].

3. Cardioprotection by combined antioxidant therapy

After reviewing the most relevant pathophysiological processes of myocardial ischemia–reperfusion injury, the central role being played by the burst of oxidative stress in the first minutes of revascularization certainly has positioned itself as a pharmacological target of choice. In the following section, we describe the molecular basis of an innovative combined antioxidant therapy, which includes a reinforcement of endogenous antioxidant defences, aimed to prevent or at least ameliorate the MRI in patients with AMI undergoing PCA.

3.1. Ascorbate

Vitamin C (ascorbic acid or ascorbate) is a potent water-soluble antioxidant in humans, which cannot be endogenously synthesized [46] and must be incorporated through vegetables and fruits [47]. Vitamin C is an electron donor and is oxidized to dehydroascorbate when acting as a reducing agent, returning to reduced form when is used by the cell [48] (**Figure 2**). A study in a group of apparently healthy adult nonsmoking population showed an inverse correlation between plasma vitamin C and products of oxidative damage to DNA, proteins and lipids [49]. Another study evaluated oxidant and antioxidant parameters in the blood of the patients with MI before and after thrombolysis and showed that the activity of superoxide dismutase (SOD), an antioxidant enzyme, was significantly reduced, whereas the activity of XO, an oxidant enzyme, together with the levels of malondialdehyde (MDA), a lipid peroxidation biomarker, significantly increased after reperfusion. These parameters improved to normal or near-normal levels when patients were supplemented with oral vitamin C postreperfusion [50], confirming the *in vivo* antioxidant capacity of vitamin C. Other properties of this compound are described in the following experiments. Ascorbic acid, together vitamin E, reverse endothelial dysfunction through a modulator effect by upregulating endothelial NOS (eNOS) and downregulating NOX on the vascular wall [51]. In essential hypertensive patients, impaired endothelium-dependent vasodilation improved with vitamin C supplementation, an effect that can be reversed by a NOS inhibitor, suggesting a restoration of NO availability and oxidative stress-mediated endothelium impairment in this pathology [52]. Pretreatment with vitamin C prevents vascular function damage and release of IL-6 induced by endothelin-1 in humans [53]. Intracellular vitamin C in human cell lines and primary endothelial cells, together with cell cultures in medium with dehydroascorbic acid, showed significantly decreased TNFα-induced NF-κB activation [54].

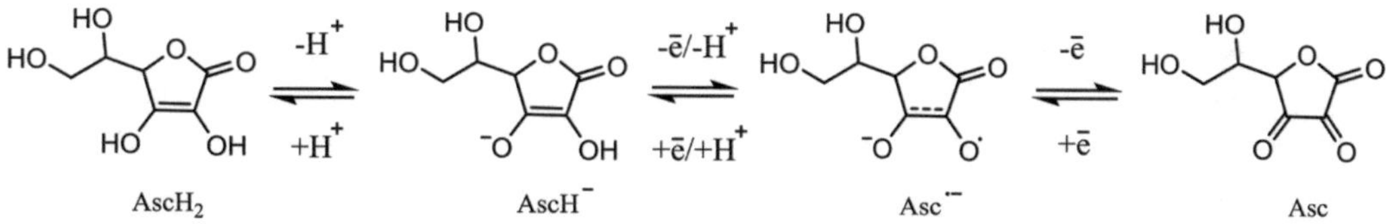

Figure 2. Oxidation of ascorbate ($AscH^-$) to dehydroascorbic acid (Asc) for the loss of two electrons in succession, through the formation of ascorbyl radical intermediate ($Asc^{\bullet-}$). Importantly, ascorbate is the ionized form of ascorbic acid ($AscH_2$) at physiological pH (7.4).

Vitamin C has been used in I/R models. Gao et al. [55] demonstrated that in isolated rat hearts subjected to I/R, glutathione monoethyl ester (GSHme), but no ascorbic acid, administered at the onset of reperfusion exerted protective effects against MRI. Furthermore, GSHme coadministered together with ascorbic acid had enhanced protective effects, suggesting a synergistic effect between the two compounds. Another *in vivo* experimental study showed that intravenous (IV) administration of vitamin C or vitamin C plus vitamin E, prior to coronary occlusion following reperfusion, had not significant differences in infarct size compared to the control group. Besides, vitamin C alone tends to increase infarct size, whereas the vitamin combination tends to decrease [56]. The clinical trials in which vitamin C is orally administered, in combination with other vitamins, in different doses to patients with cardiovascular history showed no beneficial cardioprotective long-term effects [27]. In patients with AMI subjected to PCA, administration of vitamin C orally (2.0 g) followed by a constant infusion (20 mg/min), before reperfusion, did not suppress the rapid and transient increase in levels of urinary 8-epi-prostaglandin F2α (8-epi-PGF2α), a biomarker of oxidative stress *in vivo*, after PCA [57]. A review [14] of the cardioprotective strategies using vitamin C in combination with other vitamins in AMI followed by restoration of coronary blood flow showed variable results when administered orally, but when an infusion of vitamin C (1000 mg/12 h) was followed by oral doses (1200 mg/24 h) and vitamin E (600 mg/24 h), positive clinical outcomes were obtained within a composite endpoint. According to the latter, a study in patients undergoing elective percutaneous coronary intervention for stable angina showed that 1 g vitamin C administered by infusion (16.6 mg/min), 1 hour before of intervention, improved the impaired microcirculatory reperfusion and had significantly reduced plasma levels of oxidative stress biomarkers [58].

These results could be explained by the fact that oral administration of vitamin C shows a plasma concentration–time profile, in a dose range of 200–2500 mg/day, producing a steady-state plasma concentration approximately by 80 μmol/l (0.08 mmol/l), due to apparent saturation of tissue uptake and in less degree by function of oral bioavailability and renal excretion [59]. At these physiological concentrations, superoxide anion reacts with NO at a rate 10^4-fold greater than that at which it reacts with ascorbic acid (**Table 1A** and **C**), situation that is favored during the ROS burst in the first minutes of postischemia myocardial reperfusion because superoxide anion levels are exacerbated.

	Reaction	Rate constant (M^{-1} s^{-1})
(A)	$O_2^{\cdot -} + \cdot NO \rightarrow ONOO^-$	7×10^9
(B)	$O_2^{\cdot -} + SOD \rightarrow O_2 + H_2O_2$	2×10^9
(C)	$O_2^{\cdot -} + AscH_2 \rightarrow Products$	$2.7–3.3 \times 10^5$

$ONOO^-$, peroxynitrite; H_2O_2, hydrogen peroxide; O_2, molecular oxygen [60–62].

Table 1. Comparison of the reaction rate constants of superoxide anion ($O_2^{\bullet -}$) with nitric oxide ($^\bullet NO$), superoxide dismutase (SOD) and ascorbic acid ($AscH_2$).

Superoxide anion reacts avidly with NO to form peroxynitrite ($ONOO^-$) (**Table 1A**), an agent very reactive and toxic to biomolecules, with a constant rate higher than that of the reaction between superoxide anion and SOD (**Table 1B**). Furthermore, peroxynitrite (pKa at 37°C = 6.8) can be protonated in medium with acidotic pH during ischemia, resulting in ONOOH that is inherently unstable. Reperfusion restored the intracellular pH to physiologic levels, favoring decomposition of ONOOH to hydroxyl radical and nitrogen dioxide radical (**Figure 3**) [24], both responsible for generating oxidative stress and nitrosative stress damage to cardiomyocytes. Thus, peroxynitrite contributes to MRI generating lipid peroxidation and protein nitration in tyrosine residues, affecting the function and structure of the latter; oxidation of thiol groups related to cell antioxidant capacity; rupture of double-stranded DNA; and BH_4 NOS cofactor oxidation, which reduces the formation of NO [63].

Jackson et al. [64] demonstrated *in vitro* that supraphysiologic vitamin C concentration of 10 mmol/l is needed to overcome the competition with NO for superoxide. Consequently, only IV infusion can achieve these plasma ascorbate levels. It has been documented that the use of high doses of IV vitamin C over 10 mmol/l in patients appears to have a positive safety profile, but it should be avoided in patients with renal function impairment or glucose-6-phosphate

http://dx.doi.org/10.5772/63658

dehydrogenase deficiency [65]. Human plasma vitamin C concentration–time profile following short-term IV infusion shows peak concentrations higher than 20 mmol/l, remaining over 10 mmol/l for 3 hours [66]. It is important to note that vitamin C needs to be incorporated into the cell to exert its effects. Specific Na^+-dependent transporters for ascorbic acid (reduced form) are called SVCT1 and SVCT2, while transporters for dehydroascorbic acid (oxidized form) are members of GLUT family (GLUT1/3/4) that facilitate transport of glucose [67]. These transporters are expressed in the human myocardium [68–70].

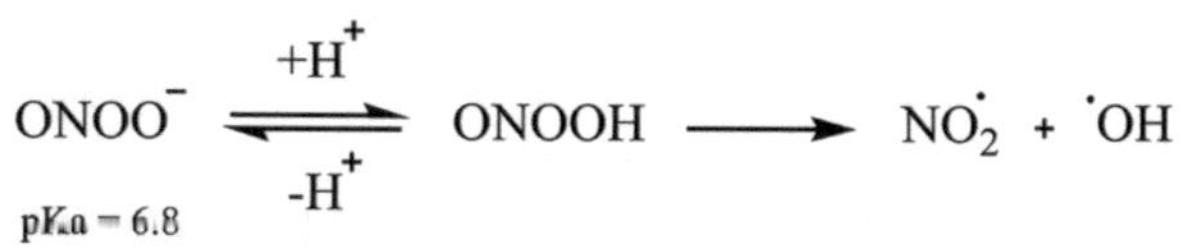

Figure 3. Formation of hydroxyl radical (•OH) and nitrogen dioxide radical (NO_2•) from peroxynitrite ($ONOO^-$) through an intermediary peroxynitrous acid (ONOOH).

3.2. N-Acetyl cysteine

When ascorbate is oxidized to dehydroascorbate, it can return to its reduced form through a reduced glutathione (GSH)-dependent recycling mechanism inside the cell, which may be direct [71] or enzyme mediated [72] (**Figure 4**) and can lead to a dehydroascorbate concentration-dependent decrease in intracellular GSH levels [71, 73, 74]. This process has been described in human erythrocytes [73], bovine aortic endothelial cells [74], among others and fulfills a function of blood antioxidant reserve [75]. Glutathione (γ-glutamyl-cysteinyl-glycine) is an endogenous agent playing a primary role of nonenzymatic antioxidant defence together with participating in metabolic processes and cellular regulation. It has a reduced form (GSH) and an oxidized form (GSSG) which are interconvertible. It is synthesized in all cell types of the organism, being mostly in the cytosol and to a lesser extent in the extracellular plasma [76].

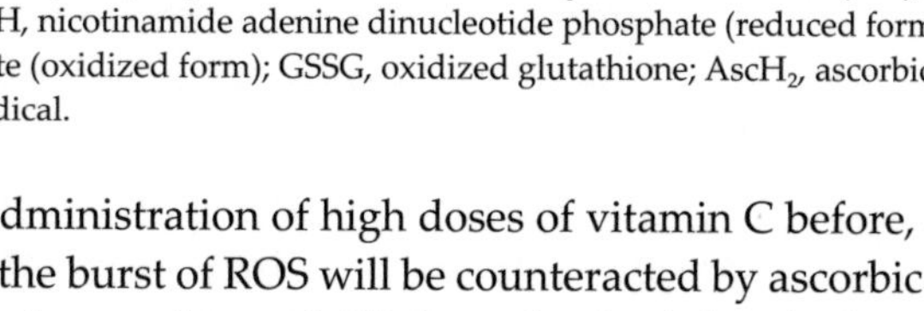

Figure 4. Reduced glutathione (GSH)-dependent reduction of dehydroascorbic acid (Asc), which may be mediated directly or by enzyme. NADPH, nicotinamide adenine dinucleotide phosphate (reduced form); $NADP^+$, nicotinamide adenine dinucleotide phosphate (oxidized form); GSSG, oxidized glutathione; $AscH_2$, ascorbic acid; RH, unsaturated fatty acid chain; R•, lipid alkyl radical.

If we consider an IV administration of high doses of vitamin C before, during and after PCA in patients with AMI, the burst of ROS will be counteracted by ascorbic acid, which generates large amounts of dehydroascorbic acid. We hypothesized that the latter interact with endogenous GSH and will cause a drop in their levels, limiting the cardioprotective effect. For this reason, we believe essential to reinforcement the endogenous antioxidant defence system with a GSH donor, such as *N*-acetyl cysteine, to optimize antioxidant therapy. Furthermore, as above-mentioned, coadministration of a GSH donor and vitamin C tend to have a synergistic protective effect on infarct size in an I/R model of isolated rat heart [56].

N-Acetyl cysteine (NAC) is a drug currently used in clinic that has demonstrated a good safety profile when administered orally, although adverse effects will be more noticeable at high doses (>3 g/day) or IV administration (e.g., for the treatment of paracetamol overdose) [77]. In experimental I/R models, high NAC dose administrated intracoronary with a radiographic contrast in pigs, at the onset of reperfusion, was safe, reduced platelet reactivity and there was a trend toward a better cardiac function at 24 h, but there was no significant difference in the myocardial infarct size and did not provide significant renal protection compared to control group [78]. On the other hand, in a rat I/R model, NAC administration by continuous infusion before, during and after reperfusion produced a significant limitation of the infarct size compared to control group, but injection of NAC bolus with the same total dose, before and at onset of reperfusion, failed to reduce it [79]. In clinical trials, group of patients undergoing coronary artery bypass and/or valve surgery treated with IV infusion of NAC, before and after of surgery, decreases the incidence of postoperative atrial fibrillation compared to control group [80]. LIPSIA-N-ACC trial [81], a randomized, single-blind, controlled trial, was designed to measure the effects of high doses of NAC on contrast-induced nephropathy (CIN) and reperfusion injury in ST-segment elevation MI patients undergoing primary angioplasty intervention (PCI) with moderate contrast volumes. CIN is the acute deterioration of renal function occurring after intravascular administration of contrast media that is not attributable to other causes, defined as increase in serum creatinine > 0.3 mg/dL or 25% above baseline levels within 48 hours after contrast administration, which is associated with increased rates of morbidity and mortality. Of the 251 patients enrolled, 126 were randomized to the NAC treated group and 125 to the placebo group. NAC was administered as an IV bolus (1200 mg) before angioplasty and twice daily for 48 hours after angioplasty. In addition, all patients and controls were hydrated with IV infusion of NaCl (0.9%), at a rate of 1 ml/kg of body weight per hour for 12 h, after PCI. Iopromide was used as a nonionic low-osmolality contrast agent for PCI. In the primary outcomes, CIN (>25% increase in serum creatinine level <72 h after randomization) occurred in 14% in the NAC-treated group and 20% in the placebo group, with no significant differences; the MRI (measured as myocardial salvage index by MRI) was also not statistically significant difference in both groups, so it is concluded that NAC not provide an additional clinical benefit to placebo with respect to CIN and MRI. However, activated oxygen protein products and oxidized low-density lipoprotein were evaluated as oxidative stress markers in blood plasma (in venous blood samples collected before, immediately after PCI, and subsequently for up to 3 days) and found that the NAC-treated group had a significant reduction (20%) of these markers, while the placebo group had no significant differences. In another study, patients with AMI that received NAC infusion (a total dose of 15 g/24 h), combined with IV nitroglycerin and streptokinase, were well tolerated together with having significantly lesser oxidative stress, a trend toward more rapid reperfusion and better preservation of left ventricular function compared to control group [82].

3.3. Deferoxamine

It has been shown in I/R models of isolated perfused heart that during a period of ischemia the amount of tissue available iron (Fe) increases in a time-dependent manner. Fe is rapidly mobilized through the perfusion fluid leading to very high Fe levels (up to 50-fold compared to pre-ischemic values) in the first small volumes of coronary flow fractions (CFF), returning to baseline over time. In addition, the levels of Fe in the CFFs correlated well with the loss of cardiac function following global ischemia of varying duration [83]. Similarly, the Fe levels increase up to 30-fold in cardiac tissue during ischemia, in a time-dependent manner, due to acidification in ischemia because this effect contributes tremendously to the mobilization of Fe from intracellular ferritin storage. After reperfusion, tissue Fe levels decrease, although it is known that the superoxide anion contributes to the mobilization of Fe from ferritin [84–86]. Langendorff models with myocardial iron overload develop different functional, biochemical and ultrastructural alterations as compared to control groups of myocardial I/R, which are prevented by deferoxamine (DFO), an iron chelator [87], realizing the harmful tissue effect of Fe high levels. The role of Fe in the postischemia MRI has been demonstrated in experimental models by the use of iron chelators at the onset of reperfusion, improving cardiac function relative to control group [88, 89]. Furthermore, a long-term study conducted in randomly selected men aged 42, 48, 54 and 60, who had no symptoms of coronary heart disease at entry, showed that elevated levels of serum ferritin (stored Fe) was a strong risk factor for developing AMI [90].

Physiologically, transition metals, such as iron, are mainly stored or complexed. However, under certain pathological conditions, the nonchelated state iron levels are increased, thus generating oxidative stress. Reduced iron (Fe^{2+}) can react with hydrogen peroxide to generate hydroxyl radical ($^{\bullet}OH$), a process known as Fenton reaction (**Table 2A**). At the same time, oxidized iron (Fe^{3+}) can react with superoxide anion to form again Fe^{2+} and oxygen (**Table 2B**). The sum of the Fenton reaction and the superoxide-mediated reduction of Fe^{3+} originates the Haber–Weiss reaction (**Table 2C**), where hydroxyl radical is generated from superoxide anion and hydrogen peroxide [24]. Thus, during myocardial I/R increase, the Fe^{2+} availability and ROS levels that favor the formation of highly harmful and reactive hydroxyl radical through these redox reactions, can significantly contribute to MRI. This allows considering the iron overload during I/R as a pharmacological target for cardioprotection.

In addition, our interest is focused on the interaction between vitamin C and iron. Ascorbate has pro-oxidant effect because of reduction of Fe^{3+} to Fe^{2+} (**Table 2D**), which is substrate to Fenton reaction leading to ROS production [92]. Under physiological conditions, *in vivo* studies with vitamin C supplementation showed predominantly reduced levels in markers of oxidative damage in DNA, lipids and proteins, even in the presence of iron. These results were correlated with *in vitro* systems, such as isolated or cultured cells and biological fluids, where the antioxidant role, or no effect of vitamin C, predominated over a pro-oxidant role [91]. Considering that iron overload occurs in postischemia myocardial reperfusion, IV infusion of high doses of vitamin C at the onset of reperfusion could generate a strong interaction with iron, which not only decrease the concentration of ascorbate available in blood to counteract the burst of oxidative stress, reducing its antioxidant effect, but also favor pro-oxidant effects and ROS production. Thus, use of an iron chelator, as DFO, as adjuvant to antioxidant therapy with vitamin C should be considered to reduce deleterious effects and maximize cardioprotection in patients with AMI being subjected to PCA. A experimental study in pigs showed that the combined use of vitamin C (100 mg/kg) and DFO (60 mg/kg), administered as IV infusion at the beginning, during and after reperfusion postischemia, had no difference in the measured cardiac parameters compared to the control group, although it was observed a trend toward reducing infarct size [94]. However, no markers of oxidative stress, apoptosis or other biochemical parameter related to myocardial damage were measured. Another study in sheep demonstrated that administration by IV infusion of vitamin C (1.5 g) and DFO (1 g) (in combination but not separately), before reperfusion, significantly protected against the development of ventricular arrhythmias induced by I/R, compared to control group [95].

	Reaction	Rate constant ($M^{-1}\ s^{-1}$)
(A)	$Fe^{2+} + H_2O_2 \rightarrow Fe^{3+} + \cdot OH + OH^-$	76
(B)	$O_2^{\cdot -} + Fe^{3+} \rightarrow O_2 + Fe^{2+}$	$1.9 \times 10^6 - 10^4$
(C)	$O_2^{\cdot -} + H_2O_2 \rightarrow O_2 + \cdot OH + OH^-$	<2.3
(D)	$AscH^- + Fe^{3+} \rightarrow Asc^{\cdot -} + Fe^{2+} + H^+$	10^2

H_2O_2, hydrogen peroxide; Fe^{2+}, reduced iron; Fe^{3+}, oxidized iron; $^{\bullet}OH$, Hydroxyl radical; OH^-, Hydroxyl anion; $O_2^{\bullet -}$, Superoxide anion; O_2, Molecular oxygen; $AscH^-$, Ascorbate; $Asc^{\bullet -}$, Ascorbyl radical [91–93].

Table 2. Fenton (A), Haber–Weiss (C) and others redox reactions.

DFO has shown beneficial effects in experimental models of I/R. Isolated, perfused rabbit hearts treated with DFO, during ischemia and reflow, demonstrated improved functional and metabolic recovery of myocardium together a reduction in reperfusion-induced oxygen free-radical generation, compared to control group [96]. In a canine model of I/R, DFO pretreatment before ischemia, but not at the beginning of reperfusion, reduced significantly infarct size and release of GSSG into the coronary sinus during early reflow, compared to control group [97]. Decrease in infarct size by early treatment with DFO was corroborated by another independent study in canine model of I/R [98]. Regarding clinical trials, patients undergoing coronary artery bypass grafting, that received an IV infusion of DFO for 8 hours, prevented the increase in oxidative stress markers and improving ventricular functional parameters after surgery, compared to control group [99]. Other clinical trial in patients with ST-elevation MI subjected to primary percutaneous coronary intervention (PPCI) showed that administration of IV bolus of DFO (500 mg) immediately before surgery, followed by a 12-h infusion (50 mg/kg), significantly reduced in plasma F2-isoprostane levels, with no difference in infarct size, after PPCI compared to placebo group [100].

http://dx.doi.org/10.5772/63658

4. Conclusion and perspectives

In this chapter, we have reviewed the molecular processes involved in the pathophysiology of myocardial damage by postischemia reperfusion, emphasizing the central role of oxidative stress as the key mediator of this damage. Accordingly, increased ROS production can give rise to the occurrence of events ranging from inflammation, damage to biomolecules and metabolic cell impairment to even cell death. From this paradigm, a novel antioxidant therapy is proposed as cardioprotective action in patients with AMI subject to PCA. This treatment considers the use of vitamin C (sodium ascorbate) in high doses administered intravenously, combined with NAC and DFO prior to surgery so as to optimize and enhance the beneficial effects and reduce the harmful effects on myocardium occurring in this setting (**Figure 5**). However, the results from different experimental models are controversial and more studies are still lacking. On this line, it is important to note that MRI is an unsolved problem in the clinical practice. Different strategies to prevent this damage during surgery for revascularization in patients with AMI have been tried without conclusive results, and we expect that our proposal can contribute as an effective, low risk and economic alternative in the near future.

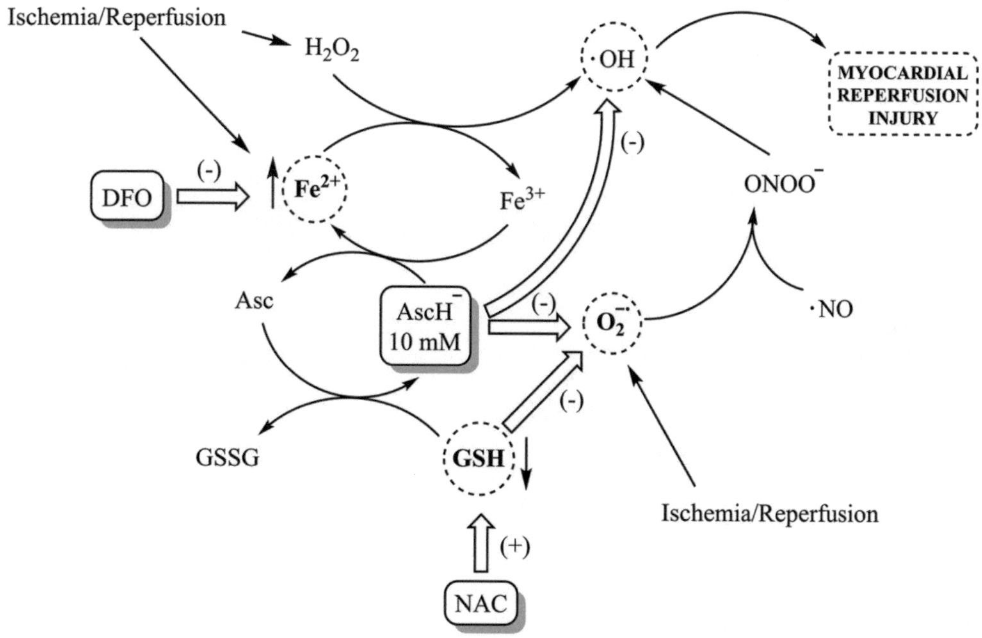

Figure 5. Diagram of the proposed combined antioxidant therapy for patients with AMI subject to PCA, which considers the use of: (i) ascorbate ($AscH^-$) in high doses to compete with nitric oxide ($^•NO$) by superoxide anion ($O_2^{•-}$); (ii) deferoxamine (DFO) to counteract reduced iron (Fe^{2+}) overload and thus prevent the Fenton reaction and interaction with $AscH^-$; (iii) *N*-acetyl cysteine (NAC) as reduced glutathione (GSH) donor to reinforce the antioxidant defense system and mitigate its interaction with dehydroascorbic acid (Asc). In this way, it counteracts directly and indirectly the hydroxyl radical ($^•OH$), which is the main mediator of myocardial damage by oxidative stress during reperfusion. H_2O_2, hydrogen peroxide; GSSG, oxidized glutathione; $ONOO^-$, Peroxynitrite; Fe^{3+}, oxidized iron.

Acknowledgements

This study was supported by the Fondo de Fomento al Desarrollo Científico y Tecnológico (FONDEF), grant ID15I10285.

Nomenclature

Asc	dehydroascorbic acid
$AscH_2$	ascorbic acid
AMI	acute myocardial infarction
ARE	antioxidant response elements
ATP	adenosine triphosphate
CFF	coronary flow fraction
DFO	deferoxamine
eNOS	endothelial nitric oxide synthase
8-epi-PGF2α	8-epi-prostaglandin F2α
GSH	reduced glutathione
GSSG	oxidized glutathione
IHD	ischemic heart disease
IL-6	interleukin 6
I/R	ischemia–reperfusion
IV	intravenous
kDA	kilo dalton
LMRI	lethal myocardial reperfusion injury
PCA	percutaneous coronary angioplasty
MDA	malondialdehyde
mETC	mitochondrial electron transport chain
MI	myocardial infarction
MRI	myocardial reperfusion injury
mPTP	mitochondrial permeability transition pore
NAC	N-acetyl cysteine
NF-κB	nuclear factor kappa B
NO	nitric oxide
NOX	NADPH oxidase
Nrf2	nuclear factor-erythroid 2-related factor 2

·OH	hydroxyl radical
$ONOO^-$	peroxynitrite
PPCI	primary percutaneous coronary intervention
ROS	reactive oxygen species
SOD	superoxide dismutase
TNFα	tumor necrosis factor alpha
XO	xanthine oxidase

Author details

Pablo Parra and Ramón Rodrigo*

*Address all correspondence to: rrodrigo@med.uchile.cl

Molecular and Clinical Pharmacology Program, Institute of Biomedical Sciences, Faculty of Medicine, University of Chile, Santiago, Chile

References

[1] World Health Organization. The Top 10 causes of death [Internet]. [Updated: 2014-05]. Available from: http://www.who.int/mediacentre/factsheets/fs310/en/ [Accessed: 2015-12-06].

[2] World Health Organization. Global status report on noncommunicable diseases 2014. Geneva, Switzerland, World Health Organization, 2014. 298 p.

[3] Garcia-Dorado D, Rodríguez-Sinovas A, Ruiz-Meana M, Inserte J. Protection against myocardial ischemia–reperfusion injury in clinical practice. Revista Española de Cardiología (English Edition). 2014;67(5):394–404. DOI: 10.1016/j.rec.2014.01.010.

[4] White HD, Chew DP. Acute myocardial infarction. Lancet. 2008;372(9638):570–584. DOI: 10.1016/S0140-6736(08)61237-4.

[5] Yellon DM, Hausenloy DJ. Myocardial reperfusion injury. New England Journal of Medicine. 2007;357(11):1121–1135. DOI: 10.1056/NEJMra071667.

[6] Hausenloy DJ, Yellon DM. Myocardial ischemia–reperfusion injury: a neglected therapeutic target. Journal of Clinical Investigation. 2013;123(1):92–100. DOI: 10.1172/JCI62874.

[7] Jolly SR, Kane WJ, Bailie MB, Abrams GD, Lucchesi BR. Canine myocardial reperfusion injury. Its reduction by the combined administration of superoxide dismutase and catalase. Cardiovascular Research. 1984;54(3):277–285. DOI: 10.1161/01.RES.54.3.277

[8] Zweier JL, Flaherty JT, Weisfeldt ML. Direct measurement of free radical generation following reperfusion of ischemic myocardium. Proceedings of the National Academy of Sciences of the United States of America. 1987;84(5):1404–1407.

[9] Ambrosio G, Weisfeldt ML, Jacobus WE, Flaherty JT. Evidence for a reversible oxygen radical-mediated component of reperfusion injury: reduction by recombinant human superoxide dismutase administered at the time of reflow. Circulation. 1987;75(1):282–291. DOI: 10.1161/01.CIR.75.1.282.

[10] Zweier JL, Rayburn BK, Flaherty JT, Weisfeldt ML. Recombinant superoxide dismutase reduces oxygen free radical concentrations in reperfused myocardium. Journal of Clinical Investigation. 1987;80(6):1728–1734. DOI: 10.1172/JCI113264.

[11] Zweier JL. Measurement of superoxide-derived free radicals in the reperfused heart. Evidence for a free radical mechanism of reperfusion injury. Journal of Biological Chemistry. 1988;263(3):1353–1357.

[12] Grill HP, Zweier JL, Kuppusamy P, Weisfeldt ML, Flaherty JT. Direct measurement of myocardial free radical generation in an in vivo model: effects of postischemic reperfusion and treatment with human recombinant superoxide dismutase. Journal of the American College of Cardiology. 1992;20(7):1604–1611. DOI: 10.1016/0735-1097(92)90457-X.

[13] Lecour S, Baouali AB, Maupoil V, Chahine R, Abadie C, Javouhey-Donzel A, et al. Demonstration of the production of oxygen-centered free radicals during electrolysis using E.S.R. spin-trapping techniques: effects on cardiac function in the isolated rat heart. Free Radical Biology and Medicine. 1998;24(4):573–579. DOI: 10.1016/S0891-5849(97)00294-3.

[14] Rodrigo R, Libuy M, Feliú F, Hasson D. Molecular basis of cardioprotective effect of antioxidant vitamins in myocardial infarction. BioMed Research International. 2013;2013:437613. DOI: 10.1155/2013/437613.

[15] Neely JR, Grotyohann LW. Role of glycolytic products in damage to ischemic myocardium. Dissociation of adenosine triphosphate levels and recovery of function of reperfused ischemic hearts. Circulation Research. 1984;55(6):816–824. DOI: 10.1161/01.RES.55.6.816.

[16] Avkiran M, Marber M. Na^+/H^+ exchange inhibitors for cardioprotective therapy: progress, problems and prospects. Journal of the American College of Cardiology. 2002;39(5):747–753. DOI: 10.1016/S0735-1097(02)01693-5.

[17] Rossi AE, Dirksen RT. Sarcoplasmic reticulum: the dynamic calcium governor of muscle. Muscle & Nerve. 2006;33(6):715–731. DOI: 10.1002/mus.20512.

[18] Sasaki M, Joh T. Oxidative stress and ischemia–reperfusion injury in gastrointestinal tract and antioxidant, protective agents. Journal of Clinical Biochemistry and Nutrition. 2007;40(1):1–12. DOI: 10.3164/jcbn.40.1.

[19] Bernardi P, Vassanelli S, Veronese P, Colonna R, Szabó I, Zoratti M. Modulation of the mitochondrial permeability transition pore. Effect of protons and divalent cations. Journal of Biological Chemistry. 1992;267(5):2934–2939.

[20] Ong SB, Samangouei P, Kalkhoran SB, Hausenloy DJ. The mitochondrial permeability transition pore and its role in myocardial ischemia reperfusion injury. Journal of Molecular and Cellular Cardiology. 2015;78:23–34. DOI: 10.1016/j.yjmcc.2014.11.005.

[21] Orchard CH, Kentish JC. Effects of changes of pH on the contractile function of cardiac muscle. American Journal of Physiology. 1990;258(6 Pt 1):C967–C981.

[22] Granger DN, Kvietys PR. Reperfusion injury and reactive oxygen species: the evolution of a concept. Redox Biology. 2015;6:524–551. DOI: 10.1016/j.redox.2015.08.020.

[23] Braunersreuther V, Montecucco F, Asrih M, Pelli G, Galan K, Frias M, et al. Role of NADPH oxidase isoforms NOX1, NOX2 and NOX4 in myocardial ischemia/reperfusion injury. Journal of Molecular and Cellular Cardiology. 2013;64:99–107. DOI: 10.1016/j.yjmcc.2013.09.007.

[24] Raedschelders K, Ansley DM, Chen DD. The cellular and molecular origin of reactive oxygen species generation during myocardial ischemia and reperfusion. Pharmacology & Therapeutics. 2012;133(2):230–255. DOI: 10.1016/j.pharmthera.2011.11.004.

[25] Vásquez-Vivar J, Martásek P, Whitsett J, Joseph J, Kalyanaraman B. The ratio between tetrahydrobiopterin and oxidized tetrahydrobiopterin analogues controls superoxide release from endothelial nitric oxide synthase: an EPR spin trapping study. Biochemical Journal. 2002;362(Pt 3):733–739. DOI: 10.1042/bj3620733.

[26] Avery SV. Molecular targets of oxidative stress. Biochemical Journal. 2011;434(2):201–210. DOI: 10.1042/BJ20101695.

[27] Rodrigo R, Prieto JC, Castillo R. Cardioprotection against ischaemia/reperfusion by vitamins C and E plus n–3 fatty acids: molecular mechanisms and potential clinical applications. Clinical Science. 2013;124(1):1–15. DOI: 10.1042/CS20110663.

[28] Gloire G, Legrand-Poels S, Piette J. NF-kappaB activation by reactive oxygen species: fifteen years later. Biochemical Pharmacology. 2006;72(11):1493–1505. DOI: 10.1016/j.bcp.2006.04.011.

[29] Perkins N1, Gilmore TD. Good cop, bad cop: the different faces of NF-kappaB. Cell Death and Differentiation. 2006;13(5):759–772. DOI: 10.1038/sj.cdd.4401838.

[30] Kucharczak J, Simmons MJ, Fan Y, Gélinas C. To be, or not to be: NF-kappaB is the answer – role of Rel/NF-kappaB in the regulation of apoptosis. Oncogene. 2003;22(56):8961–8982. DOI: 10.1038/sj.onc.1207230.

[31] Morgan MJ, Liu ZG. Crosstalk of reactive oxygen species and NF-κB signaling. Cell Research. 2011;21(1):103–115. DOI: 10.1038/cr.2010.178.

[32] Hybertson BM, Gao B, Bose SK, McCord JM. Oxidative stress in health and disease: the therapeutic potential of Nrf2 activation. Molecular Aspects of Medicine. 2011;32(4–6): 234–246. DOI: 10.1016/j.mam.2011.10.006.

[33] Zhu H, Jia Z, Misra BR, Zhang L, Cao Z, Yamamoto M, et al. Nuclear factor E2-related factor 2-dependent myocardiac cytoprotection against oxidative and electrophilic stress. Cardiovascular Toxicology. 2008;8(2):71–85. DOI: 10.1007/s12012-008-9016-0.

[34] Bond JM1, Chacon E, Herman B, Lemasters JJ. Intracellular pH and Ca^{2+} homeostasis in the pH paradox of reperfusion injury to neonatal rat cardiac myocytes. American Journal of Physiology. 1993;265(1 Pt 1):C129–C137. DOI: 10.1111/j.1749-6632.1994.tb36714.x.

[35] Lemasters JJ, Bond JM, Chacon E, Harper IS, Kaplan SH, Ohata H, et al. The pH paradox in ischemia–reperfusion injury to cardiac myocytes. Experientia Supplementum. 1996;76:99–114. DOI: 10.1007/978-3-0348-8988-9_7.

[36] Morciano G, Giorgi C, Bonora M, Punzetti S, Pavasini R, Wieckowski MR, et al. Molecular identity of the mitochondrial permeability transition pore and its role in ischemia–reperfusion injury. Journal of Molecular and Cellular Cardiology. 2015;78:142–153. DOI: 10.1016/j.yjmcc.2014.08.015.

[37] Griffiths EJ, Halestrap AP. Mitochondrial non-specific pores remain closed during cardiac ischaemia, but open upon reperfusion. Biochemical Journal. 1995;307(Pt 1):93–98. DOI: 10.1042/bj3070093.

[38] Kim JS, Jin Y, Lemasters JJ. Reactive oxygen species, but not Ca^{2+} overloading, trigger pH- and mitochondrial permeability transition-dependent death of adult rat myocytes after ischemia–reperfusion. American Journal of Physiology – Heart and Circulatory Physiology. 2006;290(5):H2024–H2034. DOI: 10.1152/ajpheart.00683.2005.

[39] Seidlmayer LK, Juettner VV, Kettlewell S, Pavlov EV, Blatter LA, Dedkova EN. Distinct mPTP activation mechanisms in ischaemia–reperfusion: contributions of Ca^{2+}, ROS, pH, and inorganic polyphosphate. Cardiovascular Research. 2015;106(2):237–248. DOI: 10.1093/cvr/cvv097.

[40] Valverde CA, Kornyeyev D, Ferreiro M, Petrosky AD, Mattiazzi A, Escobar AL. Transient Ca^{2+} depletion of the sarcoplasmic reticulum at the onset of reperfusion. Cardiovascular Research. 2010;85(4):671–680. DOI: 10.1093/cvr/cvp371.

[41] Hausenloy DJ, Maddock HL, Baxter GF, Yellon DM. Inhibiting mitochondrial permeability transition pore opening: a new paradigm for myocardial preconditioning?. Cardiovascular Research. 2002;55(3):534–543. DOI: 10.1016/S0008-6363(02)00455-8.

[42] Hausenloy DJ, Duchen MR, Yellon DM. Inhibiting mitochondrial permeability transition pore opening at reperfusion protects against ischaemia–reperfusion injury. Cardiovascular Research. 2003;60(3):617–625. DOI: 10.1016/j.cardiores.2003.09.025.

[43] Argaud L, Gateau-Roesch O, Muntean D, Chalabreysse L, Loufouat J, Robert D, et al. Specific inhibition of the mitochondrial permeability transition prevents lethal reperfusion injury. Journal of Molecular and Cellular Cardiology. 2005;38(2):367–374. DOI: 10.1016/j.yjmcc.2004.12.001.

[44] Skyschally A, Schulz R, Heusch G. Cyclosporine A at reperfusion reduces infarct size in pigs. Cardiovascular Drugs and Therapy. 2010;24(1):85–87. DOI: 10.1007/s10557-010-6219-y.

[45] Vinten-Johansen J. Involvement of neutrophils in the pathogenesis of lethal myocardial reperfusion injury. Cardiovascular Research. 2004;61(3):481–497. DOI: 10.1016/j.cardiores.2003.10.011.

[46] Nishikimi M, Yagi K. Biochemistry and molecular biology of ascorbic acid biosynthesis. In: J. Robin Harris, editor. Subcellular Biochemistry. 25th ed. New York: Springer US; 1996. p. 17–39. DOI: 10.1007/978-1-4613-0325-1_2.

[47] Haytowitz DB. Information from USDA's Nutrient Data Bank. The Journal of Nutrition. 1995;125(7):1952–1955.

[48] Padayatty SJ, Katz A, Wang Y, Eck P, Kwon O, Lee JH, et al. Vitamin C as an antioxidant: evaluation of its role in disease prevention. Journal of the American College of Nutrition. 2003;22(1):18–35. DOI: 10.1080/07315724.2003.10719272.

[49] Krajcovicová-Kudlácková M, Dusinská M, Valachovicová M, Blazícek P, Pauková V. Products of DNA, protein and lipid oxidative damage in relation to vitamin C plasma concentration. Physiological Research. 2006;55(2):227–231.

[50] Bhakuni P, Chandra M, Misra MK. Effect of ascorbic acid supplementation on certain oxidative stress parameters in the post reperfusion patients of myocardial infarction. Molecular and Cellular Biochemistry. 2006;290(1–2):153–158. DOI: 10.1007/s11010-006-9182-y.

[51] Ulker S, McKeown PP, Bayraktutan U. Vitamins reverse endothelial dysfunction through regulation of eNOS and NAD(P)H oxidase activities. Hypertension. 2003;41(3):534–539. DOI: 10.1161/01.HYP.0000057421.28533.37.

[52] Taddei S, Virdis A, Ghiadoni L, Magagna A, Salvetti A. Vitamin C improves endothelium-dependent vasodilation by restoring nitric oxide activity in essential hypertension. Circulation. 1998;97(22):2222–2229. DOI: 10.1161/01.CIR.97.22.2222.

[53] Böhm F, Settergren M, Pernow J. Vitamin C blocks vascular dysfunction and release of interleukin-6 induced by endothelin-1 in humans in vivo. Atherosclerosis. 2007;190(2): 408–415. DOI: 10.1016/j.atherosclerosis.2006.02.018.

[54] Cárcamo JM, Pedraza A, Bórquez-Ojeda O, Golde DW. Vitamin C suppresses TNF alpha-induced NF kappa B activation by inhibiting I kappa B alpha phosphorylation. Biochemistry. 2002;41(43):12995–13002. DOI: 10.1021/bi0263210.

[55] Gao F, Yao CL, Gao E, Mo QZ, Yan WL, McLaughlin R, et al. Enhancement of glutathione cardioprotection by ascorbic acid in myocardial reperfusion injury. Journal of Pharmacology and Experimental Therapeutics. 2002;301(2):543–550. DOI: 10.1124/jpet.301.2.543.

[56] Bellows SD, Hale SL, Simkhovich BZ, Kay GL, Kloner RA. Do antioxidant vitamins reduce infarct size following acute myocardial ischemia/reperfusion? Cardiovascular Drugs and Therapy. 1995;9(1):117–123. DOI: 10.1007/BF00877751.

[57] Guan W, Osanai T, Kamada T, Ishizaka H, Hanada H, Okumura K. Time course of free radical production after primary coronary angioplasty for acute myocardial infarction and the effect of vitamin C. Japanese Circulation Journal. 1999;63(12):924–928. DOI: 10.1253/jcj.63.924.

[58] Basili S, Tanzilli G, Mangieri E, Raparelli V, Di Santo S, Pignatelli P, et al. Intravenous ascorbic acid infusion improves myocardial perfusion grade during elective percutaneous coronary intervention: relationship with oxidative stress markers. JACC: Cardiovascular Interventions. 2010;3(2):221–229. DOI: 10.1016/j.jcin.2009.10.025.

[59] Graumlich JF, Ludden TM, Conry-Cantilena C, Cantilena LR Jr, Wang Y, Levine M. Pharmacokinetic model of ascorbic acid in healthy male volunteers during depletion and repletion. Pharmaceutical Research. 1997;14(9):1133–1139. DOI: 10.1023/A:1012186203165.

[60] Pryor WA, Squadrito GL. The chemistry of peroxynitrite: a product from the reaction of nitric oxide with superoxide. American Journal of Physiology. 1995;268(5 Pt 1):L699–L722.

[61] Gotoh N, Niki E. Rates of interactions of superoxide with vitamin E, vitamin C and related compounds as measured by chemiluminescence. Biochimica et Biophysica Acta (BBA) – General Subjects. 1992;1115(3):201–207. DOI: 10.1016/0304-4165(92)90054-X.

[62] Nishikimi M. Oxidation of ascorbic acid with superoxide anion generated by the xanthine–xanthine oxidase system. Biochemical and Biophysical Research Communications. 1975;63(2):463–468. DOI: 10.1016/0006-291X(75)90710-X.

[63] Kavdia M. Mathematical and computational models of oxidative and nitrosative stress. Critical Reviews in Biomedical Engineering. 2011;39(5):461–472. DOI: 10.1615/CritRevBiomedEng.v39.i5.60

[64] Jackson TS, Xu A, Vita JA, Keaney JF Jr. Ascorbate prevents the interaction of superoxide and nitric oxide only at very high physiological concentrations. Circulation Research. 1998;83(9):916–922. DOI: 10.1161/01.RES.83.9.916.

[65] Padayatty SJ, Sun AY, Chen Q, Espey MG, Drisko J, Levine M. Vitamin C: intravenous use by complementary and alternative medicine practitioners and adverse effects. PLoS One. 2010;5(7):e11414. DOI: 10.1371/journal.pone.0011414.

[66] Duconge J, Miranda-Massari JR, Gonzalez MJ, Jackson JA, Warnock W, Riordan NH. Pharmacokinetics of vitamin C: insights into the oral and intravenous administration of ascorbate. Puerto Rico Health Sciences Journal. 2008;27(1):7–19.

[67] Rivas CI, Zúñiga FA, Salas-Burgos A, Mardones L, Ormazabal V, Vera JC. Vitamin C transporters. Journal of Physiology and Biochemistry. 2008;64(4):357–375. DOI: 10.1007/BF03174092.

[68] Grover-McKay M, Walsh SA, Thompson SA. Glucose transporter 3 (GLUT3) protein is present in human myocardium. Biochimica et Biophysica Acta (BBA) – Biomembranes. 1999;1416(1–2):145–154. DOI: 10.1016/S0005-2736(98)00216-8.

[69] Savini I, Rossi A, Pierro C, Avigliano L, Catani MV. SVCT1 and SVCT2: key proteins for vitamin C uptake. Amino Acids. 2008;34(3):347–355. DOI: 10.1007/s00726-007-0555-7.

[70] Rajan DP, Huang W, Dutta B, Devoe LD, Leibach FH, Ganapathy V, et al. Human placental sodium-dependent vitamin C transporter (SVCT2): molecular cloning and transport function. Biochemical and Biophysical Research Communications. 1999;262(3):762–768. DOI: 10.1006/bbrc.1999.1272.

[71] May JM, Qu ZC, Whitesell RR, Cobb CE. Ascorbate recycling in human erythrocytes: role of GSH in reducing dehydroascorbate. Free Radical Biology and Medicine. 1996;20(4):543–551. DOI: 10.1016/0891-5849(95)02130-2.

[72] Mendiratta S, Qu ZC, May JM. Enzyme-dependent ascorbate recycling in human erythrocytes: role of thioredoxin reductase. Free Radical Biology and Medicine. 1998;25(2):221–228. DOI: 10.1016/S0891-5849(98)00060-4.

[73] May JM, Qu Z, Morrow JD. Mechanisms of ascorbic acid recycling in human erythrocytes. Biochimica et Biophysica Acta (BBA) – General Subjects. 2001;1528(2–3):159–166. DOI: 10.1016/S0304-4165(01)00188-X.

[74] May JM, Qu Z, Li X. Requirement for GSH in recycling of ascorbic acid in endothelial cells. Biochemical Pharmacology. 2001;62(7):873–881. DOI: 10.1016/S0006-2952(01)00736-5.

[75] Mendiratta S, Qu ZC, May JM. Erythrocyte ascorbate recycling: antioxidant effects in blood. Free Radical Biology and Medicine. 1998;24(5):789–797. DOI: 10.1016/S0891-5849(97)00351-1.

[76] Wu G, Fang YZ, Yang S, Lupton JR, Turner ND. Glutathione metabolism and its implications for health. Journal of Nutrition. 2004;134(3):489–492.

[77] Dodd S, Dean O, Copolov DL, Malhi GS, Berk M. N-acetylcysteine for antioxidant therapy: pharmacology and clinical utility. Expert Opinion on Biological Therapy. 2008;8(12):1955–1962. DOI: 10.1517/14728220802517901.

[78] Meyer M, Bell SP, Chen Z, Nyotowidjojo I, Lachapelle RR, Christian TF, et al. High dose intracoronary N-acetylcysteine in a porcine model of ST-elevation myocardial infarction. Journal of Thrombosis and Thrombolysis. 2013;36(4):433–441. DOI: 10.1007/s11239-013-0901-4.

[79] Abe M, Takiguchi Y, Ichimaru S, Tsuchiya K, Wada K. Comparison of the protective effect of N-acetylcysteine by different treatments on rat myocardial ischemia–reperfusion injury. Journal of Pharmacological Sciences. 2008;106(4):571–577. DOI: 10.1254/jphs.FP0071664.

[80] Ozaydin M, Peker O, Erdogan D, Kapan S, Turker Y, Varol E, et al. N-acetylcysteine for the prevention of postoperative atrial fibrillation: a prospective, randomized, placebo-controlled pilot study. European Heart Journal. 2008;29(5):625–631. DOI: 10.1093/eurheartj/ehn011.

[81] Thiele H, Hildebrand L, Schirdewahn C, Eitel I, Adams V, Fuernau G, et al . Impact of high-dose N-acetylcysteine versus placebo on contrast-induced nephropathy and myocardial reperfusion injury in unselected patients with ST-segment elevation myocardial infarction undergoing primary percutaneous coronary intervention. The LIPSIA-N-ACC (Prospective, Single-Blind, Placebo-Controlled, Randomized Leipzig Immediate PercutaneouS Coronary Intervention Acute Myocardial Infarction N-ACC) Trial. Journal of the American College of Cardiology. 2010;55(20):2201–2209. DOI: 10.1016/j.jacc.2009.08.091.

[82] Arstall MA, Yang J, Stafford I, Betts WH, Horowitz JD. N-acetylcysteine in combination with nitroglycerin and streptokinase for the treatment of evolving acute myocardial infarction. Circulation. 1995;92(10):2855–2862. DOI: 10.1161/01.CIR.92.10.2855.

[83] Berenshtein E, Mayer B, Goldberg C, Kitrossky N, Chevion M. Patterns of mobilization of copper and iron following myocardial ischemia: possible predictive criteria for tissue injury. Journal of Molecular and Cellular Cardiology. 1997;29(11):3025–3034. DOI: 10.1006/jmcc.1997.0535.

[84] Voogd A, Sluiter W, van Eijk HG, Koster JF. Low molecular weight iron and the oxygen paradox in isolated rat hearts. Journal of Clinical Investigation. 1992;90(5):2050–2055. DOI: 10.1172/JCI116086.

[85] Funk F, Lenders JP, Crichton RR, Schneider W. Reductive mobilisation of ferritin iron. European Journal of Biochemistry. 1985;152(1):167–172. DOI: 10.1111/j.1432-1033.1985.tb09177.x.

[86] Biemond P, van Eijk HG, Swaak AJ, Koster JF. Iron mobilization from ferritin by superoxide derived from stimulated polymorphonuclear leukocytes. Possible mecha-

nism in inflammation diseases. Journal of Clinical Investigation. 1984;73(6):1576–1579. DOI: 10.1172/JCI111364.

[87] Pucheu S, Coudray C, Tresallet N, Favier A, de Leiris J. Effect of iron overload in the isolated ischemic and reperfused rat heart. Cardiovascular Drugs and Therapy. 1993;7(4):701–711. DOI: 10.1007/BF00877824.

[88] Korkmaz S, Barnucz E, Loganathan S, Li S, Radovits T, Hegedus P, et al. Q50, an iron-chelating and zinc-complexing agent, improves cardiac function in rat models of ischemia/reperfusion-induced myocardial injury. Circulation Journal. 2013;77(7):1817–1826. DOI: 10.1253/circj.CJ-12-1162.

[89] van der Kraaij AM, van Eijk HG, Koster JF. Prevention of postischemic cardiac injury by the orally active iron chelator 1,2-dimethyl-3-hydroxy-4-pyridone (L1) and the antioxidant (+)-cyanidanol-3. Circulation. 1989;80(1):158–164. DOI: 10.1161/01.CIR.80.1.158.

[90] Salonen JT, Nyyssönen K, Korpela H, Tuomilehto J, Seppänen R, Salonen R. High stored iron levels are associated with excess risk of myocardial infarction in eastern Finnish men. Circulation. 1992;86(3):803–811. DOI: 10.1161/01.CIR.86.3.803.

[91] Carr A, Frei B. Does vitamin C act as a pro-oxidant under physiological conditions?. FASEB Journal. 1999;13(9):1007–1024.

[92] Buettner GR, Jurkiewicz BA. Catalytic metals, ascorbate and free radicals: combinations to avoid. Radiation Research. 1996;145(5):532–541.

[93] Buettnera GR, Dohertya TP, Patterson LK. The kinetics of the reaction of superoxide radical with Fe(III) complexes of EDTA, DETAPAC and HEDTA. FEBS Letters. 1983;158(1):143–146. DOI: 10.1016/0014-5793(83)80695-4.

[94] Chatziathanasiou GN, Nikas DN, Katsouras CS, Kazakos ND, Bouba V, Vougiouklakis T, et al. Combined intravenous treatment with ascorbic acid and desferrioxamine to reduce myocardial reperfusion injury in an experimental model resembling the clinical setting of primary PCI. Hellenic Journal of Cardiology. 2012;53(3):195–204.

[95] Karahaliou A, Katsouras C, Koulouras V, Nikas D, Niokou D, Papadopoulos G, et al. Ventricular arrhythmias and antioxidative medication: experimental study. Hellenic Journal of Cardiology. 2008;49(5):320–328.

[96] Williams RE, Zweier JL, Flaherty JT. Treatment with deferoxamine during ischemia improves functional and metabolic recovery and reduces reperfusion-induced oxygen radical generation in rabbit hearts. Circulation. 1991;83(3):1006–1014. DOI: 10.1161/01.CIR.83.3.1006.

[97] Lesnefsky EJ, Repine JE, Horwitz LD. Deferoxamine pretreatment reduces canine infarct size and oxidative injury. Journal of Pharmacology and Experimental Therapeutics. 1990;253(3):1103–1109.

[98] Reddy BR, Kloner RA, Przyklenk K. Early treatment with deferoxamine limits myocardial ischemic/reperfusion injury. Free Radical Biology & Medicine. 1989;7(1):45–52. DOI: 10.1016/0891-5849(89)90099-3.

[99] Paraskevaidis IA, Iliodromitis EK, Vlahakos D, Tsiapras DP, Nikolaidis A, Marathias A, et al. Deferoxamine infusion during coronary artery bypass grafting ameliorates lipid peroxidation and protects the myocardium against reperfusion injury: immediate and long-term significance. European Heart Journal. 2005;26(3):263–270. DOI: 10.1093/eurheartj/ehi028.

[100] Chan W, Taylor AJ, Ellims AH, Lefkovits L, Wong C, Kingwell BA, et al. Effect of iron chelation on myocardial infarct size and oxidative stress in ST-elevation-myocardial infarction. Circulation. Cardiovascular Interventions. 2012;5(2):270–278. DOI: 10.1161/CIRCINTERVENTIONS.111.966226.